The Skin Microbiome Manual

Antti Lauerma · Nanna Fyhrquist ·
Howard I. Maibach · Bernhard Homey
Editors

The Skin Microbiome Manual

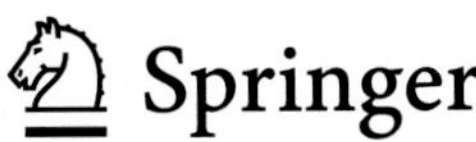 Springer

Editors
Antti Lauerma
Department of Dermatology
University of Helsinki
Helsinki, Finland

Howard I. Maibach
University of California San Francisco
San Francisco, CA, USA

Nanna Fyhrquist
Institute of Environmental Medicine
Karolinska Institute
Stockholm, Sweden

Bernhard Homey
Department of Dermatology
Heinrich Heine University
Düsseldorf, Nordrhein-Westfalen, Germany

ISBN 978-3-031-82691-7   ISBN 978-3-031-82689-4   (eBook)
https://doi.org/10.1007/978-3-031-82689-4

This Springer imprint is published by the registered company Springer Nature Switzerland AG
The registered company address is: Gewerbestrasse 11, 6330 Cham, Switzerland

If disposing of this product, please recycle the paper.

Contents

Chapter 1
Effects of Cream Application in Childhood on Skin Barrier and Development of Atopic Diseases

Helen A. Brough, Sayantani B. Sindher, Maeve M. Kelleher, Didem Sanver,
Mohamed H. Shamji, Vanitha Sampath, Shifaa Alkotob, Gideon Lack,
and Kari Nadeau

Abstract Dry skin and atopic dermatitis are early manifestations of skin barrier dysfunction and inflammation and are the first step in the atopic march leading to food and respiratory allergies through environmental exposure to allergens. The lipid composition of the outermost layer of the skin (the stratum corneum) is crucial in the development of skin barrier dysfunction and has an important interplay with the skin pH, hydrophobic properties and rheological properties. In the first section of this chapter, we review the lipid structure of the stratum corneum and emollient properties that influence barrier function including ceramides, free fatty acids and cholesterol. In the second section, we review petrolatum-based and trilipid emollients in the primary prevention of atopic dermatitis and food allergy; despite promising pilot study data where petrolatum-based emollients were shown to improve stratum corneum hydration, they did not have effects on preventing, delaying or reducing

H. A. Brough (✉) · G. Lack
Evelina London Children's Hospital, Guy's and St Thomas' NHS Foundation Trust, Children's
Allergy Service, King's College London, Department of Women and Children's Health, School of
Life Course Sciences and School of Immunology and Microbial Sciences, 2nd Floor, Stairwell B,
South Wing, St Thomas' Hospital, Westminster Bridge Road, London SE1 7EH, England
e-mail: helen.brough@gstt.nhs.uk

S. B. Sindher · S. Alkotob
Sean N. Parker Center for Asthma and Allergy Research, Stanford School of Medicine, Palo Alto,
CA, USA

M. M. Kelleher · D. Sanver · M. H. Shamji
National Heart and Lung Institute, Section of Inflammation, Repair, Development, Imperial
College of London, London, England

D. Sanver
Department of Food Engineering, Faculty of Engineering and Architecture, Necmettin Erbakan
University, 42090 Konya, Turkey

V. Sampath · K. Nadeau
Department of Environmental Health, Harvard T.H. Chan School of Public Health, Boston, MA,
USA

the severity of atopic dermatitis and in one study increased risk of skin infections and showed a trend towards increased food allergy. Primary prevention with trilipid emollients shows promising pilot data but results from larger randomized controlled trials are awaited. The third section outlines other topical therapies, including vitamin D, probiotics, calcineurin inhibitors, and corticosteroids. These have beneficial effect in the management of eczema, and proactive topical steroid application in early infancy has been shown to reduce IgE, and potentially reduce allergic march sequelae, but further research is ongoing in this field.

Keywords Atopic dermatitis · Emollient · Primary prevention · Secondary prevention · Atopic march · Food allergy · Probiotics · Vitamin D · Topical steroids

1.1 Introduction

Dry skin condition is a common dermatological problem that primarily affects young children. It has been observed that AD in infancy is associated with an increase in food allergy, inhalant allergies, and rhinitis (Goksör et al. 2016; Tsakok et al. 2016). Early onset of AD, typically defined as having the first clinical presentation of AD before 6 months has a strong association with IgE-mediated food allergy (Martin et al. 2015). Normal skin, which is not dry, or inflamed prevents the passage of allergens through the skin. Dry and inflamed skin allows the passage of allergens through the skin, leading to an inflammatory Th2 response, and epicutaneous sensitization to food and potentially inhalant allergens. Thus, dry skin and atopic dermatitis may be the first step in the atopic march leading to food and respiratory allergies. One would therefore hypothesize that creams that repair and maintain skin barrier properties may potentially have anti-inflammatory effects on the skin thus counteracting these effects.

Individuals with dry skin have a reduced barrier function of the stratum corneum (SC, the outermost layer of the epidermis), which helps to hydrate and retain water. Water loss from the skin is associated with impaired barrier function. Changes in lipid composition and organization in the SC are associated with impaired skin barrier. For example, several advanced biophysical techniques such as Fourier transform infrared spectroscopy (FTIR) and small and wide-angle X-ray scattering (SAXS/WAXS) have compared the lipid composition and lateral lipid organization in both healthy individuals and those with atopic dermatitis (AD) and show healthy individuals have SC lipids densely packed with an orthorhombic orientation (Van Smeden et al. 2014a, b). There is evidence that shows SC of AD has a lower level of total lipids and ceramides (CERs), which is associated with a reduced skin barrier function. Delivering densely packed lipids to the skin via skin creams is an effective way to relieve the symptoms of dry skin and improve the skin barrier. Therefore, it is important to better understand the biophysical and biochemical properties of lipids that support the use of skin cream formulations. The first section of this chapter details the stratum corneum lipids, then moves to biophysical and biochemical properties of the emollients, and finally, compare the mechanisms of different emollients. The insight and knowledge generated from lipid studies will then allow us to make more informed decision about the formulation of more effective emollients.

Atopic dermatitis (AD) is an important clinical manifestation of an impaired skin barrier. Genetic determinants of the skin barrier, such as FLG mutation, are strongly associated with AD, food allergy, and asthma. This association with asthma, is only in the setting of clinical AD (Irvine et al. 2011). The second section of this chapter will review topical therapies that that been used in the primary prevention of AD and whether this is effective in preventing subsequent atopic march sequelae. The third section details topical therapies in children with established AD to reduce the severity and duration of AD and evaluate whether they can reduce the onset of subsequent allergic diseases.

1.2 Biophysical Properties of the Skin and Emollients

1.2.1 Biophysical Characterization of Stratum Corneum Lipid Profile in Healthy Subjects and Atopic Dermatitis Patients

1.2.1.1 The Structure and Composition of the Stratum Corneum

The stratum corneum (SC), the outermost layer of the human epidermis (Fig. 1.1a) with a thickness of 9–13 μm, is the main barrier that controls the penetration of substances. It consists of approximately 10 to 25 tightly-packed, well-hydrated corneocyte layers surrounded by intercellular SC lipid matrix. The corneocytes are flattened protein-rich dead cells, which are nearly parallel to the skin surface (Harding 2004). Instead of the normal cell membrane, they possess an inner envelope of cross-linked proteins, the cornified envelope (CE). The corneocytes contain a mixture of water-soluble natural moisturizing factors (NMF), whose primary role is to maintain skin hydration. In healthy SC, the lipid matrix envelops the NMF and prevents its loss from the corneocytes. Shown in Fig. 1.1b, the SC is analogous to a "bricks in mortar" structure, where the bricks represent the corneocytes, and the mortar represents the lipids. The SC lipid matrix contains multi-lamellar stacks of planar lipid bilayers (Fig. 1.1c) enriched in ceramides (CERs), cholesterol (CHOL), and free fatty acids (FFAs) at equimolar ratios (33 mol% each) (Fig. 1.1e). By weight, this molar ratio is equal to 45–50 wt% CERs, 25 wt% CHOL, 10–15 wt% FFAs, and each of other lipids < 5 wt% of the total lipid dry mass of the lipid matrix (Harding 2004). The lipids in the SC lipid matrix are oriented in repeating lamellar structure. Electron microscopy as well as neutron diffraction studies reveal no swelling of the lipid lamellar or no free unbound water in the deepest layers of the SC, indicating that water transport through the SC is physically inhibited and in turn, water loss is minimized (Bouwstra et al. 2003). Since the intercellular lipid matrix is the main

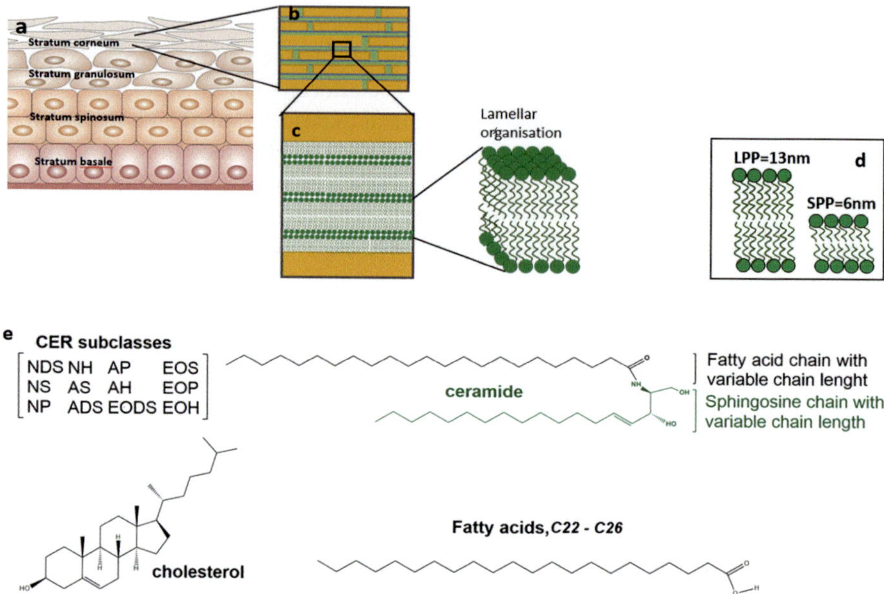

Fig. 1.1 Lipid organization in the stratum corneum (SC) showing the outermost layer of the epidermis (**a**), the stratum corneum (SC) (**b**), Schematic representation of the SC, "bricks and mortar" structure, where the corneocytes represent the bricks and the lipids represent the mortar (**c**), lamellar arrangement of the intercellular lipids of the SC (**d**), long and short repeat distances of the lamellar repeat phases, referred to as the LPP (~13 nm) or SPP (~6 nm), respectively (**e**) structure of the major skin lipids of SC including ceramides (CER), cholesterol (CHOL) and free fatty acids (FFA)

pathway for cutaneous penetration of substances, lipids play a vital role in the skin barrier function. Therefore, it is important to understand the SC lipid composition and organization to more fully explain skin barrier function.

Advances in analytical techniques such as gas or liquid chromatography coupled with mass spectrometry (GC/MS) or (LC/MS) have helped identify the structure of SC lipids and identify the 12 subclasses of CERs (Janssens et al. 2012). In all classes, CER molecules are composed of the double-tailed hydrophobic chains that are made up of a sphingosine tail (S-chain) coupled to a fatty acid tail (N-chain) via an amide bond. The fatty acid chain of CERs is longer than the sphingoside chain with a higher polydispersity in length and hydrogen bonding. The polydispersity of chain lengths in each CER subclass, the varying number of hydroxyl (OH) groups in the acyl chain and the presence of an unsaturated bonding help form a diverse range of CER molecules in SC. The SC lipids possess different physicochemical properties than the cellular lipids. Considering the structural properties, 12 CER subclasses are denoted as: [NdS], [NS], [NP], [NH] (the non-hydroxy fatty acid, [N] classes), [AdS] [AS], [AH], [AP] (α-hydroxy fatty acid, [A] classes) and [EOP], [EOH], [EOdS], [EOS] (esterified ω-hydroxy fatty acid in the omega position, [EO] subclasses). In this letter code-based nomenclature, the first letter (e.g. [N], [A]) defines the type of fatty acid modification present, while the last letter (the third for [EO]) marks the type of sphingoid base. This means, [S] stands for sphingosine with a 4,5-double bond, [H] stands for 6-hydroxy-sphingosine with a 6-OH, 4,5-double bond, and [P] stands for phytosphingosine with a 4-OH. The CER composition and content within the SC were reported to be significant to maintain skin barrier function. FFAs consist of a single carbon chain and exhibit a similar length polydispersity to CERs with a varying chain length between 12 and 36C. However, long-chain FFAs, mainly C22, C24, and C26, are more dominant in human SC compared with shorter chain lengths with 16, 18 and 20 carbon atoms (Groen et al. 2011). The main sterol in the SC is cholesterol, which plays a crucial role in the correct lipid organization of the SC and skin barrier function. Also, cholesterol is responsible for the fluidity of lipid bilayers.

1.2.1.2 Lipid Organization in Human Stratum Corneum

Lipid organization in human SC exhibits a unique arrangement: the lipids are organized into two co-existing crystalline lamellae that are oriented nearly parallel to the surface of the corneocytes. As well as the lamellar organization, the lateral organization is a vital parameter for skin barrier function. Lipids within the plane of the lamellae are perpendicular to the lamellar lipid organization, known as the lateral organization. Three possible lateral lipid organizations have been identified in healthy human SC: (i) the very densely packed, orthorhombic arrangement; (ii) the less dense, hexagonal organization; and (iii) the liquid organization. Both lamellar organization and lateral packing play an essential role in the skin barrier function (Van Smeden et al. 2014a, b).

1.2.1.3 Lamellar and Lateral Lipid Organization

Visualization of the intercellular lipid matrix in human SC show the lipid organization in lamellar sheets that are stacked on top of each other in a regular arrangement. As depicted in Fig. 1.1(d), further studies in human SC using Small Angle X-ray Scattering (SAXS) revealed two co-existing lamellar phases within the lipid matrix, with well-defined repeat distances of 13 nm (long periodicity phase—LPP) and 6 nm (short periodicity phase—SPP) (Van Smeden et al. 2014a, b). To gain an in-depth understanding regarding the SC lipid matrix constituents, model membrane architectures were developed from isolated skin lipids and their mixtures to mimic the lipid composition and organization in the SC in a simplified setting. Because the interactions within the lipid matrix are complex and dynamic, these models allow us to better evaluate and document the role of individual CER species and other lipids on the epidermal barrier function. Mimicking the SC lipid behavior indicated the crucial role of CER and CHOL in the emergence of these two phases. The studies suggest that LPP is an important parameter that contributes to the cutaneous barrier function.

The lamellar organization in SC of healthy and diseased skin revealed by X-ray scattering (SAXS) showed differences in LPP formation, which could be related to increased permeability of the skin barrier (Janssens et al. 2011), and hence may contribute to a reduced skin barrier function. Several studies also explored the way the lipids arrange themselves within the lamellae, the lateral organization, which used advanced biophysical techniques such as Wide-angle X-ray Scattering (WAXS) and Fourier Transform Infrared Spectroscopy (FTIR) to explore the lateral packing in both isolated human SC and mice (Babita et al. 2006; Bouwstra and Ponec 2006). The findings suggest the predominant presence of very dense orthorhombic lipid organization in healthy human SC, with small domains of hexagonal organization, and even low-density disordered, liquid state (Damien and Boncheva 2010). It was also reported that long-chain FFAs are responsible for orthorhombic lateral packing since they enhance the packing density (van Smeden et al. 2014a, b). It is important to gain a deeper understanding regarding the role of lipid behavior, e.g. its organization and composition, to elucidate the mechanism of skin barrier function in healthy and diseased skin. This understanding will provide insight into the relationship between SC lipids and skin diseases, and in turn, inform treatments for skin diseases. An early study investigated the effect of lateral orthorhombic lipid packing on the permeability of benzoic acid (BA) using both excised human SC and a model that mimics SC lipid composition and barrier function (Groen et al. 2011). This model was also used to examine the effect of shorter chain FFA on the barrier function. For this purpose, diffusion studies were performed over a range of temperature between 15 to 45 °C. In terms of permeability to BA, excised human SC and model SC revealed a significant similarity, which correlates well with other studies. This showed that the lipid model closely mimicked the permeation properties of human SC. The study also refuted previous studies regarding water permeation through human SC, suggesting no noticeable difference between orthorhombic and hexagonal lateral packing in diffusivity of BA. However, when skin lipids were modelled with short-chain FFA, the lamellar organization was significantly altered, and in turn, increased permeability. These results show how the formation of ordered lamellar phases influence on the SC barrier function, compared with the way lipids pack laterally.

1.2.1.4   Lamellar and Lateral Lipid Organization in Atopic Dermatitis

Lipid composition and the lamellar structure were also investigated in diseased skin, e.g. atopic dermatitis (AD), to determine whether the altered lipid behavior contributed to the reduced skin barrier function. AD or atopic eczema describes the chronic, autoimmune pruritic inflammatory skin condition with an estimated prevalence of up to 15% to 20% of children and 1% to 3% of adults in developed countries. AD is characterized by a defective skin barrier. Several influencing factors from genetic susceptibility to cutaneous inflammation are risk factors for AD. Although the mechanism behind the pathological process of AD is not fully explored, filaggrin (FLG) is accepted as one of the most influential genes in predisposing AD.

For example, up to 50% of Northern European kindreds and a considerable proportion of Asian subjects with AD have either single or double allele loss-of-function mutations in the gene encoding for FLG (Elias and Wakefield 2014). The initial product of FLG is pro-FLG, which is a highly cationic phosphoprotein enriched in hydrophobic amino acids. During the cornification process from pro-FLG to FLG in healthy nonatopic humans, these amino acids are proteolytically removed from the proteins and deaminated into polycarboxylic acids, also known as natural moisturizing factors (NMF). Disruption in this process results in the loss of all by-products including NMF, which accounts for the SC hydration and acidification. As a result, the SC is poorly formed and becomes prone to water loss. Filaggrin deficiency-associated AD is linked to abnormalities in lipid content, distribution, and lamellar lipid organization in lesional skin. This can eventually lead to a defective epidermal barrier (Elias and Wakefield 2014).

Early studies of AD reported a decrease in total SC lipid content, and the ratio of the SC lipid classes (CERs, FFAs and CHOL) in both lesional and non-lesional skin. The decrease was more evident for certain CER classes, i.e. CER[NP] and CER[EOS]. On the other hand, an increased level of CER[AS] was also observed. In terms of lateral organization of lipids, SC of AD skin revealed a higher level of lipids forming a hexagonal lateral packing compared with control skin (Janssens et al. 2012). The full CER profile of AD patients were characterized by CER composition, chain length distribution, and FLG mutations and the skin barrier function monitored by transepidermal water loss (TEWL) (Ishikawa et al. 2010). This study was the first to uncover the importance of lipid chain length distribution in AD patients. The findings showed an increase (around threefold) in the level of short-chain CERs (CER[NS]), together with a significantly reduced level of long-chain acyl-CER (around 50%) in SC lipid profile of AD patients, which correlated substantially with the skin barrier function showing an increase in TEWL values (Ishikawa et al. 2010). It was also reported that the observed changes in CER composition were not associated with FLG mutations, suggesting that the differences could arise from AD-effects. Further studies including control samples also correlated with the finding that altered lipid composition in SC of AD patients is not related to FLG mutations, and other parameters such as inflammation or antimicrobial activity in AD patients may influence the alterations in lipid composition, hence skin barrier function (Janssens et al. 2012).

A limited number of studies also investigated the FFA composition in AD skin, which reported a considerable decrease in the level of long fatty acid chains (≥ 24 carbon atoms), along with an increase in the shorter FFA with C16 and C18 (Van Smeden et al. 2014a, b). As in the case of CER chain length, the modulations in FFA profile were more pronounced in lesional skin. FFA alterations in SC were also reported to arise from inflammation or antimicrobial activity. Given that FFAs are the building blocks for the CERs, it was suggested a reduced CER chain length reported in AD arises from a reduced FFA chain length.

All these studies clearly indicate that there is a close relationship between modulations in SC lipids and defective barrier function in AD skin. Moreover, barrier abnormalities have not only been associated with the development of AD but also suggested to be critical for the development of later allergies, including allergic rhinitis, and food allergies. Therefore, even though the modulations in lipid properties are not directly causative for the disease, it is important to obtain an in-depth information on the mechanisms behind these modulations. As a result of the reduced concentrations of the key lipids of SC, as well as the disruptions of SC lamellar lipid organization in AD, barrier abnormalities may occur, which are associated with an increased risk of skin diseases (Van Smeden et al. 2014a, b). Disrupted lipid composition and weakened barrier in AD increase TEWL through the skin. This results in xerotic skin with severely dry and itchy skin. To alleviate these symptoms and maintain the normal function of skin, several emollient formulations have been designed with each targeting a different mechanism: (i) incorporation of humectants such as glycerine into formulation promotes desquamation by retaining moisture in the surface layers of the SC and (ii) inclusion of occlusive ingredients such as petrolatum-based white soft paraffin (WSP), or lipid-based ceramides in the formulation prevents transepidermal water escaping via skin occlusion with ingredients (Bulsara et al. 2017). With this in mind, several studies aimed to design effective formulations using occlusive ingredients that can mimic key features of barrier lipids in SC. For this purpose, occlusive agents were initially screened via in vitro water vapor transmission rate (WVTR) testing, and further characterized using Fourier transform infrared (FTIR) spectroscopy and X-ray diffraction (XRD) methods. Biophysical characterization using such sophisticated techniques provide in depth picture of lateral packing of molecules and thickness of the lamellar system. These characteristics of the formulations show their design efficacy in terms of mimicking the structural features of human SC.

In addition to these studies with ceramides, other studies concentrated on characterizing formulations with cheaper occlusive agents such as phospholipids and fatty acids, which can mimic the behavior of the SC lipid matrix. Using these agents, studies aimed to avoid the high-cost and formulation challenges associated with ceramides. The behavior of several fatty acids including behenic acid and cetostearyl alcohol, and phosphatidylcholines with a chain length between C14-C22 were evaluated for their ability to mimic the structural characteristics of the SC lipid matrix. The parameters considered to choose these agents were based on the extent of acyl chain saturation and their length, which determine how tightly these lipids pack. However, this chapter will mainly concentrate on petrolatum-based emollients which consist of petrolatum or other ingredients like paraffin, and lipid-based emollients with CER, FFAs and CHOL. The insight and knowledge generated from lipid studies will provide valuable information to the formulation industry to make more informed development decisions with reduced costs. Understanding the role of lipids in SC will help designing topically applied substances with desired effects to improve skin barrier function (Bulsara et al. 2017).

1.2.2 Biophysical Characterization of Emollients

In the literature, the terms 'emollients' and 'moisturizers' are often used together. Moisturizer is a more commonly used term by the general public, whereas emollient is often a technical term. It is also often seen in literature that moisturizers are referred to as emollients (Penzer 2013). It has been established that applying skincare products may influence the barrier properties of the skin. However, the mechanism underlying the improvement in skin barrier function is not fully understood. The pH of the products and their composition are two important parameters that influence the skin barrier function.

Classification of emollients

To address the best emollient type for individuals with AD, a panel of clinical experts from the UK developed recommendations (Moncrieff et al. 2013). According to their classification, *occlusive emollient creams* are oil-in-water emulsions and *occlusive emollient ointments* are water-in-oil emulsions (or 100% lipid). While the creams form a thin lipid film barrier on the skin, ointments provide a thicker lipid barrier to prevent the water loss. Therefore, creams are recommended for moderately dry skin, whereas ointments are recommended for more severe AD. For very severe AD, *occlusive ointment with no water content* that includes white soft paraffin (WSP), liquid paraffin (LP), or a 50:50 ratio of the WSP/ LP can be considered. The mechanism of action of occlusive is generally based on their ability to physically block TEWL from the skin by forming a layer on the skin surface (Purnamawati et al. 2017). *Humectant containing emollients* was recommended for patients with psoriasis, where petrolatum-based emollients are not effective. Humectants are low molecular hygroscopic substances such as urea, glycerine, and sorbitol. In combination with occlusive ingredients, they help to hydrate the SC by attracting water into the SC from the dermis. The last category of *antipruritic emollients* are products with antipruritic agents, which are used as the first-line therapy for pruritus as well as in all dry-skin conditions. The panel also came to an agreement for not prescribing aqueous cream BP since it contains 1% of sodium lauryl sulfate (SLS) which increases skin pH, TEWL, and removes skin lipids. Other alternative pharmaceutical presentations for AD are categorized as oils, gels, and lotions, which all affect the skin in different ways (Eichenfield et al. 2014). Emollient gels usually contain high concentrations of oily ingredients in semisolid aqueous systems. Lotions generally lack the hydrating properties necessary for treating atopic dermatitis.

1.2.2.1 Skin pH, Hydrophilic Index and Stratum Corneum Barrier

The natural pH of adult SC ranges from 4 to 6, in the acidic range. Maintaining pH balance of natural skin is important to maintaining the overall functions of human skin such as the structural integrity of the SC and proper hydration of the epidermis. The correct pH is also important to keep resident flora and maintain enzyme (protease) function. An increase in the pH of the SC into the neutral and basic range can disrupt enzyme activity which involves barrier restoration, breaking down filaggrin and decreasing the production of natural moisturizing factor (NMF). An increased pH also corresponds to an increased TEWL, one of the most important biophysical indicators of the epidermal barrier function. Moreover, the skin pH has also been reported to play a role correctly organizing matrix lipids, i.e., fluctuations in the pH could alter the composition and spatial structure of the intracellular lipids, which dry the skin. Such a barrier-dependent increase in pH is seen with AD patients, with the highest value for lesional skin of patients with AD (Schmid-Wendtner and Korting 2006).

Several skincare products are applied on the skin to balance the skin pH and prevent dryness. Studies revealed a pH-dependent barrier recovery; that is, exposing perturbed skin sites to neutral pH buffers delay the recovery of barrier permeability. Therefore, it is essential to consider the pH of these products used daily. To address this, three skincare products with pH values of 3, 5 and 8 were applied twice a day for 5 weeks in healthy volunteers to investigate the influence of pH on the physical properties of skin (Kim et al. 2009). The alkaline product (pH 8) significantly increased TEWL reading and impaired the skin barrier, which became more sensitive to external exposures such as 1% (w/v) SLS (sodium lauryl sulphate). Hence, it is important to understand the role of pH in AD to gain a better understanding how the products are used in eczema restore pH balance.

A comprehensive study (Shi et al. 2012) measured the Hydrophilic Index (HI) of 31 emollients and utilized this parameter as an indication of "greasiness" to help select an appropriate emollient and avoid confusion from the textural differences between different emollients. The study also measured the pH of the skin moisturizers and explored a link between HI index and pH and their ability to restore SC acid milieu. pH of selected products varied between 3.73 and 8.19. Most of the products remained in the acidic range with values between 4 to 6. The HI values were reported between 26.84 and 100.00, with almost 2/3 of them exhibiting a HI < 50, suggesting that most products exhibit high lipid content. Based on the pH and HI measurements, the authors recommended 22 products of the original 31 that have low pH values for AD patients. However, 7 of these were reported to be quite hydrophilic. The hydration effect of these hydrophilic products was reported to be mainly limited to the superficial layers of the SC rather than deeper layers in the SC. Therefore, they did not benefit the lipid metabolism in the deeper SC, and were not judged suitable for patients with mild-to-severe AD (Caussin et al. 2009). Hydrophobic emollients on the other hand retained water both on the skin surface and deeper SC. They have also been reported to change the lamellar lipid organization of the membrane bilayer in deeper SC, preventing water loss from the epidermis (Caussin et al. 2007, 2008). Despite their benefits, an unwanted greasy feeling may be reported upon application of these emollients.

1.2.2.2   The Physicochemical Characteristics of the Emollients

Along with pH and HI, rheological properties of emollients such as hardness, adhesiveness, and spreadability have also been investigated (Kitagawa et al. 2016; Douguet et al. 2017). The ideal emollient should not include any ingredient that could be irritating to the skin, and should be odorless, easily spreadable on the skin, and cost-effective for people with AD (van Zuuren, Fedorowicz et al. 2017). For patients with AD, investigations of emollients are mainly limited to steroid ointments and their mixtures with other cream formulations. For example, in one study, the effect of surfactants on the rheological properties of 3 steroid ointments and their generic ointments were compared (Kitagawa et al. 2016). Authors reported that generic and brand name steroid ointments are bioequivalent, their rheological properties such as hardness, adhesiveness, and spreadability show noticeable differences depending upon the type of surfactants used. For example, non-ionic surfactants decreased hardness and adhesiveness while increasing spreadability of the emollients. On the other hand, when glyceryl monostearate (GMS) was used as a surfactant, hardness and adhesiveness of the emollients were higher, while spreadability was lower. Moreover, non-ionic surfactants promoted phase separation when mixed with a water-in-oil type white petrolatum-based heparinoid cream, however, the mixing combability was better in the presence of GMS. The study reported that rheological properties of ointments are strongly affected by the emulsifying capacity of the surfactants. Hydrophilic-lipohilic balance (HLB) of surfactants can be used as an effective parameter in predicting their emulsifying capacity. For example, HLB of glyceryl monostearate is 3.8, which makes it a suitable agent in preparation of water-in-oil emulsions, whereas, non-ionic surfactants of polyoxyethylene (POE) exhibit higher HLB (>10), which makes them suitable in formulating oil-in-water emulsions.

Shibata et al. compared the physical characteristics of cream and ointment steroids of the same kind. Although creams revealed higher spreadability scores, whereas mometasone furoate was significantly lower. On the other hand, mometasone furoate was found to be more viscous and odiferous compared to other emollients studied. They related the spreadability parameter to the potential of emollients to reduce mechanical irritation to lesions during topical application (Shibata et al. 2007). The rheological properties are crucial parameters to take into account when designing emollients. For example, products with high viscosity are not only more difficult to spread on the skin, but also, they can lead to adverse reactions such as skin friction. To gain a comprehensive grasp on the influence of rheological properties such as absorption, stability, viscosity, and spreadability, more studies need to be conducted.

The abnormalities in skin barrier function result in TEWL and enhance the penetration of allergens into the skin. Such barrier-impaired skin can be treated using a number of topically applied emollients. Early and daily application with emollients is the most common protective factor against developing AD. Keeping the area well-moisturized and supple prevents cracking to a great extent. Hence, it is recommended to include moisturizers (emollients) in every AD patient's treatment plan. Different emollients reveal different repair mechanism for the skin barrier and it is therefore important to choose the most appropriate emollient type based on the patient's needs. In the next section, we cover petrolatum-based emollients, trilipid emollients and others for their influence on the most critical biophysical parameters (TEWL, skin pH, epidermal hydration, and sebum excretion) that characterize the status of the epidermal barrier.

1.2.3 The Effect of Different Emollients on Biophysical Properties of Skin

The current section highlights the effect of different emollients on the skin biophysical properties such as alterations in skin pH, TEWL, and SC hydration. The subsequent section will discuss some of these studies in terms of the clinical outcome of prevention of atopic disease.

1.2.3.1 The Effect of Petrolatum-Based Emollient Formulations in AD Management

The first-ever therapeutic product developed to prevent dry skin (xerosis) is petrolatum, a mineral-oil based ingredient widely used in skincare products as an occlusive agent because of its ability to block the evaporation of water. Due to its occlusive property, petrolatum hydrates the skin by blocking TEWL (Rawlings and Lombard 2012). Therefore, it has already been established as a commonly used positive standard when assessing the skin hydration ability of other ingredients. Several studies addressed the early dryness and impaired skin function using emollients to investigate whether emollient therapy during the early stages in life could potentially improve barrier function. This hypothesis represents a novel approach in AD management.

Initial studies in this area mainly focused on daily application of petrolatum-based emollients as they are affordable and widely available over-the-counter (OTC). In one of the early pilot studies, a petrolatum-based OTC cream (Cetaphil) designed as oil-in-water emulsion was applied twice daily in 22 neonates who had a high risk of developing AD (Simpson et al. 2010). This emollient therapy resulted in similar TEWL values between control and emollient group. Because emollient use did not improve TEWL values, it was suggested that applying this standard cream to the infant skin does not correct the barrier abnormalities associated with AD. However, the risk of developing AD after 547 days was 15%, suggesting a protective effect in managing AD (Simpson et al. 2010).

1.2.4   The Effect of Petrolatum-Based Emollient Formulations in AD Prevention

In another study, authors compared petroleum jelly (petrolatum) with an emulsion emollient for their potential to reduce the risk of AD in 116 asymptomatic neonates in a randomized controlled parallel-group trial (Horimukai et al. 2014). Daily application of the emulsion-type emollient in the intervention group was compared with the control group. Both groups were prescribed petroleum jelly. Skin barrier function was measured as a function of TEWL, stratum corneum hydration (SCH) and skin pH at birth and at 4, 12, 24, and 32 weeks of life to predict AD development. Also, SC hydration in the lower leg at weeks 12 and 24 was considerably high compared with the control group. Retrospective post-hoc data analysis of the trial showed an association between skin barrier function measured through non-invasive skin tests (TEWL, SCH and skin pH) and AD development by age 32 weeks (Horimukai et al. 2016a, b). A noticeable difference was observed in TEWL readings from the forehead with values ranging between 6.4 and 8.9 $g/m^2/h$, with an optimal cutoff, 6.50 $g/m^2/h$, as well as in SCH values on the lower leg (15 AU), and on the forehead (21 AU). Compared to SCH and pH values, measurement of TEWL on the forehead within the first week of life revealed a more pronounced and more statistically significant correlation in predicting the risk of developing AD in early infancy (Horimukai et al. 2016a, b). Clinical outcomes are discussed in the section below.

Further, Yonezawa et al. conducted a randomized control trial to investigate the relationship between bathing and newborns' skin barrier function in 227 healthy Asian newborns aged between 1 week to 3 months old (Yonezawa et al. 2018). The effect of moisturizing skincare was assessed using different moisturizers. The intervention group (n = 113) used lotion daily and bathed every 2 days, and the control group (n = 114) bathed each day without applying lotion. The skin barrier function was evaluated by alterations in pH, SC hydration (SCH), TEWL, and sebum secretion at 3 months of age. Face TEWL recordings ($g/m^2/h$) revealed a lower value with intervention group (14.69 ± 7.38) compared with the control (17.08 ± 8.26), along with a higher face SCH value (60.38 ± 13.66 vs. 53.52 ± 14.55). Similarly, body SCH was higher than control SCH value (58.89 ± 12.96 vs 53.02 ± 10.08), indicating skin dryness was prevented. Moreover, a significant reduction in diaper dermatitis was observed with intervention group between birth and 1 month old, compared to the control group (6.3% vs 15.9%). Overall, this randomized parallel comparison study promoted an increase in SCH among newborns with daily skincare.

The data from the largest trial in this context—the BEEP randomized controlled trial—with 1394 high-risk infants was recently published (Chalmers et al. 2020). To understand the influence of these two emollients on the mechanistic properties of skin, Danby et al., recruited two cohorts of volunteers with a tendency to a defective skin barrier to investigate the effect of two different emollients, a gel-based and a cream-based (Danby et al. 2016a, b). While the first cohort (18 volunteers) was treated with a gel, the other cohort (19 volunteers) received Diprobase® cream twice daily for 4 weeks. The effect of these emollients on skin dryness, the SC hydration, skin pH and

TEWL values were determined before and after treatment. Moreover, the skin barrier recovery was also assessed after tape-stripping. The application of the emollients for four weeks did not alter TEWL values, indicating no noteworthy effect of either emollients on skin barrier function. This was also validated by the estimated SC thickness, which remained unchanged upon treatment. In contrast, both emollients considerably improved skin hydration. For example, the sites treated with gel were 42% ± 5.1% more hydrated compared with untreated controls. The cream-based emollient also increased the skin hydration 14% ± 4.8% and the less pronounced increase with the gel-based emollient was attributed to the shorter duration of this product on the skin. Interestingly, both emollients imparted a statistically significant increase in skin pH compared with the pH change of untreated skin. Normally an increase in skin pH is an indication for a skin barrier breakdown. Therefore, an ideal topical agent should not increase the skin pH.

1.2.4.1 The Effect of Trilipid-Based Emollient in AD Management

Recently, there has been a shift from classical petrolatum-based moisturizers towards more sophisticated lamellar lipid-based products with ceramides, fatty acids, and other phospholipids. These lipid-based formulations have been shown to mimic the structural character of SC lipid matrix with an ability to repair skin barrier. Electron microscopy images also showed that lipid-based emollients can penetrate into deeper SC, while typical emollients can only form a more superficial occlusive barrier.

One of the early studies investigated the effect of twice daily application of trilipids, as an alternative to commonly used moisturizers in 24 children with a mean age of 6.4 years old and an average disease duration of 5 years. The moisturizers and emollients that were replaced with trilipids included petrolatum as either active or inactive ingredient in their formulation. When these emollients were all replaced by triliipids, a significant decrease in TEWL readings was seen compared to initial values before treatment. TEWL decrease continued even after 12 weeks of treatment. Moreover, SC hydration increased significantly with trilipid therapy, and reached to a clinically meaningful level at last visit (Chamlin et al. 2002). One of the most significant outcomes of this study was obtained from electron microscopy images that visualized the morphology of the membrane bilayer structure in SC, both treated with standard emollients prior to the study, and 6 weeks after switching to trilipids. The images clearly revealed a formation of extracellular lamellar bilayers in SC, which were absent in baseline SC treated with standard emollients. The formation of lamellar bilayers in SC after applying trilipids also correlated with improved barrier function. The findings suggest that, unlike commonly used standard moisturizers, trilipids improved SC ceramide deficiency.

Another study with electron microscope visualized the alterations in epidermal differentiation of barrier-damaged mouse skin upon single treatment with a trilipid cream (Man et al. 2015). Authors used trilipids as a positive control and compared this with an in-house prepared mixture of sunflower oil, glycerol, borage oil, petrolatum, and lanolin at optimum doses. Although they found no changes in skin surface pH and SC hydration with the in-house formulated mixture, they found it stimulated epidermal differentiation-related proteins, in particular involucrin, which improved permeability. The mixture was also reported to secrete lamellar body formation similar to the trilipid emollient, suggesting that the mixture formulation may improve barrier function.

Several phase I and phase II studies have also been conducted to evaluate the safety and feasibility of a trilipid-based emollient on the infant skin barrier function, as well as its effects on skin biophysical properties such as alterations in skin pH, TEWL, SC hydration. A phase I study investigated the effect of daily application of trilipid cream for 6 weeks in 10 infants (0–4 weeks of age) with a family history of allergy (Lowe et al. 2012). Follow-up assessment at 6 weeks on the biophysical parameters of the skin revealed that the application of trilipids decreased TEWL values with a mean of 9.3 $g/m^2/hr$ compared with those reported with a mean of 26 $g/m^2/hr$ for infants in this age group. Moreover, surface pH of forearm and forehead were maintained in the follow-up duration with values of 5.1 and 4.9, respectively. Following successful demonstration of parent compliance and the safety of trilipids for AD prevention in neonates, Lowe et al., also conducted a phase III trial—the PEBBLES trial—with trilipids in high-risk infants up to 12 months of age (Lowe et al. 2018a, b, c). They investigated the effect of twice-daily application of trilipids on the prevalence of AD and skin barrier function, and assessed the biophysical parameters of the skin including skin pH, hydration "oiliness" (sebum), and TEWL. Although the biophysical data was not shown, TEWL measurements imparted no noteworthy effect on skin barrier function. Clinical outcomes from this trial are discussed in the subsequent section.

A new formulation of a popular brand available OTC was enriched with ceramides species, was also investigated in adult patients with AD. In addition to CERs, the formulation included vitamin B3, which plays a role in ceramides synthesis for barrier protection, as well as NMF components, which are known as flaggrin degradation products. The formulation was designed upon a new understanding regarding the molecular abnormalities underlying AD skin, i.e. low CER levels in AD lesional skin. The aim of this study was to assess the ability of this new CRM to improve the barrier abnormalities in controlled AD patients (Simpson et al. 2013). Twice-daily treatment with CRM for a month significantly improved TEWL, skin hydration, as well as clinical dryness, compared with untreated areas of the skin ($p < 0.01$). For example, TEWL values recorded at day 28 revealed a sevenfold reduction from baseline compared with untreated area ($p = 0.002$), expressing an improved skin barrier function. Such reduction in TEWL was in line with a significant increase in SC hydration with CRM (118% from baseline), compared with untreated skin (25.42% from baseline). Moreover, with CRM, skin dryness was reduced 56% from baseline compared with untreated (22%) after 4 weeks. Raman spectroscopy of different SC depths at day 28 revealed that CRM-treated area had a significantly higher level of CER content compared with the untreated area. Raman spectroscopy also measured the alterations in NMF and pyrrolidine carboxylic acid (PCA) from days 1 to 28 upon CRM treatment and indicated that although these changes were not statistically significant, they were in favor of CRM. Similarly, although water content level with

CRM-treated area was not significantly different, its alteration correlated with an increase in skin hydration compared with untreated areas of the skin.

Recently, a skin barrier sub-study (n = 56) investigated the role of once-daily full-body application of the emollient described above in high-risk infants within 21 days of birth for alterations in biophysical parameters including TEWL, skin pH, and skin electrical capacitance at 2 months, 6 months and 12 months (McClanahan et al. 2019a, b). Interestingly, there was no noteworthy difference in TEWL and capacitance values between the intervention group (n = 32) and the control group (n = 24) at these time-points. However, skin pH was significantly increased at 2 months with intervention arm (mean 5.46, SD 0.425) compared with controls (mean 4.98 ± 0.393), although no significant difference in pH was observed at other visits. The lack of differences in skin barrier biophysical measurements was attributed to the frequent use of emollients in the control group (45%). Another reason for the lack of differences was referred to different mechanisms in emollients. That is, their protective role to improve the biophysical skin properties could be a result of different mechanisms in skin barrier properties.

Despite several studies investigating the effect of petrolatum, trilipid, and steroid-based emollients on skin barrier of both infants and adults, few studies have compared these emollients to improve skin barrier. A recent pilot study by Sindher et al. compared the TEWL readings upon daily application of trilipids and paraffin-based emollient on different arms in children aged 0–5 years old for five weeks (Sindher et al. 2020a, b). Compared with a paraffin-based emollient, they found that trilipids reduced TEWL in infants/children with dry skin/AD or FA.

Another study compared the effect of a commercially available emollient containing 5% urea, ceramide NP and lactate (test emollient) to an alternative emollient without these additives (control emollient) on the properties of the skin barrier in older people (Danby et al. 2016a, b). Two cohorts of 21 volunteers aged > 60 years with dry skin were recruited. The first applied the test emollient twice daily for 28 days to one forearm and no treatment to the other for 28 days. The second compared the test emollient to the control emollient observing the same parameters. Effects on the skin barrier were determined by measuring skin barrier function, hydration, skin surface pH and by analyzing Fourier transform infrared spectra before and after treatment. A third cohort of 6 young adults was recruited to investigate the effect of a single treatment with the test emollient on the molecular structure of the skin barrier at greater depths by employing the tape-stripping technique. The test emollient hydrated the skin to a significantly greater extent and for a longer period of time compared with the control emollient, an effect associated with a significant elevation of carboxylate groups (a marker of natural moisturizing factor content) within the SC. Furthermore, the test emollient had additional benefits to the structure and function of the skin barrier not exhibited by the control emollient. Thus, the test emollient addressed the pathological features of xerotic aged skin, supporting its use as first-line therapy for xerotic skin conditions in this population.

1.2.4.2   Other Types of Emollients in AD Management

There is also another type of topical emollient—a heparinoid-containing moisturizer Hirudoid® —which is frequently used in Japan for treating AD. The active ingredient of this moisturizer is mucopolysaccharide polysulphate (MPS) at 0.3% w/w. From the structural point of view, MPS's are long unbranched polysaccharides with repetitive disaccharide units, which allow forming hydrogen bonding with neighboring water molecules to a great extent. This, in turn, retain water molecules and hydrates the surrounding tissues. Moreover, MPS has also been suggested to replenish the lamellar structure of the membrane (Hayama et al. 2015). As a result, a body of literature suggests that heparinoid-containing creams could improve the water content of the SC in AD patients. An early study explored the biophysical properties of a heparinoid-containing moisturizer applied twice daily for 5 days for its ability to alter TEWL and the hydration state of the skin surface in both healthy individuals and patients with AD. The effect of the heparinoid-based moisturizer on these biophysical parameters was also compared with the effect of other products including petrolatum, JP hydrophilic ointment containing glycosaminoglycans, which contains 10% urea and other humectants, and another mineral oil-based emollient with glycerol. TEWL recordings imparted no noteworthy differences in the water barrier function of the SC upon treatment with these emollients. However, assessing the hydration state of the skin surface through electrical measurements showed a significant increase in the hydration levels of the SC, with a more pronounced effect with the product containing heparinoid and JP hydrophilic ointment containing glycosaminoglycans (Tabata et al. 2000). The same group also compared these emollients using an xerotic animal skin model, which have been shown to successfully mimic human skin in terms of clinical and histopathological appearance. The once-daily treatment with heparinoid-containing moisturizers for 5 days revealed a stronger effect on skin hydration than the other topical agents in the skin of miniature swine, which lasted over 3 weeks after discontinuation of the treatment (O'Goshi et al. 2000).

Another study compared the effect of heparinoid-containing cream with a synthetic ceramide (CER) for its ability to alter TEWL and capacitance values upon their application to non-lesional skin of adult patients with AD. Upon three times daily treatment for 2–4 weeks with CER cream, TEWL values and capacitance values at 2 and 4 weeks were significantly increased. Moreover, there was a significant decrease in the clinical symptom scores, including dryness, scaling, and itchiness with the CER treatment. HIRU-containing cream also revealed a similar response to CER cream, with a less pronounced effect. In addition, the reduction in TEWL recording values (20.47 ± 8.61—before treatment) were also less noticeable with HIRU-containing product (13.64 ± 5.32) compared with the CER treatment (10.29 ± 5.41). Such a significant decrease in TEWL values with CER treatment suggested that CER cream was better at recovering the barrier function than the HIRU cream. Capacitance values (27.03 ± 11.10 before treatment) were also increased similarly by both products. That is, CER treatment increased capacitance (42.48 ± 13.06) compared with HIRU treatment (34.95 ± 12.45). Authors also suggested that barrier-replenishing effect in non-lesional skin is a critical parameter compared with water deficiency because skin barrier function improved to a greater extent than water deficiency (Matsuki et al. 2004).

To our knowledge, there is no published data regarding the effect of heparinoid containing products on the biophysical parameters of infant skin. However, a heparinoid containing ointment is currently under investigation in an controlled trial (PACI) investigating the effectiveness of early aggressive treatment for infant AD to prevent the development of later food allergy (Yamamoto-Hanada et al. 2018).

1.2.5 Take-Home Messages

- A large body of evidence connects alterations in the SC lipid environment, particularly CERs with impaired barrier and skin conditions. An ideal occlusive emollient would need to restore the healthy SC features, i.e. the presence of long periodicity phase, and a high degree of lateral order (rich in orthorhombic packing).
- More studies are needed to exert the molecular mechanisms of different CER classes.
- Different emollients, e.g. petrolatum-based and lipid-based emollients, reveal the different modes of action. Petrolatum-based, standard emollients do not necessarily prevent sensitization events. However, they hydrate the skin better.
- Future research in this context should focus on designing new products that might potentially exert a protective effect.
- Different biophysical techniques such as FTIR and SAXS can be used in future RCTs to elucidate the effect of the creams of interest on the composition and organization of the SC lipids to unravel their moisturizing capabilities.

1.3 Primary Prevention of Atopic Diseases

The skin barrier in an infant changes over the first few months of life. Just after birth, the skin barrier must adapt from an aqueous environment, having been surrounded by amniotic fluid in utero. Infant skin is drier, has a thinner epidermis and stratum corneum, and contains less lipids than in older children and adults (Stamatas et al. 2011). In prospective studies, skin changes in infancy precede the development of atopic dermatitis (Horimukai et al. 2016a, b).

As discussed above, in AD and dry skin, skin creams such as emollients have been the mainstay of treatment. Emollients themselves are used alone for mild AD alongside other treatments such as topical corticosteroids for more moderate and severe AD. Use of emollients has shown to decrease the time between flares in patients with AD (Ring et al. 2012). Because emollients can repair the skin barrier of those with AD, and in some children, skin barrier changes can be seen prior to the development of clinical AD, it was proposed that emollients could be a tool to prevent AD, and potentially other allergic conditions (Fig. 1.2).

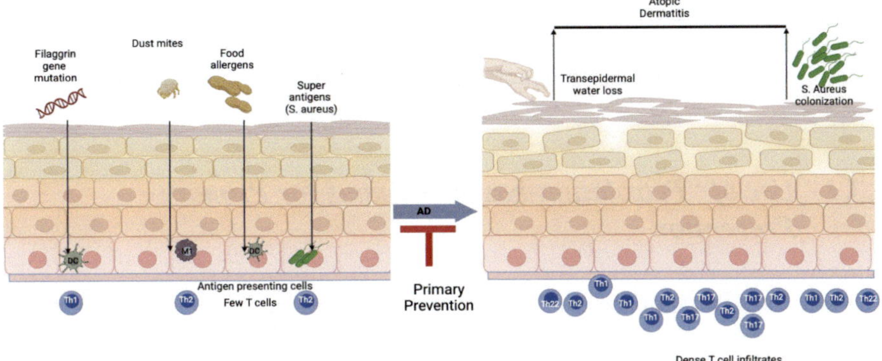

Fig. 1.2 Genetic predisposition, allergens and pathogens lead to disruption of the skin barrier and subsequent epicutaneous sensitization and allergy. It is hypothesized that application of cream barrier could prevent onset of atopic dermatitis, which is primary prevention of AD. https://help. biorender.com/hc/en-gb/articles/17605511350685-How-to-cite-your-BioRender-figure. Created in BioRender. Sampath, V. (2025) https://BioRender.com/j24j268

The journey for evidence for the primary prevention of atopic diseases with skin cream application is ongoing. It began with two pilot trials looking at the use of emollients as a primary prevention for AD in infants with a family history of atopic disease. These trials were published separately in 2014, both showing a significant reduction in AD at 6 months, in infants who had emollients applied to them in early infancy. In Simpson et al., 124 infants from the US and UK, were randomized to be treated within 3 weeks of birth with daily all-over skin treatment. This treatment was a parent choice of one of two common emollients, 50:50 cream or gel-based emollient, or sunflower seed oil. The intervention was shown to reduce AD at 6 months, with a relative risk reduction of 50% (relative risk, 0.50; 95% CI, 0.28–0.9; P = 0.017) (Simpson et al. 2014). In Horimukai et al., 118 infants from Japan were randomized to once-daily over all "emulsion" commenced within 7 days of birth. This intervention showed a 30% reduction in AD at 32 weeks (hazard ratio, 0.48; 95% CI, 0.27–0.86) (Horimukai et al.).

The success of these two pilot studies paved the way for larger trials to assess the efficacy of skin barrier interventions for primary prevention of AD and other allergic diseases. There are currently multiple studies ongoing, attempting to determine whether skin-care interventions in early infancy can prevent eczema and allergic disease (Kelleher et al. 2020). The original pilot trials had both looked at children with a family history of atopic disease. However, with a suspected petrolatum-based intervention, which appears safe in a disease that is common, some studies have looked at not just infants with "high" risk of allergy, but also infants with no family history of allergic disease. Examining different aspects of primary prevention of allergic disease through skin creams in infancy is underway. These include the effectiveness of the intervention in a pragmatic setting, the use of different types of skin creams such as those with added ceramide, or more lipid-based, where on the body the skin cream was applied, and the use of skin intervention in multifactorial studies alongside early introduction of food or symbiotic products. There is no standardized classification of emollients; they vary by both their constituents, and their consistency.

1.3.1 Use of "Petrolatum-based" Creams for Primary Prevention

The success of the Simpson pilot study led to a large-scale pragmatic study looking at the effectiveness of the same intervention in the UK population. Infants with a "high risk" of AD, i.e.,those with a family history of AD, were randomized to daily all over emollient (gel or cream based emollient) from infancy to 1 year. The primary outcome of the study was prevalence of AD at 2 years of age. The pragmatic intervention was designed to mirror real-life use of the intervention, as at that stage in the UK many parents were already using emollient or cream on their newborns, and the results of the pilot trial were very encouraging. The full study was published in January 2020, and unfortunately showed no effect of the intervention on the primary outcome of AD at 2 years, and was similarly not significant for many secondary outcomes using different measures for AD diagnosis (Chalmers et al. 2020).

PreventADALL was a large factorial designed trial looking at skin interventions and early food introduction to reduce AD (Skjerven et al. 2020). This was a combination skin care intervention, with a daily petroleum- based emollient to the face along with daily oil baths. Their primary outcome was AD at 1 year and food allergy at 3 years. At one year, the skin care intervention did not influence the development of AD, with a risk difference of 3.1% (95% CI -0·3 to 6·5). Their three-year food allergy outcomes are awaited.

Petrolatum-based creams were also used by Yonezawa et al., in a study of 227 newborns who were randomly assigned to a "milk lotion" to be used on the whole body at least daily (Yonezawa and Haruna 2019). The outcome of this study was skin barrier function at 3 months measured by transepidermal water loss, with a secondary outcome of diaper dermatitis (Yonezawa et al. 2018). These authors reported a significant decrease of TEWL on the face, but not the body of infants in the intervention group. There was also a reduction in "dry skin" at 3 months, and in diaper dermatitis. A follow up questionnaire study, of this same group, showed no difference in AD or food allergy at 2 years, between the control and intervention group. However, they did report an association between short term "skin problems" in the first couple of months of life, with AD and food allergy at 2 years.

1.3.2 Use of Lipid-Based Creams for Primary Prevention

The breakdown of constituents of emollient is an important factor to consider in the prevention of AD and allergic disease. An emollient may contain different amounts of ceramides, fatty acids and cholesterol, or even contain all three. These specialized emollients may be more effective in repairing skin barrier, and a recent small study showed that compared with "regular" emollient, a "trilipid" emollient even reduced total immunoglobulin E (Sindher et al. 2020a, b). Please see section on secondary prevention.

Dissanyake et al. used a lipid-based emollient for their primary prevention study. In this factorial study, 549 infants were randomly assigned to emollient, symbiotic, or a combination of both (Dissanayake et al. 2019). The emollient used for this group contained ceramide, cholesterol, and free fatty acids. Participants were advised to apply the emollient to their face twice a day, and to the rest of body if they wished. The primary outcome for this study was AD at 1 year, and neither the symbiotic nor the skin intervention impacted on the risk of AD development.

Two further pilot studies examining all over body lipid creams have been published. The first, PEBBLES, is a pilot study of 80 infants, examined the use of a "ceramide dominant" cream for prevention of atopic dermatitis. At 6 months, there was a risk reduction seen of 0.54 (95% CI 0.17–1.7) but confidence intervals were wide (Lowe et al. 2018a, b, c). A second pilot randomized trial of an emollient with pseudoceramide-5 and Filaggrin breakdown product showed a trend towards a decrease prevalence of AD at 1 year, but this was not significant (intervention group 13.2% vs. control group of 25.0% at 12 months (P = 0.20) (McClanahan et al. 2019a, b).

The final phases of these studies of both trials are still ongoing (Lowe et al. 2019; Eichner et al. 2020). Some caution in expectation for the full trial results should be taken, given how pilot trials for "petrolatum-based" emollients were also successful, but similar results were not seen in full studies. It is also worth remembering that specialized emollients are more expensive, which may impact the effectiveness of such an intervention, if use is decreased secondary to cost.

1.3.3 Impact on Food Sensitization and Allergy

With early onset AD being such a strong risk factor for food allergy, (Stamatas et al. 2011), it was expected that preventing eczema with skin creams would also reduce food sensitization. The main study examining food sensitization and allergy, has been the BEEP study, which took as a secondary outcome food sensitization based on skin prick test, and food allergy based both on oral food challenge, and expert diagnosis. In this study, there was no impact on cream from early infancy on AD rates. At two years, all children were offered skin prick testing to egg, milk and peanut, along with food allergy diagnostics. For skin prick testing, there was a trend towards increased rate of positive skin test in the intervention group (intervention 58/487 (12%), control 44/498 (9%) (adjusted RR 1·36, 95% CI 0·94 to 1·95). This was an important but unexpected finding. Smaller studies have also looked at food sensitization based on serum specific IgE and at earlier time points, and have not shown any significant impact on food sensitization rates (Horimukai et al., Lowe et al. 2018a, b, c, Dissanayake et al. 2019). This trial measured food allergy by oral food challenge, or if oral food challenge was not conducted, by an expert panel review who took skin test result, food consumption history and any report of food allergic reaction symptoms into account. There was no difference in food allergy rates to milk, egg, or peanut 41/547 (7%) in the emollient group and 29/568 (5%) in the control group (adjusted RR 1·47, 95% CI 0·93–2·33). The mechanism for how daily emollient *may* increase food sensitization needs to be elucidated and results from further studies should aid towards this.

1.3.4 Impact on Inhalant Allergies

Though most of the current studies using skin creams for primary prevention of allergy have focused on AD, and secondarily on food allergy, sensitization to inhaled allergens has been recorded in two studies. In Dissanayake et al. children were tested for sensitization to house dust mite, and to cat, with no difference described between intervention and control groups (Dissanayake et al. 2019). In the BEEP study (Chalmers et al. 2020), children underwent skin prick test to cat, dog, and grass pollen alongside the food allergy panel with no difference between the groups. There was also no change in prevalence of parent reported allergic rhinitis, or parent reported wheeze between control or intervention.

1.3.5 Potential Side Effects

Though adverse events are collected differently in all studies, the BEEP study did show a significant increase in skin infection in the intervention group (Chalmers et al. 2020). Potential for slippages due to using a lot of emollient on small infants was recorded in the BEEP and other studies It would be sensible to continue to advise any guardian to exercise caution while the infant has emollients on their skin.

1.3.6 Summary

Observational studies and pilot studies suggest that the use of skin creams on infants from early infancy could reduce the prevalence of eczema. However, two recently published, well conducted large studies with "petrolatum-based" creams and bathing interventions, have shown no impact of skin creams in decreasing the prevalence of eczema. Pilot trials of more complex creams have shown a trend towards a decrease of eczema, though this is not significant, and results of larger trials are awaited. Applying skin creams is associated with an increased risk of skin infections. Unexpectedly, applying skin creams to infants from the first few weeks of life may also increase the risk of food sensitization, though ongoing studies will clarify this further.

1.3.7 Highlights

- Skin emollients are used to manage established eczema.
- Early pilot studies suggested that emollients may prevent eczema in infants.
- Recent large trials show "petrolatum-based" emollients do not prevent eczema.
- "Petrolatum-based" emollients in prevention studies are associated with increased skin infection and may increase the risk of food sensitization.
- The results of ongoing trials with lipid-based emollients for eczema prevention are awaited

1.4 Secondary Prevention of Atopic Diseases

In the context of atopic dermatitis, secondary prevention would be defined under two categories. One would be to prevent the worsening/exacerbation of the existing AD and the second would be to prevent the onset/progression of the atopic march (Spergel and Paller 2003) shown in Fig. 1.3. In this section, we will discuss only *topical* treatments that have been tested in the hope of halting AD progression and, thereby the atopic march. Most studies we refer to focus on grading AD severity and parameters and a few examined outcomes on the development of food allergies, asthma, and allergic rhinitis with the use of topicals as such studies usually have systemic therapies as the drug under investigation.

1.4.1 Probiotics, Vitamin D, Sodium Cromoglycate For Atopic Dermatitis

1.4.1.1 Topical Probiotics

Many have investigated the skin microbiome, specifically the correlation between colonization by Staph aureus and incidence and severity of AD and many have explored the role of ingested probiotics in the treatment of AD. However, few studies have studied topical probiotics for AD. One study in Germany explored the effect of a lotion containing heat-treated Lactobacillus johnsonii NCC 533 (HT La1) on S.

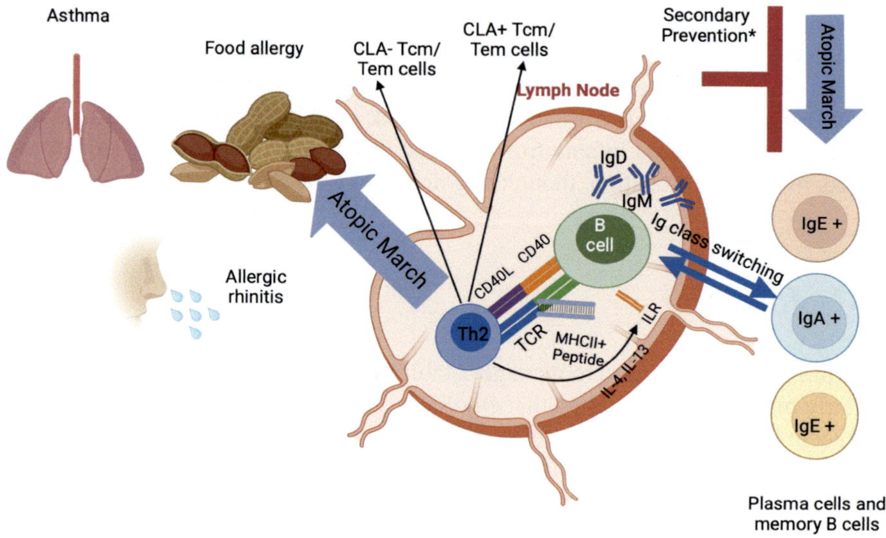

Fig. 1.3 Prevention of AD and the atopic march. Early antigen penetration occurs through an impaired epidermal barrier in high-risk infants. Thus primary prevention to inhibit AD development should focus on barrier-targeted approaches. Should primary prevention fail, overt AD ensues, including increased TEWL, S aureus colonization, disrupted epidermal barrier, and dense T-cell skin infiltration. Hyperplastic barrier, excessive CD31 T-cell infiltration, and increased FCεRI expression are all seen in lesional and nonlesional pediatric AD skin. These full-blown immune and barrier changes subsequently trigger B-cell IgE skewing, T-cell migration, and promotion of the atopic march, including FA, allergic rhinitis, and asthma. https://help.biorender.com/hc/en-gb/articles/17605511350685-How-to-cite-your-BioRender-figure. Created in BioRender. Sampath, V. (2025) https://BioRender.com/n81f129

aureus colonization in AD patients (Blanchet-Rethore et al. 2017). They enrolled 31 participants and sampled and tested for S. aureus after which the lotion was applied twice daily for 3 weeks to lesional skin. They found that both local SCORAD and S. aureus load decreased and high baseline levels of S. aureus were found to be associated with a good response to the lotion. A second study in the U.S. assessed the safety and efficacy of Roseomonas mucosa microbiome transplant for AD (Myles et al. 2018). The authors initially sampled healthy volunteers in a previous study and found that this commensal bacterium improved AD outcomes in mouse and cell models. For the human study, they enrolled 15 participants (including 5 children). Sucralose solutions containing escalating doses of R. mucosa were topically applied twice weekly for 6 weeks (adults) or 16 weeks (children). For the adults, antecubital-specific SCORAD, subjective regional pruritis, objective intensity, and steroid usage all decreased. However, treatment of the hands was not associated with improvement even in those with improvements in the antecubital area. For the pediatric cohort, SCORAD, pruritis, and steroid usage all showed a significant decrease. There was also a decrease in the S. aureus culture burden. A third study assessed the efficacy of a cream containing a 5% lysate of Vitreoscilla filiformis (Gueniche et al. 2008). It was a 2-arm study of 75 participants with AD aged 6 to 70 in a prospective, randomized, double-blind, placebo-controlled study to receive the V. filiformis containing cream or the vehicle placebo. They showed a significant decrease in pruritis, SCORAD, and loss of sleep. There was also a significant decrease in S. aureus colonization and improvement in TEWL values. These pilot studies show promising results for safety and efficacy of topical probiotics in AD whether formulated in creams or in the form of a microbiome transplant but larger-scale studies need to validate these results.

1.4.1.2 Topical Vitamin D

While topical vitamin D (Vit D) derivatives are well-established treatments for psoriasis, the same could not be said for AD. In fact, contrasting literature on the effect of topical vit D in murine models and on human subjects with AD exists. Several studies have shown that topical vit D application in murine models induces thymic stromal lymphopoietin in keratinocytes triggering AD (Li et al. 2006, 2009; Turner et al. 2013). A contrasting study by Katayama et al. demonstrated that topical vit D application downregulates biphasic IgE mediated cutaneous reactions in a murine model and suggested that topical vit D could be used in human cutaneous disorders beyond keratinizing disorders (Katayama et al. 1996). In humans, treatment of hyperkeratotic palmoplantar eczema with a vit D3 derivative (calcipotriol 50 µg/g or maxacalcitol 25 µg/g ointments) has been successful where 4 of 5 subjects had an almost complete remission and the 5th showed a significant improvement in 2 to 8 weeks of treatment (Yang and Chang 2015). Another group reported 3 subjects with chronic hand eczema treated with Daivobet ointment containing the vit D3 derivative calcipotriol (50 µg/g) and ultrapotent corticosteroid betamethasone (0.5 mg/g) (Simonsen et al. 2004; Yang and Chang 2015). The 3 participants were 33–45 year old males of which 2 showed almost complete remission of lesions with 1 showing significant improvement in 5–24 weeks of treatment. While these small human studies are promising, the results are not generalizable due to the specific and complex pathophysiology of these eczema subtypes and the small size of the cohorts.

1.4.1.3 Topical Sodium Cromoglycate

Contrasting data exists on the use of sodium cromoglycate (also known as sodium cromoglicate or cromolyn sodium). An older study using 20 participants with moderate AD treated with 5% sodium cromoglycate cream to one side of the body on lesional areas versus the vehicle cream on the other side demonstrated deterioration in 15 participants by the end of 4 weeks (Thirumoorthy et al. 1983). A contrasting study performed on 26 pediatric patients with cromolyn sodium inhalation solution mixed into a water-based emollient cream to a final concentration of 0.21% showed a clinically significant decrease in severity scores in moderate to severe AD (Moore et al. 1998). A newer and larger-scale study on 208 pediatric participants using a 4%

SCG cutaneous emulsion in vehicle for 12 weeks showed a statistically significant difference in reduction of SCORAD in the SCG group vs. placebo (Berth-Jones et al. 2015). They also demonstrated a statistically significant reduction in topical steroid use. On the other hand, another similar-scale study (177 children) with the same form of sodium cromoglicate (4% SCG emulsion) showed no significant difference in SCORAD or other secondary outcomes after 12 months of use (Edwards et al. 2015).

1.4.2 Inflammatory Response and How Topical Steroids and Tacrolimus Help with AD

AD, or atopic eczema, is a chronic relapsing–remitting inflammation of the epidermis characterized by pruritus and skin inflammation, often starts in childhood (~85% of cases) and affects much of the body; severity may change into adolescence and adulthood (Tollefson et al. 2014). AD may lead to hay fever or asthma. Scratching worsens AD and increases infection risk. Causes of AD are unknown but involve genetics, immune system dysfunction, environmental exposure (Watson and Kapur 2011), and altered permeability of the skin and exposure to certain chemicals like detergents or frequent hand washing makes symptoms worse (Tollefson et al. 2014).

Applying an emollient like petrolatum is effective in preventing skin from drying out and decrease the need for medications (Varothai et al. 2013). However, petrolatum-based skin emollients often are not effective and topical steroids such as hydrocortisone are effective in managing AD (Berke et al. 2012). In contrast, trilipid creams have been shown to reduce SCORAD at equivalent efficacy to topical steroid creams (Sugarman and Parish 2009). If topical corticosteroids and moisturizers fail, short-term treatment with topical calcineurin inhibitors like tacrolimus or pimecrolimus are indicated. (Berke et al. 2012). A meta-analysis showed that topical pimecrolimus is not as effective as corticosteroids and tacrolimus (Ashcroft et al. 2007). However a later meta-analysis indicated that topical tacrolimus and pimecrolimus were more effective than low-dose topical corticosteroids, and the **study found no evidence for increased risk of malignancy** or skin atrophy (Cury Martins et al. 2015). Topical corticosteroids have potent anti-inflammatory activity in maintaining treatment as well as in the crisis intervention (Peserico et al. 2008; Glazenburg et al. 2009) but their long-term use is known to be associated with cutaneous adverse events such as skin atrophy (Hengge et al. 2006; Aschoff et al. 2011; Jensen et al. 2012).

The mechanisms of action of topical corticosteroids differ. Topical glucocorticoids such as triamcinolone suppress immune pathways in keratinocytes (Norris 2005) and negatively affect viability, maturation and immune function of inflammatory cells (Hoetzenecker et al. 2004). Glucocorticoids possess numerous functions such as anti-inflammatory, antimitotic, apoptotic, vasoconstrictive and immunomodulatory activities. These properties are closely associated with their efficacy in skin disease treatment (Cruess 1991). In AD, impaired skin barrier, modifications of the immune system, and genetic elements direct the course of the disease. Macrophages and monocytes play a pivotal role in enhanced susceptibility to cutaneous infections and act as central connecting components in the pathogenesis of AD on the cellular level. In AD, macrophages are known to accumulate in acutely and chronically inflamed skin. During the early and short inflammatory phase, macrophages exert proinflammatory functions like antigen-presenting phagocytosis and the production of inflammatory cytokines and growth factors that facilitate the resolution of inflammation. However, persistence of pro-inflammatory activity and altered function of macrophages result in the development of chronic inflammatory diseases such as AD (Kasraie and Werfel 2013).

As seen in Fig. 1.4, glucocorticoids repress genes encoding the multiple inflammatory cytokines and chemokines that amplify and perpetuate allergic inflammation. The molecular mechanisms of suppression of inflammatory genes involve an interaction of glucocorticoid receptors (GRs) activated by corticosteroids interacting with transcription factors that have been activated by inflammatory stimuli (Barnes 2001). Corticosteroids suppress the transcription of these inflammatory genes by reversing histone acetylation, in part by recruiting histone deacetylases to the transcription start site, thus repressing inflammatory genes (Cash et al. 1986). This mechanism accounts for many of the therapeutic effects of corticosteroids in the treatment of AD and other atopic disorders. The expression and activity of several cytokines relevant to inflammatory diseases may be inhibited by treatment with glucocorticoids, including IL-1, IL-2, IL-3, IL-6, IL-11, TNF-α, GM-CSF, and chemokines that "call" inflammatory cells to the site of inflammation. Topical corticosteroids are the first-line therapy for AD; however, they are also not indicated for long-term treatment (> 4 weeks), and only a few are approved in children younger than 2 years. They also have a skin-thinning potential and possible rebound and tachyphylaxis effects, none of which are seen in tacrolimus-treated skin (Ingelman-Sundberg et al. 1981).

Tacrolimus differs from those of topical corticosteroids in that this agent inhibits the activation of pro-inflammatory cells such as T lymphocytes and mast calls (de Paulis et al. 1992; Sakuma et al. 2001) and prevents the progression of cytokine-driven inflammation (Ohtsuki et al. 2018). Topical tacrolimus is an immunomodulator and has a more selective action compared with topical corticosteroids. As seen in Fig. 1.2, topical tacrolimus acts by inhibiting calcineurin, thus, inhibiting T-cell proliferation and the production of many inflammatory cytokines, such as interleukin (IL)-2, IL-3, IL-4, IL-12, tumor necrosis factor (TNF), and interferon (IFN)-γ (Ingelman-Sundberg et al. 1981). Specifically, tacrolimus is a microbial product isolated from the organism *Streptomyces tsukubaensis* that binds to calcineurin and inhibits the calcineurin pathway, which stimulates the nuclear factor of activated T-cells (NFAT), a small but important family of transcription factors in T cells. Inhibiting calcineurin and NFAT impairs transcription of cytokines like IL-2. In this regard, the action of tacrolimus resembles that of cyclosporine (both drugs are calcineurin inhibitors), although the cellular receptors differ. In particular, tacrolimus inhibits the synthesis of interleukin-2 (IL-2), which results in decreased activation

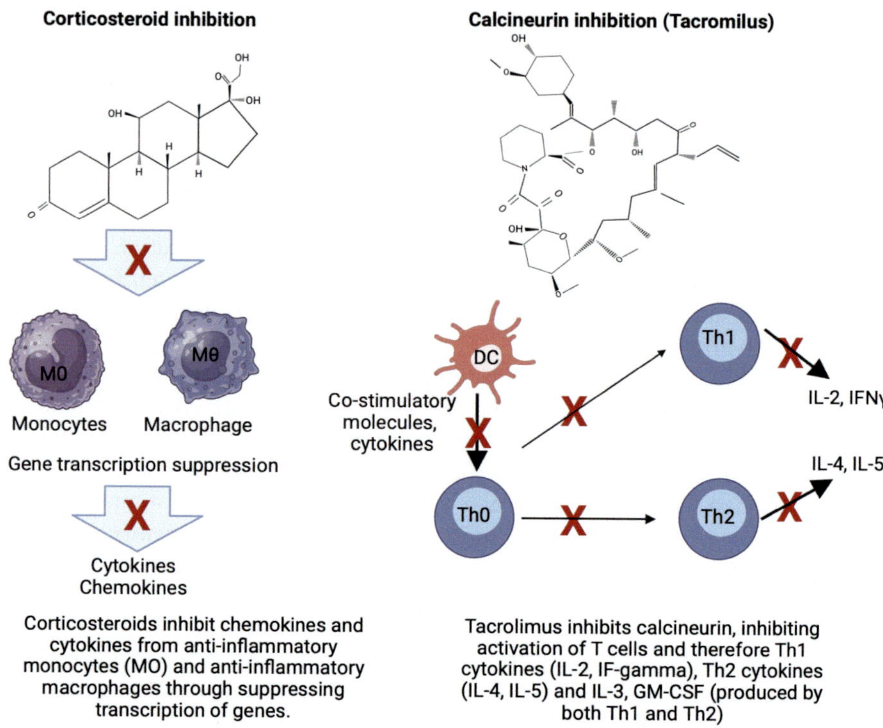

Fig. 1.4 Mechanism of action for topical corticosteroids and calcineurin. https://help.biorender.com/hc/en-gb/articles/17605511350685-How-to-cite-your-BioRender-figure. Created in BioRender. Sampath, V. (2025) https://BioRender.com/h51x324

of T-lymphocytes. Tacrolimus also inhibits release of mast cell and basophil mediators and decreases inflammatory mediator expression. Thus, Th1 release of IL-2 and IFN-g and Th2 release of IL-4 and IL-5 are inhibited (Thomson et al. 1995).

An important advantage of tacrolimus is that, unlike steroids, it does not cause skin atrophy or other steroid-related side effects. Tacrolimus is applied on the active skin lesions until they heal but may also be used continuously in low doses (twice a week), and applied to the thinner skin over the face and eyelids.

Other medications used for AD include systemic immunosuppressants such as ciclosporin, methotrexate, interferon gamma 1-beta, mycophenolate mofetil, and azathioprine (Berke et al. 2012; Yarbrough et al. 2013). In 2016, crisaborole was approved as a topical treatment for mild-to-moderate eczema. In 2017, the biologic agent dupilumab was approved to treat moderate-to-severe eczema. Leukotriene inhibitors such as montelukast are of unclear benefit as of 2018 (Ferguson et al. 2018). There is some initial but tentative evidence that allergy immunotherapy is effective in AD, but the quality of the evidence is low (Tam et al. 2016).

1.4.3 Effect of Treatment of Eczema and Long-Term Development of Rhinitis, Asthma, and Food Allergy (Secondary Intervention and Tertiary Prevention)

Targeting the skin to prevent AD or reduce the duration and severity of AD could prevent the development of FA and other atopic conditions. As previously noted, AD is often associated with the subsequent development of FA, asthma, or AR which is defined as the atopic march (Dharmage et al. 2014; Lowe et al. 2018a, b, c; Davidson et al. 2019) The timing of AD, such as early onset (particularly within the first 3 months), and severe AD markedly increases the risk of FA (Martin 2015, Hill 2018, Hill 2008). In the HealthNuts study, children with early onset severe AD had a 50% rate of challenge proven egg, peanut or sesame seed allergy by 12 months of age. In the LEAP screening study (Du Toit et al. 2013) there was a dose dependent increase in food sensitizations with increasing SCORAD levels in children between 4–11 months of age. In the Swedish population-based birth cohort, BAMSE study conducted in 4089 children, Ballardini et al. found that infantile eczema and those with persistent symptoms were at a higher risk of developing asthma (OR 2.22; 95% CI, 1.65–2.98) or rhinitis (OR 2.69; 95% CI, 2.22–3.26) in preadolescence compared to children who did not have infantile asthma (Ballardini et al. 2012). Furthermore, in addition to timing of onset, duration of untreated AD has also been shown to increase the risk of FA for each month of untreated AD (Miyaji et al. 2020). It has been postulated that this is due to the length of time that the disrupted skin is exposed to environmental food allergens, such as peanut in household dust (Brough et al. 2014); by reducing the severity and duration of AD leading to peanut sensitization and allergy (Fig. 1.5).

Numerous studies, as described previously, have explored whether prevention of AD altogether (primary prevention) can decrease the incidence of subsequent

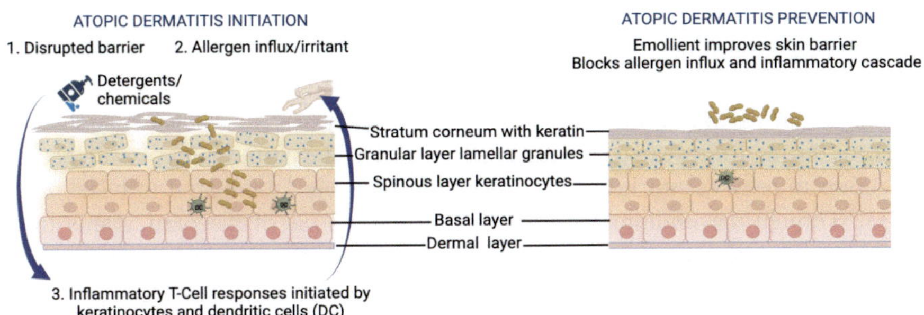

Fig. 1.5 Peanut allergens are present in the home environment (e.g. in household dust) and have been shown to increase the risk of peanut allergy in children with a disrupted skin barrier. It is postulated that by repairing the skin and reducing inflammation that this may prevent the influx of peanut allergens through the skin, and prevent epicutaneous peanut sensitization. https://help. biorender.com/hc/en-gb/articles/17605511350685-How-to-cite-your-BioRender-figure. Created in BioRender. Sampath, V. (2025) https://BioRender.com/l85x893

atopy such as food allergy (see Sect. 1.2). However, some studies have also shown that aggressive treatment of already active AD can also be beneficial in disrupting atopic march. Topical calcineurin inhibitors and topical corticosteroids (TCSs) ointments are the mainstream of pharmacotherapy to suppress skin inflammation associated with AD. The approach for use of TCSs in AD is either reactive or proactive management.

The Study of Atopic March (SAM), a large longitudinal study of development of asthma and allergies in patients with AD was conducted from 2003 to 2008 (Boguniewicz et al. 2007; Schneider et al. 2016). The study tested the effect of treatment with pimecrolimus versus placebo in 1091 infants aged 3–18 months with a history of AD for at least 3 months and atopic family history at enrollment. The goal of the study was to determine whether early intervention with pimecrolimus abrogates the atopic march. The infants were randomized 1:1 to twice-daily pimecrolumus 1% cream or placebo for the first 3 years followed by open-label pimecrolimus for 3 additional years. No significant differences between pimecrolimus- and placebo-treated groups were found in the percentage of patients who developed asthma, allergic rhinitis, food allergy, or allergic conjunctivitis by the end of the study. The study experienced a 48% discontinuation rate which considerably reduced the power of the analysis. However, baseline total IgE was higher in patients with moderate compared to mild AD. Additionally, the authors did find that allergic rhinitis and food allergy developed more significantly in infants with greater AD severity at baseline. This study was able to effectively demonstrate the safety of pimecrolimus in infants.

In 2010, Mandelin et al. described the first study in adolescents and adults suggesting long-term improvement in respiratory symptoms and serum IgE 6 years after a 4-year intervention with topical tacrolimus for the treatment of AD (Mandelin et al. 2010). During the initial trial, 65 participants aged 13–56 years and with moderate-severe eczema were enrolled in an open trial. Participants were advised to treat AD flares with 0.1% tacrolimus twice daily until 7 days after clearance of lesions (Reitamo et al. 2008). Participants were subsequently recruited 10 years later to further assess eczema control, asthma symptoms, as well and allergic sensitization via skin prick tests and serum total IgE levels. Patients who had active asthma and rhinitis during the initial study at baseline displayed a significant reduction in symptoms during follow-up (p = 0.02 and p = 0.01). The participants also displayed a reduction in total serum IgE during the follow-up visit compared to baseline (p = 0.002 Though the findings were promising, only 77% of the participants from the parent trial participated in the follow-up study and there was no control-group, therefore more rigorous blinded studies are needed.

Fukuie et al. performed a 2-year retrospective cohort study of patients with moderate to severe AD to investigate whether proactive management changes serum IgE level compared to reactive management (Fukuie et al. 2010). Participants were enrolled and advised to use betamethasone valerate 0.12% twice daily until resolution of AD flare followed by once weekly or twice weekly (titrated based on symptoms) proactive maintenance therapy for 2 years. Patients who continued maintenance proactive therapy for the duration of study were assigned to the 'proactive treatment group' (n = 25), whereas If a participant discontinued treatment then they were assigned to the 'reactive treatment group' (n = 20). Serum total IgE titer was significantly decreased in the proactive treatment group compared to the reactive treatment group (p < 0.01). This was the first study to associate proactive treatment of AD with a reduction in total IgE levels.

In a hospital-based retrospective cohort study, Miyaji et al. in 2019 studied 142 infants less than 12 months of age with AD and demonstrated that shortening the duration of eczema with aggressive treatment resulted in a subsequent decrease in the development of FA (Miyaji et al. 2020). A total of 75 infants initiated treatment for their eczema within 4 months of onset and were placed in the early treatment group. Sixty-seven infants initiated treatment more than 4 months after the onset of eczema and placed in the delayed treatment group. All of these infants had previously received reactive therapy with topical corticosteroids that were milder than betamethasone valerate before enrollment. Reactive therapy was defined as administration of steroids only during AD flares. For aggressive therapy, the researchers used betamethasone valerate (medium potency) followed by proactive maintenance therapy. Proactive therapy was defined as intermittent application of topical steroids even after resolution of flare. Logistic regression analysis showed that timing of initiating treatment and duration of AD was a risk factor for food allergy (aOR: 3.8, 95% confidence interval: 1.5, 9.6, p = 0.004) and so was the SCORAD score at first visit (aOR:1.3, 95% CI:1.1, 1.5; p = 0.009). This initial study led to the development of a randomized controlled trial (PACI study) to validate the above results.

The PACI trial was a novel multi-center, two-parallel group RCT to examine the efficacy of early aggressive treatment of AD and the development of food allergy (Yamamoto-Hanada et al. 2018). Aggressive treatment and intervention in new-onset AD versus conventional treatment was assessed in 650 infants (7–13 weeks old) who developed a pruritic rash in the previous 28 days. Infants were enrolled and randomized 1:1 to receive either aggressive or conventional intervention and its effect on the development of egg allergy at 28 weeks of age was assessed. Participants in both groups were treated with daily emollient therapy with a heparinoid ointment. In the aggressive treatment group, participants were treated with aclometasone dipropionate for face and betamethasone valerate to the whole the body twice daily (including lesional and non-lesional skin) for 14 days followed by 2 days a week twice daily until 28 weeks of life. Additional flares were treated with the same topical steroids twice daily until remission. In the conventional treatment group participants received the same topical steroids but only once daily until symptom resolution, with no maintenance steroid therapy in between flares. Although there was a significant reduction in challenge proven egg allergy in children in the intervention arm (31.4% vs 41.9%, P = 0.0028), there was also a significant reduction in weight (mean difference: − 422 g, 95% CI: − 553 to − 292 g) and length (mean difference: − 0.8 cm, 95% CI: − 1.22 to − 0.33 cm) at 28 weeks of age. The Stopping Eczema and Allergy (SEAL) (NCT03742414) is a multicenter randomized controlled study recruiting infants with dry skin of eczema (until 12 weeks of age). The intervention arm is being treated with twice-daily emollient (trilipid cream or petrolatum-based cream) and, if required, proactive topical steroids (only once daily to lesional areas, not non lesional areas) versus standard of care. Food sensitization and allergy is being assessed at two years follow-up.

Taken together, the studies reported above show the efforts behind strategies to disrupt the atopic march and reduce/prevent the development of atopy. Although topical vitamin D, probiotics and sodium cromoglycate have been shown to improve AD, they have not been explored in the setting of long-term allergy outcomes. In the studies described above, AD has already developed and aggressive intervention with corticosteroids and calcineurin inhibitors has shown some promise in reducing IgE titers, decrease in asthma and rhinitis symptoms, and decreased incidence of FA.

1.5 Overview Conclusion

An impaired skin barrier and AD have been shown to increase the risk of FA, and respiratory allergies. In order to prevent this, several topical therapies have been investigated in both primary prevention strategies before the onset of clinical AD and secondary/tertiary prevention once AD is established. In the first section of this chapter we have reviewed the vital importance of lipid components in the SC, in preventing water loss and maintaining barrier function within the SC lipid environment that lead to impaired skin barrier and skin conditions such as AD. The ideal emollient would need to have the same features as healthy SC i.e. the presence of long periodicity phase, and a high degree of lateral order (rich in orthorhombic packing) and well as support different CER classes in the skin. Different emollient properties are important considerations for skin barrier restoration in AD, such as pH, hydrophobic index and rheological (hardness, adhesiveness, and spreadability) properties. For example, petrolatum-based, standard emollients can hydrate the skin but may not necessarily prevent sensitization events. Whereas early pilot studies suggested that emollients may prevent eczema in infants, recent large trials show "petrolatum-based" emollients do not prevent eczema, sensitization or FA. Trilipid creams (ceramides (CERs), cholesterol (CHOL), and free fatty acids (FFAs)) have been shown to have beneficial effect on barrier function and are in the same ratio to healthy SC. Results of preventative emollient therapy using trilipid creams are awaited. Other topical therapy such as vitamin D, probiotics and sodium cromoglycate creams have been shown to improve AD, but their impact on allergic outcomes has not been assessed. Targeting inflammation in established AD with aggressive intervention with corticosteroids and calcineurin inhibitors shows promise both in the prevention of food and respiratory allergies.

References

Aschoff R, Schmitt J, Knuschke P, Koch E, Brautigam M, Meurer M. Evaluation of the atrophogenic potential of hydrocortisone 1% cream and pimecrolimus 1% cream in uninvolved forehead skin of patients with atopic dermatitis using optical coherence tomography. Exp Dermatol. 2011;20(10):832–6.

Ashcroft DM, Chen LC, Garside R, Stein K, Williams HC. Topical pimecrolimus for eczema. Cochrane Database Syst Rev. 2007;4:CD005500.

Babita K, Kumar V, Rana V, Jain S, Tiwary AK. Thermotropic and spectroscopic behavior of skin: relationship with percutaneous permeation enhancement. Curr Drug Deliv. 2006;3(1):95–113.

Ballardini N, Kull I, Lind T, Hallner E, Almqvist C, Ostblom E, Melen E, Pershagen G, Lilja G, Bergstrom A, Wickman M. Development and comorbidity of eczema, asthma and rhinitis to age 12: data from the BAMSE birth cohort. Allergy. 2012;67(4):537–44.

Barnes PJ. Corticosteroids, IgE, and atopy. J Clin Invest. 2001;107(3):265–6.

Berke R, Singh A, Guralnick M. Atopic dermatitis: an overview. Am Fam Phys. 2012;86(1):35–42.

Berth-Jones J, Pollock I, Hearn RM, Lewis-Jones S, Goodfield M, Griffiths CE, Gulati R, McHenry P, Abdullah A, Ott J, Wright A, Walker B, Stevens MT, Edwards AM. A randomised, controlled trial of a 4% cutaneous emulsion of sodium cromoglicate in treatment of atopic dermatitis in children. J Dermatolog Treat. 2015;26(3):291–6.

Blanchet-Rethore S, Bourdes V, Mercenier A, Haddar CH, Verhoeven PO, Andres P. Effect of a lotion containing the heat-treated probiotic strain Lactobacillus johnsonii NCC 533 on Staphylococcus aureus colonization in atopic dermatitis. Clin Cosmet Investig Dermatol. 2017;10:249–57.

Boguniewicz M, Schneider L, Leung DY, Hultsch T. The allergic profile of infants in the SAM study: a large longitudinal study of development of asthma and allergies in patients with atopic dermatitis. J Allergy Clin Immunol. 2007;119:S209.

Bouwstra JA, de Graaff A, Gooris GS, Nijsse J, Wiechers JW, van Aelst AC. Water distribution and related morphology in human stratum corneum at different hydration levels. J Investig Dermatol. 2003;120(5):750–8.

Bouwstra JA, Ponec M. The skin barrier in healthy and diseased state. Biochimica et Biophysica Acta (BBA)-Biomembranes. 2006;1758(12):2080–2095.

Brough HA, Simpson A, Makinson K, Hankinson J, Brown S, Douiri A, Belgrave DC, Penagos M, Stephens AC, McLean WH, Turcanu V, Nicolaou N, Custovic A, Lack G. Peanut allergy: effect of environmental peanut exposure in children with filaggrin loss-of-function mutations. J Allergy Clin Immunol. 2014;134(4): 867–875 e861.

Bulsara P, Varlashkin P, Dickens J, Moore D, Rawlings A, Clarke M. The rational design of biomimetic skin barrier lipid formulations using biophysical methods. Int J Cosmet Sci. 2017;39(2):206–16.

Cash R, Raisman R, Lanfumey L, Ploska A, Agid Y. Cellular localization of adrenergic receptors in rat and human brain. Brain Res. 1986;370(1):127–35.

Caussin J, Rozema E, Gooris GS, Wiechers JW, Pavel S, Bouwstra JA. Hydrophilic and lipophilic moisturizers have similar penetration profiles but different effects on SC water distribution in vivo. Exp Dermatol. 2009;18(11):954–61.

Caussin J, Groenink HW, Graaff AMd, Gooris GS, Wiechers JW, Van Aelst AC, Bouwstra JA. Lipophilic and hydrophilic moisturizers show different actions on human skin as revealed by cryo scanning electron microscopy. Experim Dermatol. 2007;16(11): 891–898.

Caussin J, Gooris GS, Bouwstra JA. FTIR studies show lipophilic moisturizers to interact with stratum corneum lipids, rendering the more densely packed. Biochimica et Biophysica Acta (BBA)-Biomembranes. 2008;1778(6):1517–1524.

Chalmers JR, Haines RH, Bradshaw LE, Montgomery AA, Thomas KS, Brown SJ, Ridd MJ, Lawton S, Simpson EL, Cork MJ, Sach TH, Flohr C, Mitchell EJ, Swinden R, Tarr S, Davies-Jones S, Jay N, Kelleher MM, Perkin MR, Boyle RJ, Williams HC. Daily emollient during infancy for prevention of eczema: the BEEP randomised controlled trial. Lancet. 2020;395(10228):962–72.

Chamlin SL, Kao J, Frieden IJ, Sheu MY, Fowler AJ, Fluhr JW, Williams ML, Elias PM. Ceramide-dominant barrier repair lipids alleviate childhood atopic dermatitis: changes in barrier function provide a sensitive indicator of disease activity. J Am Acad Dermatol. 2002;47(2):198–208.

Cruess R. Special report on Quebec creates controversy. CMAJ. 1991;145(8):917–20.

Cury Martins J, Martins C, Aoki V, Gois AF, Ishii HA, da Silva EM. Topical tacrolimus for atopic dermatitis. Cochrane Database Syst Rev. 2015;7:CD009864.

Damien F, Boncheva M. The extent of orthorhombic lipid phases in the stratum corneum determines the barrier efficiency of human skin in vivo. J Invest Dermatol. 2010;130(2):611.

Danby S, Chalmers J, Brown K, Williams H, Cork M. A functional mechanistic study of the effect of emollients on the structure and function of the skin barrier. Br J Dermatol. 2016a;175(5):1011–9.

Danby SG, Brown K, Higgs-Bayliss T, Chittock J, Albenali L, Cork MJ. The effect of an emollient containing urea, ceramide NP, and lactate on skin barrier structure and function in older people with dry skin. Skin Pharmacol Physiol. 2016b;29(3):135–47.

Davidson WF, Leung DYM, Beck LA, Berin CM, Boguniewicz M, Busse WW, Chatila TA, Geha RS, Gern JE, Guttman-Yassky E, Irvine AD, Kim BS, Kong HH, Lack G, Nadeau KC, Schwaninger J, Simpson A, Simpson EL, Spergel JM, Togias A, Wahn U, Wood RA, Woodfolk JA, Ziegler SF, Plaut M. Report from the national institute of allergy and infectious diseases workshop on "Atopic dermatitis and the atopic march: mechanisms and interventions." J Allergy Clin Immunol. 2019;143(3):894–913.

de Paulis A, Stellato C, Cirillo R, Ciccarelli A, Oriente A, Marone G. Anti-inflammatory effect of FK-506 on human skin mast cells. J Invest Dermatol. 1992;99(6):723–8.

Dharmage SC, Lowe AJ, Matheson MC, Burgess JA, Allen KJ, Abramson MJ. Atopic dermatitis and the atopic march revisited. Allergy. 2014;69(1):17–27.

Dissanayake E, Tani Y, Nagai K, Sahara M, Mitsuishi C, Togawa Y, Suzuki Y, Nakano T, Yamaide F, Ohno H, Shimojo N. Skin care and synbiotics for prevention of atopic dermatitis or food allergy in newborn infants: a 2 × 2 factorial, randomized, non-treatment controlled trial. Int Arch Allergy Immunol. 2019;1–10.

Douguet M, Picard C, Savary G, Merlaud F, Loubat-Bouleuc N, Grisel M. Spreading properties of cosmetic emollients: use of synthetic skin surface to elucidate structural effect. Colloids Surf, B. 2017;154:307–14.

Du Toit G, Roberts G, Sayre PH, Plaut M, Bahnson HT, Mitchell H, Radulovic S, Chan S, Fox A, Turcanu V, Lack G, Learning Early About Peanut Allergy Study T. Identifying infants at high risk of peanut allergy: the learning early about peanut allergy (LEAP) screening study. J Allergy Clin Immunol. 2013;131(1): 135–143 e131–112.

Edwards AM, Bibawy D, Matthews S, Tongue N, Arshad SH, Lodrup Carlsen K, Oymar K, Pollock I, Clifford R, Thomas A, Gamanya R, Vyas J, Stevens MT, Carlsen KH. Long-term use of a 4% sodium cromoglicate cutaneous emulsion in the treatment of moderate to severe atopic dermatitis in children. J Dermatolog Treat. 2015;26(6):541–7.

Eichenfield LF, Tom WL, Berger TG, Krol A, Paller AS, Schwarzenberger K, Bergman JN, Chamlin SL, Cohen DE, Cooper KD. Guidelines of care for the management of atopic dermatitis: section 2. Management and treatment of atopic dermatitis with topical therapies. J Am Acad Dermatol. 2014;71(1):116–32.

Eichner B, Michaels LAC, Branca K, Ramsey K, Mitchell J, Morris CD, Fagnan LJ, Dolor RJ, Elder N, Hahn DL, Nease DE, Lapidus J, Cibotti R, Block J, Simpson EL. A community-based assessment of skin care, allergies, and eczema (CASCADE): an atopic dermatitis primary prevention study using emollients-protocol for a randomized controlled trial. Trials. 2020;21(1):243.

Elias PM, Wakefield JS. Mechanisms of abnormal lamellar body secretion and the dysfunctional skin barrier in patients with atopic dermatitis. J Allergy and Clinical Immunol. 2014;134(4): 781–791. e781.

Ferguson L, Futamura M, Vakirlis E, Kojima R, Sasaki H, Roberts A, Mori R. 2018. Leukotriene receptor antagonists for eczema. Cochrane Database Syst Rev. 2018;10: CD011224.

Fukuie T, Nomura I, Horimukai K, Manki A, Masuko I, Futamura M, Narita M, Ohzeki T, Matsumoto K, Saito H, Ohya Y. Proactive treatment appears to decrease serum immunoglobulin-E levels in patients with severe atopic dermatitis. Br J Dermatol. 2010;163(5):1127–9.

Glazenburg EJ, Wolkerstorfer A, Gerretsen AL, Mulder PG, Oranje AP. Efficacy and safety of fluticasone propionate 0.005% ointment in the long-term maintenance treatment of children with atopic dermatitis: differences between boys and girls? Pediatr Allergy Immunol. 2009;20(1):59–66.

Goksör E, Loid P, Alm B, Åberg N, Wennergren G. The allergic march comprises the coexistence of related patterns of allergic disease not just the progressive development of one disease. Acta Paediatr. 2016;105(12):1472–9.

Groen D, Poole DS, Gooris GS, Bouwstra JA. Is an orthorhombic lateral packing and a proper lamellar organization important for the skin barrier function?. Biochimica et Biophysica Acta (BBA)-Biomembranes. 2011;1808(6): 1529–1537.

Gueniche A, Knaudt B, Schuck E, Volz T, Bastien P, Martin R, Rocken M, Breton L, Biedermann T. Effects of nonpathogenic gram-negative bacterium Vitreoscilla filiformis lysate on atopic dermatitis: a prospective, randomized, double-blind, placebo-controlled clinical study. Br J Dermatol. 2008;159(6):1357–63.

Harding CR. The stratum corneum: structure and function in health and disease. Dermatol Ther. 2004;17:6–15.

Hayama K, Takano Y, Tamura J, Tagami H, Terui T. Effectiveness of a heparinoid-containing moisturiser to treat senile xerosis. Australas J Dermatol. 2015;56(1):36–9.

Hengge UR, Ruzicka T, Schwartz RA, Cork MJ. Adverse effects of topical glucocorticosteroids. J Am Acad Dermatol. 2006;54(1): 1–15; quiz 16–18.

Hoetzenecker W, Meingassner JG, Ecker R, Stingl G, Stuetz A, Elbe-Burger A. Corticosteroids but not pimecrolimus affect viability, maturation and immune function of murine epidermal Langerhans cells. J Invest Dermatol. 2004;122(3):673–84.

Horimukai K, Morita K, Narita M, Kondo M, Kitazawa H, Nozaki M, Shigematsu Y, Yoshida K, Niizeki H, Motomura K-i. Application of moisturizer to neonates prevents development of atopic dermatitis. J Allergy and Clinical Immunol. 2014;134(4): 824–830. e826.

Horimukai K, Morita K, Narita M, Kondo M, Kitazawa H, Nozaki M, Shigematsu Y, Yoshida K, Niizeki H, Motomura K-i, Sago H, Takimoto T, Inoue E, Kamemura N, Kido H, Hisatsune J, Sugai M, Murota H, Katayama I, Sasaki T, Amagai M, Morita H, Matsuda A, Matsumoto K, Saito H, Ohya Y (2014) Application of moisturizer to neonates prevents development of atopic dermatitis. J Allergy and Clinical Immunol. 2014;134(4): 824–830.e826.

Horimukai K, Morita K, Narita M, Kondo M, Kabashima S, Inoue E, Sasaki T, Niizeki H, Saito H, Matsumoto K. "Transepidermal water loss measurement during infancy can predict the subsequent development of atopic dermatitis regardless of filaggrin mutations. Allergol Int. 2016;65(1): 103–108.

Horimukai K, Morita K, Narita M, Kondo M, Kabashima S, Inoue E, Sasaki T, Niizeki H, Saito H, Matsumoto K, Ohya Y. Transepidermal water loss measurement during infancy can predict the subsequent development of atopic dermatitis regardless of filaggrin mutations. Allergol Int. 2016;65(1): 103–108.

Ingelman-Sundberg A, Rosen J, Gustafsson SA, Carlstrom K. Cytosol estrogen receptors in the urogenital tissues in stress-incontinent women. Acta Obstet Gynecol Scand. 1981;60(6):585–6.

Irvine AD, McLean WHI, Leung DYM. Filaggrin mutations associated with skin and allergic diseases. N Engl J Med. 2011;365(14):1315–27.

Ishikawa J, Narita H, Kondo N, Hotta M, Takagi Y, Masukawa Y, Kitahara T, Takema Y, Koyano S, Yamazaki S, Hatamochi A. Changes in the ceramide profile of atopic dermatitis patients. J Investig Dermatol. 2010;130(10):2511–4.

Janssens M, van Smeden J, Gooris GS, Bras W, Portale G. Lamellar lipid organization and ceramide composition in the stratum Corneum of patients with atopic eczema. J Investig Dermatol. 2011;131(10):2136–8.

Janssens M, van Smeden J, Gooris GS, Bras W, Portale G, Caspers PJ, Vreeken RJ, Hankemeier T, Kezic S, Wolterbeek R. Increase in short-chain ceramides correlates with an altered lipid organization and decreased barrier function in atopic eczema patients. J Lipid Res. 2012;53(12):2755–66.

Jensen JM, Scherer A, Wanke C, Brautigam M, Bongiovanni S, Letzkus M, Staedtler F, Kehren J, Zuehlsdorf M, Schwarz T, Weichenthal M, Folster-Holst R, Proksch E. Gene expression is differently affected by Pimecrolimus and betamethasone in Lesional skin of atopic dermatitis. Allergy. 2012;67(3):413–23.

Kasraie S, Werfel T. Role of macrophages in the pathogenesis of atopic dermatitis. Mediators Inflamm. 2013;2013: 942375.

Katayama I, Minatohara K, Yokozeki H, Nishioka K. Topical vitamin D3 downregulates IgE-mediated murine biphasic cutaneous reactions. Int Arch Allergy Immunol. 1996;111(1):71–6.

Kelleher MM, Cro S, Cornelius V, Axon E, Lodrup Carlsen KC, Skjerven HO, Rehbinder EM, Lowe A, Dissanayake E, Shimojo N and et al. Skincare interventions in infants for preventing eczema and food allergy. Cochrane Database of Systemat Rev. 2020:(2).

Kim E, Kim S, Nam G, Lee H, Moon S, Chang I. The alkaline pH-adapted skin barrier is disrupted severely by SLS-induced irritation. Int J Cosmet Sci. 2009;31(4):263–9.

Kitagawa S, Yutani R, Kodani R-I, Teraoka R. Differences in the rheological properties and mixing compatibility with heparinoid cream of brand name and generic steroidal ointments: the effects of their surfactants. Results in Pharma Sci. 2016;6:7–14.

Li M, Hener P, Zhang Z, Kato S, Metzger D, Chambon P. Topical vitamin D3 and low-calcemic analogs induce thymic stromal lymphopoietin in mouse keratinocytes and trigger an atopic dermatitis. Proc Natl Acad Sci USA. 2006;103(31):11736–41.

Li M, Hener P, Zhang Z, Ganti KP, Metzger D, Chambon P. Induction of thymic stromal lymphopoietin expression in keratinocytes is necessary for generating an atopic dermatitis upon application of the active vitamin D3 analogue MC903 on mouse skin. J Invest Dermatol. 2009;129(2):498–502.

Lowe AJ, Tang ML, Dharmage SC, Varigos G, Forster D, Gurrin LC, Robertson CF, Abramson MJ, Allen KJ, Su J. A phase I study of daily treatment with a ceramide-dominant triple lipid mixture commencing in neonates. BMC Dermatol. 2012;12(1):3.

Lowe A, Su J, Allen K, Abramson M, Cranswick N, Robertson C, Forster D, Varigos G, Hamilton S, Kennedy R. A randomized trial of a barrier lipid replacement strategy for the prevention of atopic dermatitis and allergic sensitization: the PEBBLES pilot study. Br J Dermatol. 2018a;178(1):e19–21.

Lowe AJ, Leung DYM, Tang MLK, Su JC, Allen KJ. The skin as a target for prevention of the atopic march. Ann Allergy Asthma Immunol. 2018b;120(2):145–51.

Lowe AJ, Su JC, Allen KJ, Abramson MJ, Cranswick N, Robertson CF, Forster D, Varigos G, Hamilton S, Kennedy R, Axelrad C, Tang MLK, Dharmage SC. A randomized trial of a barrier lipid replacement strategy for the prevention of atopic dermatitis and allergic sensitization: the PEBBLES pilot study. Br J Dermatol. 2018c;178(1):e19–21.

Lowe A, Su J, Tang M, Lodge CJ, Matheson M, Allen KJ, Varigos G, Sasi A, Cranswick N, Hamilton S, Robertson CF, Hui J, Abramson M, O'Brien S, Dharmage S. PEBBLES study protocol: a randomised controlled trial to prevent atopic dermatitis, food allergy and sensitisation in infants with a family history of allergic disease using a skin barrier improvement strategy. BMJ Open. 2019;9(3): e024594.

Man G, Cheung C, Crumrine D, Hupe M, Hill Z, Man M-Q, Elias PM. An optimized inexpensive emollient mixture improves barrier repair in murine skin. Dermatol Sin. 2015;33(2):96–102.

Mandelin JM, Remitz A, Virtanen HM, Malmberg LP, Haahtela T, Reitamo S. A 10-year open follow-up of eczema and respiratory symptoms in patients with atopic dermatitis treated with topical tacrolimus for the first 4 years. J Dermatolog Treat. 2010;21(3):167–70.

Martin PE, Eckert JK, Koplin JJ, Lowe AJ, Gurrin LC, Dharmage SC, Vuillermin P, Tang MLK, Ponsonby AL, Matheson M, Hill DJ, Allen KJ, for the HealthNuts Study I. Which infants with eczema are at risk of food allergy? Results from a population-based cohort. Clinical and Experim Allergy 2015;45(1): 255–264.

Matsuki H, Kiyokane K, Matsuki T, Sato S, Imokawa G. Reevaluation of the importance of barrier dysfunction in the nonlesional dry skin of atopic dermatitis patients through the use of two barrier creams. Exog Dermatol. 2004;3(6):293–302.

McClanahan D, Wong A, Kezic S, Samrao A, Hajar T, Hill E, Simpson E. A randomized controlled trial of an emollient with ceramide and filaggrin-associated amino acids for the primary prevention of atopic dermatitis in high-risk infants. J Eur Acad Dermatol Venereol. 2019a;33(11):2087–94.

McClanahan D, Wong A, Kezic S, Samrao A, Hajar T, Hill E, Simpson EL. A randomized controlled trial of an emollient with ceramide and filaggrin-associated amino acids for the primary prevention of atopic dermatitis in high-risk infants. J Eur Acad Dermatol Venereol. 2019.

Miyaji Y, Yang L, Yamamoto-Hanada K, Narita M, Saito H, Ohya Y. Earlier aggressive treatment to shorten the duration of eczema in infants resulted in fewer food allergies at 2 years of age. J Allergy Clin Immunol Pract. 2020;8(5): 1721–1724 e1726.

Moncrieff G, Cork M, Lawton S, Kokiet S, Daly C, Clark C. Use of emollients in dry-skin conditions: consensus statement. Clin Exp Dermatol. 2013;38(3):231–8.

Moore C, Ehlayel MS, Junprasert J, Sorensen RU. Topical sodium cromoglycate in the treatment of moderate-to-severe atopic dermatitis. Ann Allergy Asthma Immunol. 1998;81(5):452–8.

Myles IA, Earland NJ, Anderson ED, Moore IN, Kieh MD, Williams KW, Saleem A, Fontecilla NM, Welch PA, Darnell DA, Barnhart LA, Sun AA, Uzel G, Datta SK. First-in-human topical microbiome transplantation with Roseomonas mucosa for atopic dermatitis. JCI Insight 2018;3(9).

Norris DA. Mechanisms of action of topical therapies and the rationale for combination therapy. J Am Acad Dermatol. 2005;53(1 Suppl 1):S17-25.

O'Goshi K-I, Tabata N, Sato Y, Tagami H. Comparative study of the efficacy of various moisturizers on the skin of the ASR miniature swine. Skin Pharmacol Physiol. 2000;13(2):120–7.

Ohtsuki M, Morimoto H, Nakagawa H. Tacrolimus ointment for the treatment of adult and pediatric atopic dermatitis: review on safety and benefits. J Dermatol. 2018;45(8):936–42.

Penzer R. Prescribing emollients for dry skin conditions. Nurse Prescribing. 2013;11(6):276–83.

Peserico A, Stadtler G, Sebastian M, Fernandez RS, Vick K, Bieber T. Reduction of relapses of atopic dermatitis with methylprednisolone aceponate cream twice weekly in addition to maintenance treatment with emollient: a multicentre, randomized, double-blind, controlled study. Br J Dermatol. 2008;158(4):801–7.

Purnamawati S, Indrastuti N, Danarti R, Saefudin T. The role of moisturizers in addressing various kinds of dermatitis: a review. Clin Med Res. 2017;15(3–4):75–87.

Rawlings A, Lombard K. A review on the extensive skin benefits of mineral oil. Int J Cosmet Sci. 2012;34(6):511–8.

Reitamo S, Rustin M, Harper J, Kalimo K, Rubins A, Cambazard F, Brenninkmeijer EE, Smith C, Berth-Jones J, Ruzicka T, Sharpe G, Taieb A, Tacrolimus Ointment Long-term Follow-up Study G. A 4-year follow-up study of atopic dermatitis therapy with 0.1% tacrolimus ointment in children and adult patients. Br J Dermatol. 2008;159(4): 942–951.

Ring J, Alomar A, Bieber T, Deleuran M, Fink-Wagner A, Gelmetti C, Gieler U, Lipozencic J, Luger T, Oranje AP, Schäfer T, Schwennesen T, Seidenari S, Simon D, Ständer S, Stingl G, Szalai S, Szepietowski JC, Taïeb A, Werfel T, Wollenberg A, Darsow U. Guidelines for treatment of atopic eczema (atopic dermatitis) part I. J Eur Acad Dermatol Venereol. 2012;26(8):1045–60.

Sakuma S, Higashi Y, Sato N, Sasakawa T, Sengoku T, Ohkubo Y, Amaya T, Goto T. Tacrolimus suppressed the production of cytokines involved in atopic dermatitis by direct stimulation of human PBMC system. (Comparison with steroids). Int Immunopharmacol. 2001;1(6):1219–26.

Schmid-Wendtner M-H, Korting HC. The pH of the skin surface and its impact on the barrier function. Skin Pharmacol Physiol. 2006;19(6):296–302.

Schneider L, Hanifin J, Boguniewicz M, Eichenfield LF, Spergel JM, Dakovic R, Paller AS. Study of the atopic march: development of atopic comorbidities. Pediatr Dermatol. 2016;33(4):388–98.

Shi VY, Tran K, Lio PA. A comparison of physicochemical properties of a selection of modern moisturizers: hydrophilic index and pH. J Drugs in Dermatol: JDD. 2012;11(5):633–6.

Shibata Y, Ikeda H, Kihira K. Investigation of patients' satisfaction in using potent topical corticosteroid preparations. Hiroshima J Med Sci. 2007;56(3/4):33.

Simonsen L, Hoy G, Didriksen E, Persson J, Melchior N, Hansen J. Development of a new formulation combining calcipotriol and betamethasone dipropionate in an ointment vehicle. Drug Dev Ind Pharm. 2004;30(10):1095–102.

Simpson EL, Berry TM, Brown PA, Hanifin JM. A pilot study of emollient therapy for the primary prevention of atopic dermatitis. J Am Acad Dermatol. 2010;63(4):587–93.

Simpson E, Böhling A, Bielfeldt S, Bosc C, Kerrouche N. Improvement of skin barrier function in atopic dermatitis patients with a new moisturizer containing a ceramide precursor. J Dermatol Treat. 2013;24(2):122–5.

Simpson EL, Chalmers JR, Hanifin JM, Thomas KS, Cork MJ, McLean WHI, Brown SJ, Chen Z, Chen Y, Williams HC. Emollient enhancement of the skin barrier from birth offers effective atopic dermatitis prevention. J Allergy Clin Immunol. 2014;134(4):818–23.

Sindher S, Alkotob SS, Shojinaga MN, Brough HA, Bahnson T, Lack G, Leung D, Nadeau K. Pilot study measuring transepidermal water loss (TEWL) in children suggests trilipid cream is more effective than a paraffin-based emollient. Allergy. 2020.

Sindher S, Alkotob SS, Shojinaga MN, Hamilton R, Chan S, Cao S, Bahnson HT, Brough HA, Lack G, Leung DYM, Nadeau KC. Increases in plasma IgG4/IgE with trilipid vs paraffin/petrolatum-based emollients for dry skin/eczema. Pediatr Allergy Immunol. 2020.

Skjerven HO, Rehbinder EM, Vettukattil R, LeBlanc M, Granum B, Haugen G, Hedlin G, Landrø L, Marsland BJ, Rudi K, Sjøborg KD, Söderhäll C, Staff AC, Carlsen KH, Asarnoj A, Bains KES, Carlsen OCL, Endre KMA, Granlund PA, Hermansen JU, Gudmundsdóttir HK, Hilde K, Håland G, Kreyberg I, Olsen IC, Mägi CO, Nordhagen LS, Saunders CM, Skrindo I, Tedner SG, Værnesbranden MR, Wiik J, Jonassen CM, Nordlund B, Carlsen KCL. Skin emollient and early complementary feeding to prevent infant atopic dermatitis (PreventADALL): a factorial, multicentre, cluster-randomised trial. Lancet. 2020;395(10228):951–61.

Van Smeden J, Janssens M, Gooris G, Bouwstra J. The important role of stratum corneum lipids for the cutaneous barrier function. Biochimica et Biophysica Acta (BBA)-Molecular and Cell Biol Lipids. 2014;1841(3): 295–313.

Spergel JM, Paller AS. Atopic dermatitis and the atopic march. J Allergy Clin Immunol. 2003;112(6 Suppl):S118-127.

Stamatas GN, Nikolovski J, Mack MC, Kollias N. Infant skin physiology and development during the first years of life: a review of recent findings based on in vivo studies. Int J Cosmet Sci. 2011;33(1):17–24.

Sugarman JL, Parish LC. Efficacy of a lipid-based barrier repair formulation in moderate-to-severe pediatric atopic dermatitis. J Drugs Dermatol. 2009;8(12):1106–11.

Tabata N, O'Goshi K, Zhen Y, Kligman A, Tagami H. Biophysical assessment of persistent effects of moisturizers after their daily applications: evaluation of corneotherapy. Dermatology. 2000;200(4):308–13.

Tam H, Calderon MA, Manikam L, Nankervis H, Garcia Nunez I, Williams HC, Durham S, Boyle RJ. Specific allergen immunotherapy for the treatment of atopic eczema. Cochrane Database Syst Rev 2016;2: CD008774.

Thirumoorthy T, Giam YC, Rajan VS. Topical sodium Cromoglycate cream in atopic eczema. Singapore Med J. 1983;24(2):102–3.

Thomson AW, Bonham CA, Zeevi A. Mode of action of tacrolimus (FK506): molecular and cellular mechanisms. Ther Drug Monit. 1995;17(6):584–91.

Tollefson MM, Bruckner AL, Section On D. Atopic dermatitis: skin-directed management. Pediatrics. 2014;134(6):e1735-1744.

Tsakok T, Marrs T, Mohsin M, Baron S, du Toit G, Till S, Flohr C. Does atopic dermatitis cause food allergy? A systematic review. J Allergy Clin Immunol. 2016;137(4):1071–8.

Turner MJ, Dasilva-Arnold SC, Yi Q, Mehrotra P, Kaplan MH, Travers JB. Topical application of a vitamin D analogue exacerbates atopic dermatitis and induces the atopic dermatitis-like phenotype in Stat6VT mice. Pediatr Dermatol. 2013;30(5):574–8.

van Smeden J, Janssens M, Kaye EC, Caspers PJ, Lavrijsen AP, Vreeken RJ, Bouwstra JA. The importance of free fatty acid chain length for the skin barrier function in atopic eczema patients. Exp Dermatol. 2014b;23(1):45–52.

Varothai S, Nitayavardhana S, Kulthanan K. Moisturizers for patients with atopic dermatitis. Asian Pac J Allergy Immunol. 2013;31(2):91–8.

van Zuuren EJ, Fedorowicz Z, Christensen R, Lavrijsen AP, Arents BW. Emollients and moisturisers for eczema. Cochrane Database of Systemat Rev. 2017;2.

Watson W, Kapur S. Atopic dermatitis. Allergy Asthma Clin Immunol. 2011;7(Suppl 1):S4.

Yamamoto-Hanada K, Kobayashi T, Williams HC, Mikami M, Saito-Abe M, Morita K, Natsume O, Sato M, Iwama M, Miyaji Y, Miyata M, Inagaki S, Tatsuki F, Masami N, Nakayama SF, Kido H, Saito H, Ohya Y. Early aggressive intervention for infantile atopic dermatitis to prevent development of food allergy: a multicenter, investigator-blinded, randomized, parallel group controlled trial (PACI Study)-protocol for a randomized controlled trial. Clin Transl Allergy. 2018;8:47.

Yang M, Chang JM. Successful treatment of refractory chronic hand eczema with calcipotriol/betamethasone ointment: a report of three cases. Exp Ther Med. 2015;10(5):1943–6.

Yarbrough KB, Neuhaus KJ, Simpson EL. The effects of treatment on itch in atopic dermatitis. Dermatol Ther. 2013;26(2):110–9.

Yonezawa K, Haruna M. Short-term skin problems in infants aged 0–3 months affect food allergies or atopic dermatitis until 2 years of age, among infants of the general population. Allergy Asthma Clin Immunol. 2019;15:74.

Yonezawa K, Haruna M, Matsuzaki M, Shiraishi M, Kojima R. Effects of moisturizing skincare on skin barrier function and the prevention of skin problems in 3-month-old infants: a randomized controlled trial. J Dermatol. 2018;45(1):24–30.

Chapter 2
The Human Skin Microbiome

L. B. Noerreslet, M. L. Clausen, and T. Agner

Abstract A complex and diverse community of bacteria, fungi, viruses and mites densely colonises the human skin. The entire collection of all microbial genes in a community of a given habitat is usually referred to as the microbiome and will for the sake of consistency be used throughout this chapter. The human skin microbiome is individually unique in composition and shaped by several factors in close relation to the skin barrier. Current research strives to establish common characteristics of the healthy skin microbiome from which to detect alterations associated with skin diseases. Studying the human skin microbiome composition may be valuable in elucidating the aetiology of various, common skin diseases with the hope of therapeutic approaches targeting the skin microbiome. Based on current knowledge, this chapter gives an introduction to the human skin microbiome, primarily the bacterial, and explains factors of importance for the healthy and diseased skin microbiome composition.

Keywords Microbiome · Microbiota · Bacteria · Microorganisms

2.1 Introduction

Early evidence determined the importance of the protective skin barrier in maintenance of a healthy skin. In this millennium this understanding is supplemented by increasing knowledge of the essential role of the skin microbiome. Using traditional culture-dependent methods, several specific microorganisms (microbes) were early on suggested to be a central role in the pathogenesis of different inflammatory skin

L. B. Noerreslet (✉) · M. L. Clausen · T. Agner
Department of Dermatology, Bispebjerg University Hospital, 2400 Copenhagen NV, Denmark
e-mail: line.brok.norreslet@rsyd.dk

M. L. Clausen
e-mail: mlclausen@gmail.com

T. Agner
e-mail: tove.agner@regionh.dk

A. Lauerma et al. (eds.), *The Skin Microbiome Manual*,
https://doi.org/10.1007/978-3-031-82689-4_2

diseases, such as *Staphylococcus aureus* (*S. aureus*) in atopic dermatitis (AD) and *Cutibacterium acnes* (*C. acnes*) in acne vulgaris. Culture-based methods continue to play an important role in research of cutaneous microorganisms. However, culturing only allows for identification of certain bacterial species, and the true relative abundance of different species can be difficult to investigate from cultures. With new methods for DNA sequencing developed in the late 1990s, "next-generation", high-throughput sequencing methods revolutionised and accelerated the complex investigation of the microbiome composition. Today's culture-independent skin microbiome research explores the entire composition of the microbial environment of the skin and a more detailed understanding of mechanisms shaping and influencing the skin microbiome is continuously evolving. To date, most of the research regarding the skin microbiome has focused on the bacterial community composition, and the causal link to skin diseases is yet to be discovered (Costello et al. 2009; Grice et al. 2009, 2008; Oh et al. 2016).

2.2 The Skin as a Habitat for Microorganisms

2.2.1 Skin Structure and Barrier Functions

The human skin microbiome composition is influenced by numerous endogenous and environmental factors and also heavily influenced by a close interaction with the skin immune system. An understanding of the skin physiology and the skin barrier function is essential to establish a foundation from which to understand the composition of the skin microbiome. The defensive functions of the human skin barrier include both a physical barrier, a chemical barrier, and an immunological barrier, and they all have great impact on the microorganisms inhabiting a specific region of the skin (Fig. 2.1). The barrier functions are primarily mediated by the outermost layer of the epidermis, stratum corneum (Fig. 2.1). The two-component structure of stratum corneum with corneocytes embedded in lipid-enriched extracellular matrix (Elias 2006) enables the epidermis to serve as a permeable barrier for the movement of water and electrolytes, as well as providing protection from mechanical stress and penetration of harmful substances and microorganisms. Moreover, the stratum corneum functions as a chemical and immune barrier with ongoing metabolic activity, generating osmotically active humectants and adapting to external or internal perturbations. Thus, together with the physical and chemical skin barrier, immunological defence and environmental factors, the microbial barrier serves to protect against pathogenic microorganisms. The relatively low skin surface temperature of 29–34 °C and an acidic pH of 4.5–5.5 are both unfavourable for the growth of most pathogenic bacteria. Furthermore, a variety of innate and adaptive immune cells, particularly the keratinocytes and leukocytes, supports the maintenance of a healthy skin barrier by frontline protection against invading pathogens (Heath and Carbone 2013).

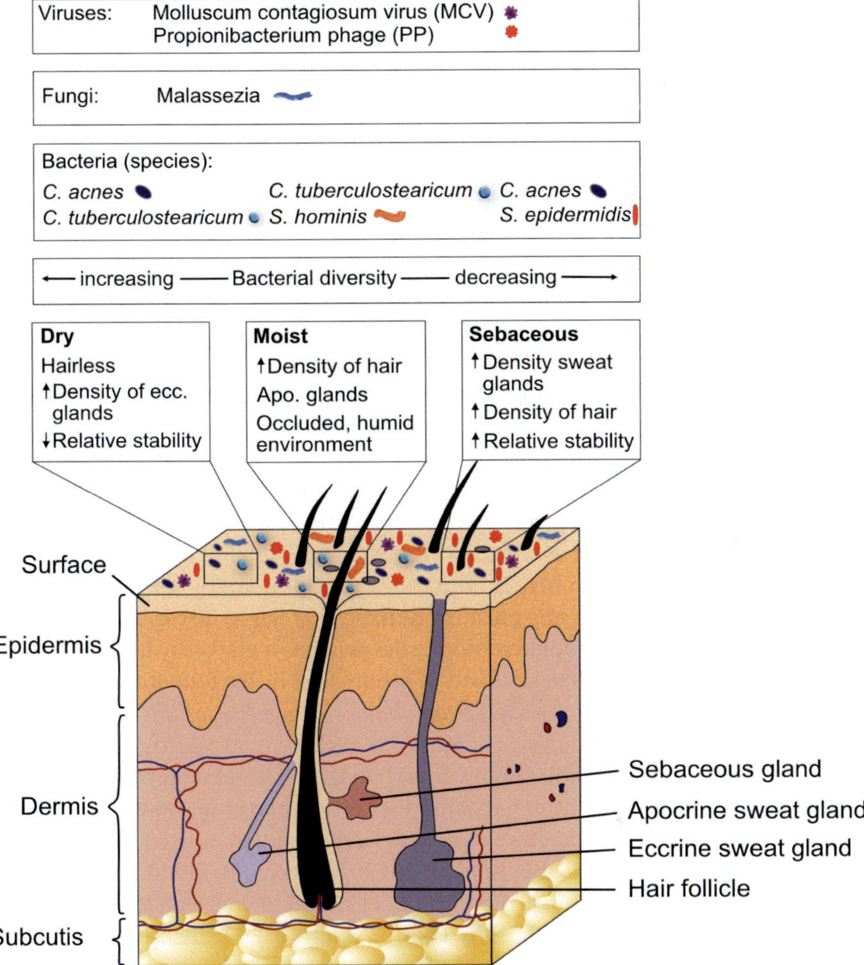

Fig. 2.1 Schematic model of the skin with most abundant viruses, fungi and bacteria on the human skin surface of dry, moist and sebaceous skin (Byrd et al. 2018; SanMiguel and Grice 2015; Grice and Segre 2011)

In the dermis, hair follicles, sebaceous glands and sweat glands are topographically unevenly distributed and influence the microorganisms situated in relation to these structures and at the skin surface. Through secretion of a lipid-rich sebum to the skin, the sebaceous glands protect skin and hair from dehydration and the sebum has antibacterial properties. The sweat glands are categorised into eccrine and apocrine glands, of which the eccrine glands are the most abundant and secrete odourless, translucent liquid. The apocrine glands are located only in the axillary, breast, and anogenital regions, where the milky and viscous liquid is secreted into hair follicles, triggered by androgen stimulation (Wilke et al. 2007; Wood and Kelly 2010). These variations in the human skin create unique microenvironments for microorganisms across body sites.

Classification

The bacterial microorganisms are categorised according to their function. Commensals are residents on the normal, healthy skin, usually harmless or even protective as they can interact in a mutualistic relationship with the host immune system (Gallo and Nakatsuji 2011). Pathogenic microorganisms, also termed transients, are typically temporarily colonising the skin and have the potential to act harmfully.

The systematic classification of microorganisms is described by phylogeny and/ or taxonomy. Phylogeny is the study of the evolutionary development of microorganisms, based on the hypothesis that all life is derived from a common ancestor, and is often illustrated with a phylogenetic tree. Taxonomy is a hierarchical classification system for naming microorganisms based on characteristics, e.g. phylogeny characteristics. Considering classical biology taxonomy, cellular microorganisms can be categorised into three domains; archaea; bacteria, and; eukaryotes (including fungi), whereas viruses for now are considered non-living and not part of any domain. Inferior to the domain level is kingdom followed by phylum, class, order, family, genus, species and strain (subtypes) (Fig. 2.2). Bacteria are by far the most abundant domain of microorganisms on skin (Belkaid and Segre 2014; Oh et al. 2014). However, compared to the gut microbiome, the skin has a markedly higher representation of viruses and fungi (Oh et al. 2014). On human skin, the four dominant bacteria phyla are *Actinobacteria, Firmicutes, Proteobacteria*, and *Bacteroidetes* (Grice et al. 2009). The bacterial community composition varies greatly across body sites at genus, species and strain level. On the other hand, the fungal community composition, sometimes referred to as the mycobiome, is dominated by multiple species of the genus *Malassezia*, and therefore with a lower diversity compared to the bacterial composition (Findley et al. 2013; Jo et al. 2017; Nguyen and Soulika 2019; Edslev et al. 2020). Viral genes, called the virome, is the least investigated, and to date no core reference from normal healthy control skin is established; however, sparse baseline references do exist (Oh et al. 2016; Hannigan et al. 2015). Viral communities are particularly complex to characterise due to technical limitations and can be assessed using whole genome metagenomics in which the entire DNA from a sample is sequenced. Considering the relatively sparse literature on skin fungal and viral genomes in contrast to the bacterial genomes, this may induce bias of our current understanding of the overall microbiome composition.

The diversity of the microbiome is determined based on DNA sequencing data (generated by next-generation sequencing, NGS), either amplicon sequencing of a target gene (e.g. the *16S rRNA* gene for bacteria analysis) or shut-gun sequencing for metagenomics. Amplicon sequences can be assigned into operational taxonomic units (OTU's), using a sequence similarity clustering method (often with a similarity threshold of 97% or higher), or into amplicon sequence variants (ASV's) (Callahan et al. 2016), which is a clustering free method (Fig. 2.2). Diversity can be referred to as α-diversity or β-diversity. Alpha-diversity represents the average species diversity in a habitat or specific area, sometimes considered as the intra-individual (within sample)

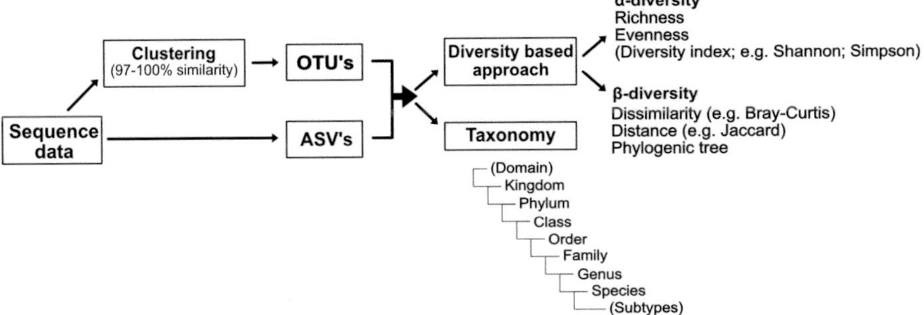

Fig. 2.2 Classification of microorganisms using an DNA amplicon-based approach. Target genes are amplified by PCR and sequenced. Sequence data can be used to assess diversity and identify taxa in samples

diversity, and is described by richness, which is the number of OTU's or ASV's, and evenness, which is a term for the relative abundance. Taken together, richness and evenness can be expressed in a diversity index (e.g. Shannon's or Simpson's). Beta-diversity represents the diversity of species between two habitats or regions, also occasionally considered as inter-individual diversity or diversity between two samples. Beta-diversity can be examined by a dissimilarity or similarity index (e.g. Bray–Curtis or Jaccard), optionally in combination with phylogenetic analysis.

The human skin microbiome is largely stable over time, at both short-term and up to two years (Costello et al. 2009; Grice et al. 2009; Oh et al. 2016; Hannigan et al. 2015), though less stable than the microbiome of the gut (Flores et al. 2014). The degree of temporal variability is considered to be dependent on the individual, topography and phylogeny (Costello et al. 2009; Grice et al. 2009; Oh et al. 2016). The temporal variation of the bacterial microbiome is higher interpersonally compared with the variability within specific skin site across time (Costello et al. 2009; Grice et al. 2009), and dry skin sites are less stable over time compared with sebaceous skin sites.

Most studies have investigated the skin microbiome at the surface of epidermis, while the dermal microbiome is sparsely studied (Nakatsuji et al. 2013). Whereas the epidermal microbiome is largely influenced by environmental conditions and topography, the dermal microbiome is characterised by less bacterial community composition variability and richness, is less influenced by exogenous factors and topography, and distinctly different from that of the epidermis (Bay et al. 2020; Prast-Nielsen et al. 2019). Differences may arise from sampling methods, as the epidermal (surface) microbiome is most often sampled using swabs, whereas the dermal microbiome is examined using biopsies.

2.3 Influential Factors

Numerous conditions have the potential to influence the microbiome composition on human skin. Apart from the temporal variability of the microbiome, various endogenous (host) and exogenous (environmental) factors are of importance, though the level of evidence for each factor varies and the mechanisms are poorly understood (Fig. 2.3). Naturally, the factors co-occur and interact with each other, complicating the evaluation of each factor's independent influence on the skin microbiome. The skin microbiome has been described as a 'microbial fingerprint' due to exclusive individual characteristics (Oh et al. 2016). In the following, important factors influencing the microbiome composition, in particular the bacterial microbiome, are covered based on present literature.

Topography

The composition of the microbiome is largely dependent on skin-site characteristics, which vary at different anatomical sites (Costello et al. 2009; Grice et al. 2009). Physiological conditions of the skin include lipid and sebum composition, pH, hydration, temperature and immunological factors such as expression of antimicrobial peptides (AMPs). The microenvironment of the skin determines the bacterial communities composition, whereas viruses and fungi seem to be less site-specific (Oh et al. 2016; Byrd et al. 2018). The composition of the microbiome has shown some distinct differences related to the skin being dry, moist or sebaceous (Fig. 2.1) (Costello et al. 2009; Grice et al. 2009). Dry skin, e.g. hand and forearm, harbour many phyla including the four dominant types *Actinobacteria, Proteobacteria, Firmicutes* and *Bacteriodetes*

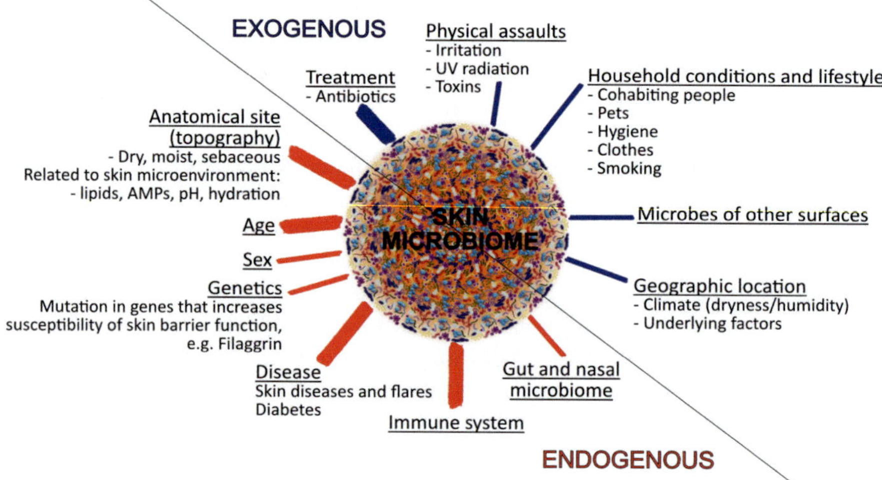

Fig. 2.3 Endogenous and exogenous factors of importance for the human skin microbiome composition. Thick branches represent relatively higher level of literature supporting its association with the human skin microbiome

(Grice et al. 2009) (Fig. 2.1). Moist skin, e.g. the elbow crease, mainly comprises the genera *Staphylococcus (Firmicutes)* and *Corynebacteria (Actinobacteria),* whereas sebaceous skin, e.g. the face (T-zone) and upper torso, is dominated by *Propionibacterium (Actinobacteria)* and *Staphylococcus* spp. (*Firmicutes*). In other words, greatest bacterial diversity of the skin microbiome composition is found on dry skin, whereas sebaceous skin sites express least diversity.

Age

Age is another important endogenous factor shaping the skin microbiome composition. The microbiome changes greatly throughout life, from birth to old age, primarily associated with dynamic changes in skin barrier structure in addition to the maturation of the host immune system. At birth, infants are covered with vernix caseosa; a white, lipid-rich liquid containing AMPs (IL-37 and lysozyme), which is of great importance regarding cutaneous innate immunity in the neonate (Marchini et al. 2002; Tollin et al. 2005). Depending on birth delivery method, the skin rapidly gets colonised with microorganisms during or immediately after birth. Whereas vaginally delivered infants share skin microbiome composition similarly to the vaginal flora of their mother (predominantly *Lactobacillus*), the skin of caesarean section delivered infants is significantly different, comparable to that of their mother's skin (*Staphylococcus, Streptococcus, Corynebacterium* and *Propionibacterium*) (Chu et al. 2017; Dominguez-Bello et al. 2010). The rapid microbial skin colonisation from early life is thought to critically affect the development of the skin immune function. Throughout the infantile period, the skin and immune system mature, and the skin microbiome composition continuously changes. In contrast to adults, the skin microbiome composition of infants is not influenced by topography. In puberty, the production of sebum and sebum-related products increase (Leyden et al. 1975), and at the same time the microbiome composition goes in the direction of that of adults (Shi et al. 2016; Oh et al. 2012). Overall, younger children express higher levels of *Proteobacteria* and *Firmicutes*, whereas adolescents and young adults are dominated by more lipophilic *Corynebacteriaceae, Propionibacteriaceae* and *Corynebacterium* (Oh et al. 2012).

In adult populations of different ages, sparse evidence points towards a correlation of skin microbiome and skin aging. Certain corynebacterial taxa have been suggested to reflect physiological aging processes, as the relative abundance increased with age (Dimitriu et al. 2019). However, to date, age in relation to the skin microbiome is insufficiently investigated.

Sex

Influence of sex on the microbiome composition and bacterial diversity is thought to arise indirectly from sex hormone production, affecting the skin differently in males and females (Giacomoni et al. 2009). Sex hormones are essential in regulation of epidermal thickness, which is thicker in males compared with females (Dao and Kazin 2007). Moreover, sex hormones influence immune responses and thus ultimately the skin microbiome. Skin surface pH is generally slightly more acidic in males (Giacomoni et al. 2009; Dao and Kazin 2007). Sweat rate and sebum production from glands located in the dermis are doubled in males compared with females.

Lastly, body hair growth, subcutaneous fat and use of cosmetics differ between sexes. Several studies have examined sex differences in relation to the skin microbiome with heterogeneous results, primarily dependent on which anatomic site was investigated (SanMiguel and Grice 2015).

Genetics

Mutations in genes which lead to increased susceptibility of the skin barrier may contribute to differences in the skin microbiome composition. In focus for this is the filaggrin gene (*FLG*). Filaggrin is a filament-aggregating protein of major epidermal structural importance, as it aligns keratin filaments and contributes to the hydration of the SC (McAleer and Irvine 2013; Rawlings and Harding 2004; Oord and Sheikh 2009), and thereby healthy skin (Sandilands et al. 2009). Inherited loss-of-function mutations in *FLG* are strongly associated with a diagnosis of AD (Palmer et al. 2006), and found in around one third of patients with moderate-to-severe AD. Moreover, a decreased bacterial diversity profile of the overall skin microbiome has been linked to AD-patients with *FLG*-mutations compared to those without (Clausen et al. 2018). Meanwhile, lowered expression of filaggrin has been observed in AD patients with wild type *FLG* alleles, suggesting that filaggrin levels can also be regulated by host immune functions (Howell et al. 2009; Kezic et al. 2011). Furthermore, filaggrin deficiency might affect lipid formation (Vavrova et al. 2014) and enhance *S. aureus* growth (Miajlovic et al. 2010). A recent study associated filaggrin deficient skin in both healthy individuals and AD-patients with marked shifts in microbiome composition expressed by reduced α-diversity compared to those without filaggrin deficient skin (Baurecht et al. 2018).

Immune System

The understanding of the cutaneous immune defence system in relation to skin microbiome composition is complex and limited, though evolving. A variety of cell types are situated in the skin and provide the front-line immune defence against invading pathogens. Keratinocytes have a key role in detection and defence against pathogens (Gallo and Nakatsuji 2011; Kuo et al. 2013) through expression of pattern recognition receptors. These include Toll-like receptors recognising pathogenic microorganisms, and Nod-like receptors, reacting to bacterial peptidoglycan. Keratinocyte expression of other pattern recognition receptors responds to certain viral and fungal components. Furthermore, keratinocytes can secrete substances such as AMPs, either directly as a response to microbial detection or indirectly via cytokine (interleukin) or chemokine activation. Keratinocytes are the main source of AMPs in normal skin. However, as a result of diseased, inflamed skin the recruited leukocytes take over most of the AMP production. With an antibiotic-like function, AMPs can be targeted to inhibit pathogenic growth of specific bacterial strains, and thereby be crucial in the skin homeostasis (Gallo and Nakatsuji 2011; Clausen and Agner 2016; Hanson et al. 2019). An interaction between host AMPs and AMPs secreted from the bacteria might influence growth and living conditions, hence influencing the microbiome composition. The relationship between host immune response and skin bacteria is crucial for obtaining the right symbiosis and dominance of commensal and beneficial bacteria yet fighting the pathogenic bacteria.

Diseases

Several skin diseases have been associated with distinct alterations in the skin microbiome, and will be discussed later (Byrd et al. 2018; Clausen et al. 2018; Baurecht et al. 2018; Kong et al. 2012; Findley and Grice 2014; Lee et al. 2019; Nakatsuji et al. 2018; Nakatsuji and Gallo 2019; Picardo and Ottaviani 2014; Ring et al. 2019, 2017; Sanford and Gallo 2013). Moreover, changes in the skin microbiome have been associated with diabetes mellitus, where physical changes in the skin barrier such as increased pH and dryness are observed (Behm et al. 2012). Most research on the association between the microbiome and diabetes has been performed in relation to the gut, few studies suggest an altered skin microbiome in association with diabetic skin and wounds (Gardiner et al. 2017; Grice et al. 2010). In a murine study, the diabetic skin microbiome was altered in addition to a distinct host gene expression profile (Grice et al. 2010). Primary immunodeficiency patients have also been associated with decreased skin microbiome diversity (Oh et al. 2013). This patient population could be of particular interest when studying the role of microbe-host interactions in diseases, and the degree to which compromised immunity can influence the microbiome. Data on skin microbiome from patients receiving immune-modulating treatment are not available.

Gut and Nasal Microbiome

Can changes in the gut and nasal microbiome, respectively, lead to cutaneous manifestations? The 'brain-gut-skin axis' hypothesis was established almost 100 years ago, suggesting that emotional stress alters the gut microbiome, increases gut permeability and induces systemic inflammation (Stokes and Pillsbury 1930). Most studies conclude that this gut-skin connection may be a result of neurologic and immunologic responses to environmental shifts, and thereby a systemic inflammation that eventually distresses the skin (O'Neill et al. 2016; Salem et al. 2018).

Supportive of the gut-skin theory, numerous studies have investigated the gut microbiome in relation to different skin diseases. Decreased gut microbiome diversity and presence of specific species in early childhood have been associated with AD development later in life (Forno et al. 2008; Abrahamsson et al. 2012). In the gut microbiome of children, *Clostridium difficile* and *Escherichia coli,* respectively, were associated with a higher risk of AD development (Penders et al. 2007; Nimwegen et al. 2011). However, a pathophysiological understanding of how the disease manifestations in skin are related to these gut microorganisms is lacking.

In psoriasis, decreased bacterial diversity and decreased abundance of *Actinobacteria* are found in the gut microbiome, while an increased *Firmicutes/Bacteroides* ratio is suggested to relate to severity of disease (Scher et al. 2015), though results are heterogeneous (Codoner et al. 2018).

In acne vulgaris, the gut microbiome is sparsely investigated, however, an association of acne in relation to an altered gut microbiome has been reported (Yan et al. 2018; Deng et al. 2018). In brief, decreased *Actinobacteria,* increased *Proteobacteria* and lower microbiome diversity in the gut of patients with acne compared to healthy individuals were found.

In rosacea, the most studied gut microorganism is *Helicobacter pylori*, however; its role in rosacea remains controversial (Jorgensen et al. 2017).

The nasal microbiome and its connection to the skin microbiome is only sparsely investigated. In AD, the nasal microbiome might be related to that of the skin (Totte et al. 2019), associated with disease severity and distinctly different from that of healthy individuals (Clausen et al. 2018; Totte et al. 2019). A theory of cross-transmission of bacteria between gut, nose and skin is speculated (Totte et al. 2019), however; not firmly documented to date.

Exogenous Factors

Environmental exposures and direct contact to touched objects are obviously suggested to influence the skin microbiome composition, though the level of evidence is not solid. **Treatment** is another important exogenous factor. Use antibiotics reduce quantity and diversity of the microbiome, though mainly studied in relation to the gut microbiome (Dethlefsen and Relman 2011). In patients with AD, systemic antibiotics can temporarily reduce *S. aureus* skin colonisation and improve severity of skin lesions (Boguniewicz et al. 2001).

Physical assaults of the skin barrier such as irritation, ultraviolet (UV) radiation or toxins can also affect the skin microbiome. The mechanism is mainly thought to be through a mediation of immune system reactivity as a respond to impaired barrier function or the UV radiation (Patra et al. 2018).

Lifestyle factors may influence skin microbiome (Dimitriu et al. 2019). Microorganisms can be transferred directly by shaking of hands and indirectly by touching an object such as paper or glass (Neckovic et al. 2020). Cohabiting individuals express shared microbiome characteristics with each other, and with pets, linen and towels (Ross et al. 2017; Song et al. 2013; Lax et al. 2014). Microbial communities of various indoor surfaces have been found to differ significantly between homes, and to be identifiable by the family living in the home (Lax et al. 2014). Human-associated microbial communities have also been identified on office equipment (Fierer et al. 2010), mobile phones and shoes (Lax et al. 2015), collectively suggesting its future potential role in a forensic context (Neckovic et al. 2020). Hygiene naturally also influences the skin microbiome. One study found that time since last hand wash was influential of the immediate skin community composition, while overall bacterial diversity was unaffected (Fierer et al. 2008), suggesting a rapid reestablishment of bacterial communities after hand wash. Smoking has also been suggested to be influential of the epidermal skin microbiome composition and overall bacterial OTU richness (Bay et al. 2020).

Geographical variability in skin microbiome has also been observed (Blaser et al. 2013; Hospodsky et al. 2014). To date, most studies have investigated the skin microbiome of Western populations (Grice et al. 2009, 2008; Oh et al. 2016; Bay et al. 2020; Byrd et al. 2018; Consortum 2012a). Few studies of other ethnic populations suggest that the skin microbiome differs in relation to ethnicity. The first large-scale skin microbiome study of an Asian population found a distinctly different skin microbiome composition compared with that of Caucasian populations (Leung et al. 2015). Comparing hands of Tanzanian women to hands of US women, bacterial communities were found to vary (Hospodsky et al. 2014). It seems likely that the observed differences are due to underlying lifestyle differences, cultural or ethnic factors; however, the mechanisms are not fully understood. Furthermore, UV radiation varies geographically, and a corresponding microbial variability seems plausible.

2.4 Healthy Versus Diseased Skin

The healthy skin microbiome is characterised by great diversity in the microbiome composition (Consortum 2012b), temporal stability (Costello et al. 2009; Grice et al. 2009; Oh et al. 2016; Kong et al. 2012), presence of skin commensals and absence of pathogenic microorganisms, as opposed to diseased skin (Fig. 2.4).

Dysbiosis

An imbalanced microbiome is termed 'dysbiosis'. Dysbiosis is a consequence of change in abundance and diversity of the microorganisms, and often characterised by the dominance of specific pathogenic microorganisms. Generally, dysbiosis occurs due to dysregulation of the cutaneous ecosystem, as well as influence from endogenous or exogenous factors as described in the previous section. Although cause and effect are difficult to discriminate, dysbiosis clearly plays a role in the pathogenesis of many skin diseases such as AD, acne vulgaris, hidradenitis suppurativa and psoriasis. Without exception, patient populations with these inflammatory skin diseases express some kind of dysbiosis of the skin microbiome (Kong et al. 2012; Nakatsuji and Gallo 2019; Ring et al. 2017; Alekseyenko et al. 2013; Langan et al. 2019; Totte et al. 2016). In accordance with the clinically different presentation of the diseases and their predilection sites, the microbiome composition and dysbiosis differ considerably.

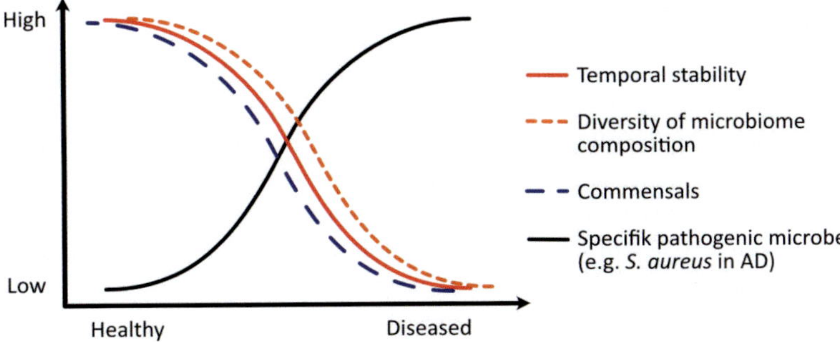

Fig. 2.4 Microbiome characteristics in healthy and diseased skin

Skin Commensals

Certain skin commensals and mutualistic microorganisms are considered essential for the microbiome stability. Two of the major commensal microorganisms inhabiting the skin and sebaceous follicles are *S. epidermidis* and *C. acnes* (formerly known as *Propionibacterium acnes*), respectively (Christensen and Bruggemann 2014). These bacteria have several modes of actions in which they protect homeostasis and protect against dysbiosis and invading pathogens. Firstly, commensals might directly inhibit pathogenic growth by competing with pathogens for habitable space and nutrients. Furthermore, *S. epidermidis* has been found to secrete antimicrobial agents (AMPs/bactericidal compounds) specifically directed to inhibit pathogenic *S. aureus'* strains (Gallo and Nakatsuji 2011; Nakatsuji et al. 2017) and *S. aureus* biofilm formation (Iwase et al. 2010). Likewise, *C. acnes* is found to inhibit MRSA colonisation in mice wounds by production of short-chain fatty acids (Shu et al. 2013). Secondly, the skin commensals enhance and educate the host immune system (Sanford and Gallo 2013; Cogen et al. 2010). Via manipulation of the host immune response, *S. epidermidis* can protect against group A *Streptococcus* colonisation (Cogen et al. 2010), suppress inflammation during wound repair (Lai et al. 2009), and has even been suggested to promote antitumor immunity (Nakatsuji et al. 2018). Thus, commensal microorganisms are thought to play an important role in maintenance of the healthy skin microbiome.

In general, *S. epidermidis* and *C. acnes* are regarded merely as commensals or mutualistic microorganisms. However, they may also act as opportunistic pathogens (Otto 2009; Cogen et al. 2008), complicating the understanding of their role in the healthy skin microbiome. *S. epidermidis* is a frequent cause of hospital-acquired infections from indwelling medical devices through biofilm formation; however, only in circumstances where the host is compromised (immune deficient, surgery, injury) (Otto 2009; Le et al. 2018; Becker et al. 2014). Several *S. epidermidis* strains have been identified, differing significantly in their capacity to express virulence factors and form biofilm. Isolates of *S. epidermidis* from healthy individuals lack a specific gene, the *ica*ADBC operon, which has frequently been found in clinical strains harvested from hospital-acquired infections (Cho et al. 2002; Kozitskaya et al. 2004). Despite of the dualistic properties of *S. epidermidis*, most evidence points towards beneficial effects of its presence, mainly due to its recognised beneficial interaction with the immune response.

Likewise, *C. acnes* is thought to have a key role in the pathogenesis of acne vulgaris (Fitz-Gibbon et al. 2013; Kurokawa et al. 2009; Leyden et al. 1998), though the causal relationship it still debated (O'Neill and Gallo 2018). As for *S. epidermidis*, specific strains of *C. acnes* are thought to be decisive of its role as either commensal or pathogenic. Several studies have sequenced *C. acnes* isolates from acne lesions and healthy skin and revealed disease-specific strains, in particular strains within the type IA-2 phylogenetic clade (subgroup) are found to be related to disease (Fitz-Gibbon et al. 2013; Kasimatis et al. 2013; McDowell et al. 2013).

A higher relative abundance of commensals like *S. epidermidis* and *C. acnes* have been associated with the microbiome in healthy skin compared with that of diseased skin in AD and acne vulgaris, respectively (Kong et al. 2012; Barnard et al. 2016; Shi et al. 2018). Altogether, the presence of strain-specific commensals and their high relative abundance are considered to be associated with healthy versus diseased skin.

Disease-Specific Pathogens and Microbiome Characteristics

Presence of pathogenic microorganisms is usually associated with lower bacterial α-diversity (Shi et al. 2018) and lower relative abundance of skin commensals (Shi et al. 2016). One of the most studied skin diseases with respect to the skin microbiome is AD. The dysbiosis observed in patients with AD is characterised by reduced bacterial α-diversity (Clausen et al. 2018; Kong et al. 2012; Byrd et al. 2017) and decreased temporal stability (Kong et al. 2012) as compared with that of healthy individuals. The association between *S. aureus* and AD was first discovered in 1974 and ever since repeatedly supported (Leyden et al. 1974). *S. aureus* is associated with AD in both lesional and non-lesional skin, and its relative abundance increases during flares (Clausen et al. 2018; Kong et al. 2012; Chng et al. 2016). The prevalence of *S. aureus* in AD lesional skin has been found to be 70%, almost 20 times that of healthy controls (Totte et al. 2016). Apart from the presence of AD, severity of the disease is also correlated with decreased bacterial α-diversity, persistent colonisation and increased abundance of *S. aureus* (Shi et al. 2016; Clausen et al. 2018; Totte et al. 2016; Byrd et al. 2017). An increased abundance of *Firmicutes*, and a decreased abundance of the genus *Acinetobacter* (*Proteobacterium*) have been observed in AD skin, which is of particular interest as *Acinetobacter* can suppress the cytokine response to *S. aureus* (Smeekens et al. 2014).

In AD, hereditary defects in the epidermal barrier like *FLG*-mutation and host immune dysregulation can favour disease susceptibility, supposedly by altered response to the skin microbiome resulting in the dominant overgrowth of *S. aureus*. Deficiency in AMP (cathelicidin, defensins, dermicidin) expression has been associated with *S. aureus* skin infections in AD (Ong et al. 2002; Rieg et al. 1950). Furthermore, *S. aureus* can modulate dermal immune cells to trigger expression of inflammatory cytokines (IL-4, IL-13, IL-22) (Nakatsuji et al. 2016). The interaction between *S. aureus* and the cutaneous immune response has been suggested to be strain-dependent (Byrd et al. 2017).

The strong link between *S. aureus* and AD is undebatable. To date, however, a causal relationship is not established, and whether *S. aureus* is an aggravating co-factor initiating flares, or a consequence of disease remains to be understood. Nevertheless, current hypotheses are that the observed dysbiosis, including *S. aureus*, in the skin microbiome of AD-patients has a of major influence on disease flares, severity and chronicity.

In other inflammatory skin diseases like hidradenitis suppurativa (HS) and psoriasis the presence of specific pathogens and/or altered microbiome composition have also been found. The predilection sites of HS are the hair follicles in intertriginous moist skin areas rich in apocrine glands, i.e. the axil, inguinal and anogential region. Though the skin microbiome of HS patients is less investigated than that of AD, studies suggest certain microbial characteristics to be present in HS such as *S. aureus* colonisation in lesions (Ring and Emtestam 2016) and differences at genus and species level compared with healthy individuals (Ring et al. 2019, 2017). The dominant genera identified in HS are *Corynebacterium*, *Porphyromonas* and *Peptoniphilus*, where the latter was found to be absent at control skin (Ring et al. 2017, 2015; Nikolakis et al. 2015). Furthermore, the genus *Propionibacterium* was relatively less abundant in HS patients (Ring et al. 2017). In psoriasis, the skin microbiome dysbiosis is not as well-documented, but decreased bacterial α-diversity and a different microbiome composition compared to healthy skin have been found (Alekseyenko et al. 2013; Langan et al. 2019). Specific pathogenic species in psoriatic lesions remain unidentified, though the relative abundance of *Streptococcus* and *Staphylococcus* might be increased in lesional compared with non-lesional skin (Lewis et al. 2019). Thus, for HS and psoriasis the presence of a single bacterial strain seems insufficient to initiate or drive the disease, although the interplay between a dysregulated immune response and a dysbiotic microbiome may trigger the pathogenic inflammation (Langan et al. 2019; Nestle et al. 2009).

2.5 Conclusion

The skin microbiome composition is highly personalised and influenced by several factors, both endogenous and exogenous. An interaction between the skin barrier and the microorganisms of the skin is thought to be of major importance regarding the skin microbiome composition. Most studies have investigated bacterial microorganisms, whereas fungi and viruses on skin are not yet as thoroughly studied. The healthy skin microbiome of humans expresses great diversity, high degree of temporal stability, presence of commensals, and absence of pathogens, whereas the microbiome of diseased skin expresses the opposite characteristics (Table 2.1).

Table 2.1 Glossary

Term	Explanation
Adaptive immune cells	B and T lymphocytes
Amplicon sequence variants (ASV's)	Also termed exact sequence variants, as the method is clustering free, as opposed to OUT's. ASV's are obtained from DNA-sequenced data
Antimicrobial peptides (AMPs)	Group of diverse molecules. Part of innate immune system. Can kill specific microorganisms
Archaea	Prokaryote (no cell nucleus) microorganisms. One of the three domains of microorganisms, different from bacteria and eukaryote
Bacteria	Prokaryote microorganisms. Constitute the largest domain considering microbiome research
Cathelicidin	Together with β-defensin one of the most studied antimicrobial peptides (AMPs)
Chemokine	Signalling protein secreted by a variety of cells. Chemokines are a specific group of cytokines that can be further subdivided. Some chemokines are inflammatory and act as chemoattractant for leukocytes, monocytes and neutrophils. Others can activate an immune response
Clade	A branch or a group (nested cluster) of organisms based on a common ancestor and its descendants
Commensal—resident	Microorganism considered neutral and part of healthy normal flora; it neither benefits (mutualistic) or causes any harm (pathogenic)
Community composition	The composition of a community characterised by species diversity (ratio between the number of species, biomass and productivity), coexistence (interaction; some microorganisms dependent on others), species dominance (the common species which are abundant with maximum biomass are dominants)
Corneocytes	The final stage of the differentiation of keratinocytes and located in stratum corneum
Culture-dependent methods	Traditional microbiological, laboratory method to visualise and multiply microbial microorganisms by placing them in predetermined culture medium. Useful for determine the type of microorganism and/or its abundance
C. acnes	A species from the genus *Cutibacterium*. Formerly known as *Propionibacterium acnes*. Mostly a commensal or mutualistic skin bacteria, but it is also dominant in acne vulgaris, and can act pathogenic
Cytokine	Signalling protein secreted by cells to affect interactions and communication between cells. Cytokine is an overall term for several types of cytokines (chemokines, lymphokines, monokines, interleukins) from different cells and with different action

(continued)

Table 2.1 (continued)

Term	Explanation
Dissimilarity (Bray–Curtis)	Difference in microbial abundance between two samples (e.g. at species level), i.e. a way of expressing β-diversity. Bray–Curtis is the name of a specific statistical index quantifying the compositional dissimilarity, ranging from 0 (the exact same species with the exact same abundance between the two sites) to 1 (none of the same species are present at both sites)
Distance (Jaccard)	Presence or absence of species (no information on abundance). Jaccard distance is a statistical measure of dissimilarity between to samples ranging from 0 (exact same species) to 1 (no species in common)
Domain	The highest taxonomic rank of cellular microorganisms considering classical biology. Divided into three; archaea; bacteria, and; eukarya
Dysbiosis	Term for imbalance of the microbiome composition, and is often associated with diseased skin, e.g. atopic dermatitis
Eukarya	Also termed eukaryote. Microorganisms with a membrane-bound nucleus (opposite from prokaryotes) and include fungal cells
Evenness	The relative abundance of species in a sample
Filaggrin	A structural, filament-aggregating protein located in the stratum corneum. Filaggrin is important for the skin hydration and barrier function. Mutations in the gene coding for filaggrin are strongly associated with dry skin and atopic dermatitis
Innate immune cells	A variety of cells: macrophages, dendritic cells, mast cells, natural killer cells, neutrophils, basophils and eosinophils
Keratinocytes	Cells originated, differentiated and migrated from epidermal stem cells at stratum basal to the stratum corneum. Keratinocytes are an important part of the skin barrier in protection from physical insults, microorganisms, and prevention of water loss
Kingdom	The second highest rank in taxonomy of microorganisms. In microbiome research the main taxonomic approach is, that kingdom is divided into bacteria, eukarya and viruses
Malassezia	A genus of fungi. By far the most abundant fungus on human skin. Usually a skin commensal, but it is also associated with different skin diseases, e.g. seborrheic dermatitis
Microbial	The entire microbial community of a given habitat is also referred to as "microbiota" or "microbiome"
Microbiome	All genetic material of a microbial community sequenced together
Microbiota	An aggregate of microorganisms. Refers to the microbial taxa associated with a given environment
Microorganism, microbe	Terms often used interchangeably. Some perceive a microbe as a microorganism *or* a virus (when virus is not considered a living organism)

(continued)

Table 2.1 (continued)

Term	Explanation
Mutualistic	Mutual beneficial relationship between two parts; microbe-microbe or host-microbe
Mycobiome	The composition of all fungal genes in a community
Next-generation sequencing methods	Also term high-throughput sequencing. Overall term for several different modern sequencing methods to describe DNA data. In microbiome research 16S rRNA and shotgun are two widely used sequencing methods
Nod-like receptor	A cytoplasmatic pattern recognition receptor that recognise bacterial peptidoglycans
Operational Taxonomic Units (OUT's)	Clusters of similar sequence variants obtained from e.g. 16S rRNA sequencing. Used to categorise bacteria based on sequence similarity, usually 97–100% similarity is used as threshold
Opportunistic pathogenic	A microorganism with the potential to cause infection or disease under certain circumstances, usually when the host's resistance is lowered e.g. by drugs or a disease
Pathogen—transient	A microorganism that can cause infection or disease to its host, also termed 'transient'
Pattern recognition receptor	Proteins that are expressed mainly by cells of the innate immune system. Detect pathogens and initiate the release of inflammatory cytokines
Phylogenetic tree	Describes the sequence distance (phylogenetic tree) and can either include or exclude information on abundance. Related to the β-diversity
Phylogeny	The study of the evolutionary development of microorganisms, based on the hypothesis that all life is derived from a common ancestor, and is often illustrated with a phylogenetic tree
Richness	Number of different species
Shannon-diversity	Statistical method which measures how evenly (abundance level) the microorganisms are distributed in a sample. Describes α-diversity
Staphylococcus aureus	Bacterial species of the genus *Staphylococcus,* usually pathogenic and strongly associated with skin infections and atopic dermatitis
Staphylococcus epidermidis	Bacterial species of the genus *Staphylococcus,* usually a skin commensal, but has the capability to act as an opportunistic pathogen causing infections or disease
Stratum corneum	The outermost layer of the epidermis
Taxonomy	Identification, naming and classification of organisms
Temporal variation	Variation over time
Toll-like receptor	Group of proteins located on the membranes of a variety of leucocytes. Toll-like receptors recognise pathogens and lead to immune responses

(continued)

Table 2.1 (continued)

Term	Explanation
Topography	In microbiome skin research topography refers to the different anatomical skin niches across the body
Virome	The composition of all viral genes in a community
Virus	An infectious agent consisting of nucleic acid surrounded by a protective protein coat, and some are also enveloped by lipids. A virus has genes, but no cellular structure and though it is debated, they are considered non-living
α-diversity	The number (species richness, OUT count) and abundance (evenness) of species in a sample
β-diversity	The difference of microbial communities from different environments. Usually expressed as the difference in taxonomic abundance profiles
β-defensin	Together with cathelicidin one of the most studied antimicrobial peptides (AMPs)

Conflicts of Interest None to declare.

References

Abrahamsson TR, Jakobsson HE, Andersson AF, Bjorksten B, Engstrand L, Jenmalm MC. Low diversity of the gut microbiota in infants with atopic eczema. J Allergy Clin Immunol. 2012;129(2):434–40, 40.e1–2.

Alekseyenko AV, Perez-Perez GI, De Souza A, Strober B, Gao Z, Bihan M, et al. Community differentiation of the cutaneous microbiota in psoriasis. Microbiome. 2013;1(1):31.

Barnard E, Shi B, Kang D, Craft N, Li H. The balance of metagenomic elements shapes the skin microbiome in acne and health. Sci Rep. 2016;6:39491.

Baurecht H, Ruhlemann MC, Rodriguez E, Thielking F, Harder I, Erkens AS, et al. Epidermal lipid composition, barrier integrity, and eczematous inflammation are associated with skin microbiome configuration. J Allergy Clin Immunol. 2018;141(5):1668-76.e16.

Bay L, Barnes CJ, Fritz BG, Thorsen J, Restrup MEM, Rasmussen L, et al. Universal dermal microbiome in human skin. mBio. 2020;11(1).

Becker K, Heilmann C, Peters G. Coagulase-negative staphylococci. Clin Microbiol Rev. 2014;27(4):870–926.

Behm B, Schreml S, Landthaler M, Babilas P. Skin signs in diabetes mellitus. J Eur Acad DermLogy Venereol: JEADV. 2012;26(10):1203–11.

Belkaid Y, Segre JA. Dialogue between skin microbiota and immunity. Science (New York, NY). 2014;346(6212):954–9.

Blaser MJ, Dominguez-Bello MG, Contreras M, Magris M, Hidalgo G, Estrada I, et al. Distinct cutaneous bacterial assemblages in a sampling of South American Amerindians and US residents. ISME J. 2013;7(1):85–95.

Boguniewicz M, Sampson H, Leung SB, Harbeck R, Leung DY. Effects of cefuroxime axetil on *Staphylococcus aureus* colonization and superantigen production in atopic dermatitis. J Allergy Clin Immunol. 2001;108(4):651–2.

Byrd AL, Belkaid Y, Segre JA. The human skin microbiome. Nat Rev Microbiol. 2018;16(3):143–55.

Byrd AL, Deming C, Cassidy SKB, Harrison OJ, Ng WI, Conlan S, et al. *Staphylococcus aureus* and Staphylococcus epidermidis strain diversity underlying pediatric atopic dermatitis. Sci Transl Med. 2017;9(397).

Callahan BJ, McMurdie PJ, Rosen MJ, Han AW, Johnson AJ, Holmes SP. DADA2: high-resolution sample inference from Illumina amplicon data. Nat Methods. 2016;13(7):581–3.

Chng KR, Tay AS, Li C, Ng AH, Wang J, Suri BK, et al. Whole metagenome profiling reveals skin microbiome-dependent susceptibility to atopic dermatitis flare. Nat Microbiol. 2016;1(9):16106.

Cho SH, Naber K, Hacker J, Ziebuhr W. Detection of the icaADBC gene cluster and biofilm formation in Staphylococcus epidermidis isolates from catheter-related urinary tract infections. Int J Antimicrob Agents. 2002;19(6):570–5.

Christensen GJ, Bruggemann H. Bacterial skin commensals and their role as host guardians. Beneficial Microbes. 2014;5(2):201–15.

Chu DM, Ma J, Prince AL, Antony KM, Seferovic MD, Aagaard KM. Maturation of the infant microbiome community structure and function across multiple body sites and in relation to mode of delivery. Nat Med. 2017;23(3):314–26.

Clausen ML, Agner T. Antimicrobial peptides, infections and the skin barrier. Curr Probl Dermatol. 2016;49:38–46.

Clausen ML, Agner T, Lilje B, Edslev SM, Johannesen TB, Andersen PS. Association of disease severity with skin microbiome and filaggrin gene mutations in adult atopic dermatitis. JAMA Dermatol. 2018;154(3):293–300.

Codoner FM, Ramirez-Bosca A, Climent E, Carrion-Gutierrez M, Guerrero M, Perez-Orquin JM, et al. Gut microbial composition in patients with psoriasis. Sci Rep. 2018;8(1):3812.

Cogen AL, Nizet V, Gallo RL. Skin microbiota: a source of disease or defence? Br J Dermatol. 2008;158(3):442–55.

Cogen AL, Yamasaki K, Muto J, Sanchez KM, Crotty Alexander L, Tanios J, et al. Staphylococcus epidermidis antimicrobial delta-toxin (phenol-soluble modulin-gamma) cooperates with host antimicrobial peptides to kill group A Streptococcus. PLoS ONE. 2010;5(1): e8557.

Consortum HMP. Structure, function and diversity of the healthy human microbiome. Nature. 2012a;486(7402):207–14.

Consortum HMP. A framework for human microbiome research. Nature. 2012b;486(7402):215–21.

Costello EK, Lauber CL, Hamady M, Fierer N, Gordon JI, Knight R. Bacterial community variation in human body habitats across space and time. Science (New York, NY). 2009;326(5960):1694–7.

Dao H Jr, Kazin RA. Gender differences in skin: a review of the literature. Gend Med. 2007;4(4):308–28.

Deng Y, Wang H, Zhou J, Mou Y, Wang G, Xiong X. Patients with acne vulgaris have a distinct gut microbiota in comparison with healthy controls. Acta Derm Venereol. 2018;98(8):783–90.

Dethlefsen L, Relman DA. Incomplete recovery and individualized responses of the human distal gut microbiota to repeated antibiotic perturbation. Proc Natl Acad Sci USA. 2011;108(Suppl 1):4554–61.

Dimitriu PA, Iker B, Malik K, Leung H, Mohn WW, Hillebrand GG. New insights into the intrinsic and extrinsic factors that shape the human skin microbiome. mBio. 2019;10(4).

Dominguez-Bello MG, Costello EK, Contreras M, Magris M, Hidalgo G, Fierer N, et al. Delivery mode shapes the acquisition and structure of the initial microbiota across multiple body habitats in newborns. Proc Natl Acad Sci USA. 2010;107(26):11971–5.

Edslev SM, Andersen PS, Agner T, Saunte DM, Ingham AC, Johannesen TB, et al. Identification of cutaneous fungi and mites in adult atopic dermatitis Submitted June 2020.

Elias PMFK. Skin barrier. New York: Taylor & Francis Group; 2006.

Fierer N, Hamady M, Lauber CL, Knight R. The influence of sex, handedness, and washing on the diversity of hand surface bacteria. Proc Natl Acad Sci USA. 2008;105(46):17994–9.

Fierer N, Lauber CL, Zhou N, McDonald D, Costello EK, Knight R. Forensic identification using skin bacterial communities. Proc Natl Acad Sci USA. 2010;107(14):6477–81.

Findley K, Grice EA. The skin microbiome: a focus on pathogens and their association with skin disease. PLoS Pathog. 2014;10(10): e1004436.

Findley K, Oh J, Yang J, Conlan S, Deming C, Meyer JA, et al. Topographic diversity of fungal and bacterial communities in human skin. Nature. 2013;498(7454):367–70.

Fitz-Gibbon S, Tomida S, Chiu BH, Nguyen L, Du C, Liu M, et al. Propionibacterium acnes strain populations in the human skin microbiome associated with acne. J Invest Dermatol. 2013;133(9):2152–60.

Flores GE, Caporaso JG, Henley JB, Rideout JR, Domogala D, Chase J, et al. Temporal variability is a personalized feature of the human microbiome. Genome Biol. 2014;15(12):531.

Forno E, Onderdonk AB, McCracken J, Litonjua AA, Laskey D, Delaney ML, et al. Diversity of the gut microbiota and eczema in early life. Clinical and Molecular Allergy: CMA. 2008;6:11.

Gallo RL, Nakatsuji T. Microbial symbiosis with the innate immune defense system of the skin. J Invest Dermatol. 2011;131(10):1974–80.

Gardiner M, Vicaretti M, Sparks J, Bansal S, Bush S, Liu M, et al. A longitudinal study of the diabetic skin and wound microbiome. PeerJ. 2017;5: e3543.

Giacomoni PU, Mammone T, Teri M. Gender-linked differences in human skin. J Dermatol Sci. 2009;55(3):144–9.

Grice EA, Segre JA. The skin microbiome. Nat Rev Microbiol. 2011;9(4):244–53.

Grice EA, Kong HH, Renaud G, Young AC, Bouffard GG, Blakesley RW, et al. A diversity profile of the human skin microbiota. Genome Res. 2008;18(7):1043–50.

Grice EA, Kong HH, Conlan S, Deming CB, Davis J, Young AC, et al. Topographical and temporal diversity of the human skin microbiome. Science (New York, NY). 2009;324(5931):1190–2.

Grice EA, Snitkin ES, Yockey LJ, Bermudez DM, Liechty KW, Segre JA. Longitudinal shift in diabetic wound microbiota correlates with prolonged skin defense response. Proc Natl Acad Sci USA. 2010;107(33):14799–804.

Hannigan GD, Meisel JS, Tyldsley AS, Zheng Q, Hodkinson BP, SanMiguel AJ, et al. The human skin double-stranded DNA virome: topographical and temporal diversity, genetic enrichment, and dynamic associations with the host microbiome. mBio. 2015;6(5):e01578–15.

Hanson MA, Dostalova A, Ceroni C, Poidevin M, Kondo S, Lemaitre B. Synergy and remarkable specificity of antimicrobial peptides in vivo using a systematic knockout approach. eLife. 2019;8.

Heath WR, Carbone FR. The skin-resident and migratory immune system in steady state and memory: innate lymphocytes, dendritic cells and T cells. Nat Immunol. 2013;14(10):978–85.

Hospodsky D, Pickering AJ, Julian TR, Miller D, Gorthala S, Boehm AB, et al. Hand bacterial communities vary across two different human populations. Microbiology (Reading, England). 2014;160(Pt 6):1144–52.

Howell MD, Kim BE, Gao P, Grant AV, Boguniewicz M, DeBenedetto A, et al. Cytokine modulation of atopic dermatitis filaggrin skin expression. J Allergy Clin Immunol. 2009;124(3 Suppl 2):R7-r12.

Iwase T, Uehara Y, Shinji H, Tajima A, Seo H, Takada K, et al. Staphylococcus epidermidis Esp inhibits *Staphylococcus aureus* biofilm formation and nasal colonization. Nature. 2010;465(7296):346–9.

Jo JH, Kennedy EA, Kong HH. Topographical and physiological differences of the skin mycobiome in health and disease. Virulence. 2017;8(3):324–33.

Jorgensen AR, Egeberg A, Gideonsson R, Weinstock LB, Thyssen EP, Thyssen JP. Rosacea is associated with Helicobacter pylori: a systematic review and meta-analysis. J Eur Acad DermLogy Venereol: JEADV. 2017;31(12):2010–5.

Kasimatis G, Fitz-Gibbon S, Tomida S, Wong M, Li H. Analysis of complete genomes of Propionibacterium acnes reveals a novel plasmid and increased pseudogenes in an acne associated strain. Biomed Res Int. 2013;2013: 918320.

Kezic S, O'Regan GM, Yau N, Sandilands A, Chen H, Campbell LE, et al. Levels of filaggrin degradation products are influenced by both filaggrin genotype and atopic dermatitis severity. Allergy. 2011;66(7):934–40.

Kong HH, Oh J, Deming C, Conlan S, Grice EA, Beatson MA, et al. Temporal shifts in the skin microbiome associated with disease flares and treatment in children with atopic dermatitis. Genome Res. 2012;22(5):850–9.

Kozitskaya S, Cho SH, Dietrich K, Marre R, Naber K, Ziebuhr W. The bacterial insertion sequence element IS256 occurs preferentially in nosocomial Staphylococcus epidermidis isolates: association with biofilm formation and resistance to aminoglycosides. Infect Immun. 2004;72(2):1210–5.

Kuo IH, Yoshida T, De Benedetto A, Beck LA. The cutaneous innate immune response in patients with atopic dermatitis. J Allergy Clin Immunol. 2013;131(2):266–78.

Kurokawa I, Danby FW, Ju Q, Wang X, Xiang LF, Xia L, et al. New developments in our understanding of acne pathogenesis and treatment. Exp Dermatol. 2009;18(10):821–32.

Lai Y, Di Nardo A, Nakatsuji T, Leichtle A, Yang Y, Cogen AL, et al. Commensal bacteria regulate Toll-like receptor 3-dependent inflammation after skin injury. Nat Med. 2009;15(12):1377–82.

Langan EA, Kunstner A, Miodovnik M, Zillikens D, Thaci D, Baines JF, et al. Combined culture and metagenomic analyses reveal significant shifts in the composition of the cutaneous microbiome in psoriasis. Br J DermLogy. 2019.

Lax S, Smith DP, Hampton-Marcell J, Owens SM, Handley KM, Scott NM, et al. Longitudinal analysis of microbial interaction between humans and the indoor environment. Science (New York, NY). 2014;345(6200):1048–52.

Lax S, Hampton-Marcell JT, Gibbons SM, Colares GB, Smith D, Eisen JA, et al. Forensic analysis of the microbiome of phones and shoes. Microbiome. 2015;3:21.

Le KY, Park MD, Otto M. Immune evasion mechanisms of Staphylococcus epidermidis biofilm infection. Front Microbiol. 2018;9:359.

Lee YB, Byun EJ, Kim HS. Potential role of the microbiome in acne: a comprehensive review. J Clin Med. 2019;8(7).

Leung MH, Wilkins D, Lee PK. Insights into the pan-microbiome: skin microbial communities of Chinese individuals differ from other racial groups. Sci Rep. 2015;5:11845.

Lewis DJ, Chan WH, Hinojosa T, Hsu S, Feldman SR. Mechanisms of microbial pathogenesis and the role of the skin microbiome in psoriasis: a review. Clin Dermatol. 2019;37(2):160–6.

Leyden JJ, Marples RR, Kligman AM. *Staphylococcus aureus* in the lesions of atopic dermatitis. Br J Dermatol. 1974;90(5):525–30.

Leyden JJ, McGinley KJ, Mills OH, Kligman AM. Age-related changes in the resident bacterial flora of the human face. J Invest Dermatol. 1975;65(4):379–81.

Leyden JJ, McGinley KJ, Vowels B. Propionibacterium acnes colonization in acne and nonacne. Dermatology (Basel, Switzerland). 1998;196(1):55–8.

Marchini G, Lindow S, Brismar H, Stabi B, Berggren V, Ulfgren AK, et al. The newborn infant is protected by an innate antimicrobial barrier: peptide antibiotics are present in the skin and vernix caseosa. Br J Dermatol. 2002;147(6):1127–34.

McAleer MA, Irvine AD. The multifunctional role of filaggrin in allergic skin disease. J Allergy Clin Immunol. 2013;131(2):280–91.

McDowell A, Nagy I, Magyari M, Barnard E, Patrick S. The opportunistic pathogen Propionibacterium acnes: insights into typing, human disease, clonal diversification and CAMP factor evolution. PLoS ONE. 2013;8(9): e70897.

Miajlovic H, Fallon PG, Irvine AD, Foster TJ. Effect of filaggrin breakdown products on growth of and protein expression by Staphylococcus aureus. J Allergy Clin Immunol. 2010;126(6):1184-90.e3.

Nakatsuji T, Gallo RL. The role of the skin microbiome in atopic dermatitis. Ann Allergy Asthma Immunol: Official Publication of the American College of Allergy, Asthma, & Immunology. 2019;122(3):263–9.

Nakatsuji T, Chen TH, Two AM, Chun KA, Narala S, Geha RS, et al. *Staphylococcus aureus* exploits epidermal barrier defects in atopic dermatitis to trigger cytokine expression. J Invest Dermatol. 2016;136(11):2192–200.

Nakatsuji T, Chiang H-I, Jiang SB, Nagarajan H, Zengler K, Gallo RL. The microbiome extends to subepidermal compartments of normal skin. Nat Commun. 2013;4(1431): https://doi.org/10.1038/ncomms2441.

Nakatsuji T, Chen TH, Narala S, Chun KA, Two AM, Yun T, et al. Antimicrobials from human skin commensal bacteria protect against *Staphylococcus aureus* and are deficient in atopic dermatitis. Sci Transl Med. 2017;9(378).

Nakatsuji T, Chen TH, Butcher AM, Trzoss LL, Nam SJ, Shirakawa KT, et al. A commensal strain of Staphylococcus epidermidis protects against skin neoplasia. Sci Adv. 2018;4(2):eaao4502.

Neckovic A, van Oorschot RAH, Szkuta B, Durdle A. Investigation of direct and indirect transfer of microbiomes between individuals. Forensic Sci Int Genet. 2020;45: 102212.

Nestle FO, Kaplan DH, Barker J. Psoriasis. N Engl J Med. 2009;361(5):496–509.

Nguyen AV, Soulika AM. The dynamics of the skin's immune system. Int J Mol Sci. 2019;20(8).

Nikolakis G, Join-Lambert O, Karagiannidis I, Guet-Revillet H, Zouboulis CC, Nassif A. Bacteriology of hidradenitis suppurativa/acne inversa: a review. J Am Acad Dermatol. 2015;73(5 Suppl 1):S12–8.

Oh J, Conlan S, Polley EC, Segre JA, Kong HH. Shifts in human skin and nares microbiota of healthy children and adults. Genome Medicine. 2012;4(10):77.

Oh J, Freeman AF, Park M, Sokolic R, Candotti F, Holland SM, et al. The altered landscape of the human skin microbiome in patients with primary immunodeficiencies. Genome Res. 2013;23(12):2103–14.

Oh J, Byrd AL, Deming C, Conlan S, Kong HH, Segre JA. Biogeography and individuality shape function in the human skin metagenome. Nature. 2014;514(7520):59–64.

Oh J, Byrd AL, Park M, Kong HH, Segre JA. Temporal stability of the human skin microbiome. Cell. 2016;165(4):854–66.

O'Neill AM, Gallo RL. Host-microbiome interactions and recent progress into understanding the biology of acne vulgaris. Microbiome. 2018;6(1):177.

O'Neill CA, Monteleone G, McLaughlin JT, Paus R. The gut-skin axis in health and disease: A paradigm with therapeutic implications. BioEssays: News and Reviews in Molecular, Cellular and Developmental Biology. 2016;38(11):1167–76.

Ong PY, Ohtake T, Brandt C, Strickland I, Boguniewicz M, Ganz T, et al. Endogenous antimicrobial peptides and skin infections in atopic dermatitis. N Engl J Med. 2002;347(15):1151–60.

Otto M. Staphylococcus epidermidis–the 'accidental' pathogen. Nat Rev Microbiol. 2009;7(8):555–67.

Palmer CN, Irvine AD, Terron-Kwiatkowski A, Zhao Y, Liao H, Lee SP, et al. Common loss-of-function variants of the epidermal barrier protein filaggrin are a major predisposing factor for atopic dermatitis. Nat Genet. 2006;38(4):441–6.

Patra V, Laoubi L, Nicolas JF, Vocanson M, Wolf P. A perspective on the interplay of ultraviolet-radiation, skin microbiome and skin resident memory TCRalphabeta+ Cells. Front Med. 2018;5:166.

Penders J, Thijs C, van den Brandt PA, Kummeling I, Snijders B, Stelma F, et al. Gut microbiota composition and development of atopic manifestations in infancy: the KOALA Birth Cohort Study. Gut. 2007;56(5):661–7.

Picardo M, Ottaviani M. Skin microbiome and skin disease: the example of rosacea. J Clin Gastroenterol. 2014;48(Suppl 1):S85–6.

Prast-Nielsen S, Tobin AM, Adamzik K, Powles A, Hugerth LW, Sweeney C, et al. Investigation of the skin microbiome: swabs versus biopsies. Br J DermLogy. 2019;181(3):572–9.

Rawlings AV, Harding CR. Moisturization and skin barrier function. Dermatol Ther. 2004;17(Suppl 1):43–8.

Rieg S, Steffen H, Seeber S, Humeny A, Kalbacher H, Dietz K, et al. Deficiency of dermcidin-derived antimicrobial peptides in sweat of patients with atopic dermatitis correlates with an impaired innate defense of human skin in vivo. J Immunol (Baltimore, Md: 1950). 2005;174(12):8003–10.

Ring HC, Emtestam L. The microbiology of hidradenitis suppurativa. Dermatol Clin. 2016;34(1):29–35.

Ring HC, Riis Mikkelsen P, Miller IM, Jenssen H, Fuursted K, Saunte DM, et al. The bacteriology of hidradenitis suppurativa: a systematic review. Exp Dermatol. 2015;24(10):727–31.

Ring HC, Thorsen J, Saunte DM, Lilje B, Bay L, Riis PT, et al. The follicular skin microbiome in patients with hidradenitis suppurativa and healthy controls. JAMA Dermatol. 2017;153(9):897–905.

Ring HC, Sigsgaard V, Thorsen J, Fuursted K, Fabricius S, Saunte DM, et al. The microbiome of tunnels in hidradenitis suppurativa patients. J Eur Acad DermLogy Venereol: JEADV. 2019.

Ross AA, Doxey AC, Neufeld JD. The skin microbiome of cohabiting couples. mSystems. 2017;2(4).

Salem I, Ramser A, Isham N, Ghannoum MA. The gut microbiome as a major regulator of the gut-skin axis. Front Microbiol. 2018;9:1459.

Sandilands A, Sutherland C, Irvine AD, McLean WH. Filaggrin in the frontline: role in skin barrier function and disease. J Cell Sci. 2009;122(Pt 9):1285–94.

Sanford JA, Gallo RL. Functions of the skin microbiota in health and disease. Semin Immunol. 2013;25(5):370–7.

SanMiguel A, Grice EA. Interactions between host factors and the skin microbiome. Cell Mol Life Sci CMLS. 2015;72(8):1499–515.

Scher JU, Ubeda C, Artacho A, Attur M, Isaac S, Reddy SM, et al. Decreased bacterial diversity characterizes the altered gut microbiota in patients with psoriatic arthritis, resembling dysbiosis in inflammatory bowel disease. Arthritis Rheumatology (Hoboken, NJ). 2015;67(1):128–39.

Shi B, Bangayan NJ, Curd E, Taylor PA, Gallo RL, Leung DYM, et al. The skin microbiome is different in pediatric versus adult atopic dermatitis. J Allergy Clin Immunol. 2016;138(4):1233–6.

Shi B, Leung DYM, Taylor PA, Li H. Methicillin-resistant *Staphylococcus aureus* colonization is associated with decreased skin commensal bacteria in atopic dermatitis. J Invest Dermatol. 2018;138(7):1668–71.

Shu M, Wang Y, Yu J, Kuo S, Coda A, Jiang Y, et al. Fermentation of Propionibacterium acnes, a commensal bacterium in the human skin microbiome, as skin probiotics against methicillin-resistant *Staphylococcus aureus*. PLoS ONE. 2013;8(2): e55380.

Smeekens SP, Huttenhower C, Riza A, van de Veerdonk FL, Zeeuwen PL, Schalkwijk J, et al. Skin microbiome imbalance in patients with STAT1/STAT3 defects impairs innate host defense responses. J Innate Immun. 2014;6(3):253–62.

Song SJ, Lauber C, Costello EK, Lozupone CA, Humphrey G, Berg-Lyons D, et al. Cohabiting family members share microbiota with one another and with their dogs. eLife. 2013;2:e00458.

Stokes JH, Pillsbury DM. The effect on the skin of emotional and nervous states: III. Theoretical and practical consideration of a gastro-intestinal mechanism. Arch DermLogy Syphilol. 1930;22(6):962–93.

Tollin M, Bergsson G, Kai-Larsen Y, Lengqvist J, Sjovall J, Griffiths W, et al. Vernix caseosa as a multi-component defence system based on polypeptides, lipids and their interactions. Cell Mol Life Sci CMLS. 2005;62(19–20):2390–9.

Totte JE, van der Feltz WT, Hennekam M, van Belkum A, van Zuuren EJ, Pasmans SG. Prevalence and odds of *Staphylococcus aureus* carriage in atopic dermatitis: a systematic review and meta-analysis. Br J Dermatol. 2016;175(4):687–95.

Totte JEE, Pardo LM, Fieten KB, Vos MC, van den Broek TJ, Schuren FHJ, et al. The nasal and skin microbiome are associated with disease severity in pediatric atopic dermatitis. Br J DermLogy. 2019.

van den Oord RA, Sheikh A. Filaggrin gene defects and risk of developing allergic sensitisation and allergic disorders: systematic review and meta-analysis. BMJ (Clinical Research Ed). 2009;339: b2433.

van Nimwegen FA, Penders J, Stobberingh EE, Postma DS, Koppelman GH, Kerkhof M, et al. Mode and place of delivery, gastrointestinal microbiota, and their influence on asthma and atopy. J Allergy Clin Immunol. 2011;128(5):948–55.e1–3.

Vavrova K, Henkes D, Struver K, Sochorova M, Skolova B, Witting MY, et al. Filaggrin deficiency leads to impaired lipid profile and altered acidification pathways in a 3D skin construct. J Invest Dermatol. 2014;134(3):746–53.

Wilke K, Martin A, Terstegen L, Biel SS. A short history of sweat gland biology. Int J Cosmet Sci. 2007;29(3):169–79.

Wood AP, Kelly DP. Skin microbiology, body odor, and methylotrophic bacteria. In: Timmis KN, editor. Handbook of hydrocarbon and lipid microbiology. Berlin, Heidelberg: Springer Berlin Heidelberg; 2010. p. 3203–13.

Yan HM, Zhao HJ, Guo DY, Zhu PQ, Zhang CL, Jiang W. Gut microbiota alterations in moderate to severe acne vulgaris patients. J Dermatol. 2018;45(10):1166–71.

Chapter 3
Tools to Explore Human Skin Microbiota

Péter Oláh and Matilda Riskumäki

Abstract The interest in studying the human skin microbiota emerged in the early twentieth century, and our knowledge on the composition and role of the skin microbiota has been growing along with the evolution of research methodologies. Traditionally, microbial samples were cultivated in various culture media, enabling the preferential growth of certain species, while hindering the identification of non-culturable microbes. During recent decades, culture-free analysis methods made possible the discovery of an astonishing taxonomic diversity of microbial life in nearly all habitats of Earth, including the human skin. This breakthrough was in large part due to the advent of molecular taxonomy, the identification of microbial species based not on phenotypical traits, but their genomic DNA content. This technological shift enables the identification of both culturable and non-culturable microbes, and at the same time opens up possibilities to discover novel species, revise taxonomic classification, and study the gene content of complete microbial communities, collectively referred to as the study of *metagenomics*. Importantly, in addition to qualitative information, metagenomics also provides the relative quantity of different taxa in a given sample and facilitates quantitative comparisons across a wide variety of conditions. In the present chapter, we are going to examine in detail the sampling methods, laboratory techniques and computational analyses required to characterize the human skin microbiome using metagenomic approaches.

Keywords Skin microbiota sampling · DNA extraction · Next generation sequencing · Data analysis

P. Oláh
Department of Dermatology, University Hospital Duesseldorf, Duesseldorf, Germany

Department of Dermatology, Venereology and Oncodermatology, Medical School, University of Pécs, Pécs, Hungary

M. Riskumäki (✉)
Human Microbiome Research Program, University of Helsinki, Helsinki, Finland
e-mail: matilda.riskumaki@helsinki.fi

A. Lauerma et al. (eds.), *The Skin Microbiome Manual*,
https://doi.org/10.1007/978-3-031-82689-4_3

Introduction

Early studies on human skin microbiota relied on culture-dependent methods to isolate and identify skin-associated microbes, thus revealing underestimated measures of the true microbial diversity of the skin. Today, the fraction of culturable microbes is estimated to be 1% (Kong and Segre 2012; Marples 1969). The course of microbial research changed in the 1970's due to establishment of the Sanger sequencing technology alongside with the discovery of the ribosomal small subunit 16S RNA gene as a tool for deciphering phylogenetic relationships between prokaryotes by Carl Woese (Heather and Chain 2016; Hugerth and Andersson 2017). The introduction of polymerase chain reaction (PCR) in the 1980's enabled generation of pure DNA template in high concentration through amplification of confined DNA sequences. Over the recent decades next generation sequencing technologies have experienced rapid development together with decrease in the running time and cost (Heather and Chain 2016; Kong et al. 2017). While sequence-based approaches can recover more information about the skin microbiota in comparison to the traditional culturing methods, the technology cannot differentiate viable microbes from non-viable. Thus, the observed microbiota composition does not directly translate into the true metabolic profile of the skin microbiota. Furthermore, extracellular DNA, that is DNA that has been released from a dying cell after rupturing of its cell wall, is also detected with the sequencing approaches, thus representing microbes that no longer exist on the skin surface (Alexeyev 2013).

3.1 Sampling Microbes from the Skin

Skin bears relatively low microbial mass, thus sampling sufficient amount of microbes for the identification of microbial community structure with the use of culture-independent methods is a considerable challenge (Kong et al. 2017). Few sampling methods, including swabbing, cup scrubbing, tape stripping, skin scraping and punch biopsies, have been established to overcome the difficulties of effectively capturing microbes from the skin. All of these methods were established as the interest towards the human skin microbiota was growing in the early and mid-twentieth century (Evans et al. 1950; Marples 1969). The choice of sampling method is affected by the preferred sampling depth (see Fig. 3.1), as well as on the ease of implementation, and the level of discomfort experienced by the study subjects (Grice et al. 2008; Kong et al. 2017; Nakatsuji et al. 2013).

3.1.1 Before Sampling

The skin microbiota composition is affected by the physiological characteristics of the skin, such as dryness and sebum secretion, and subjected to temporary fluctuations

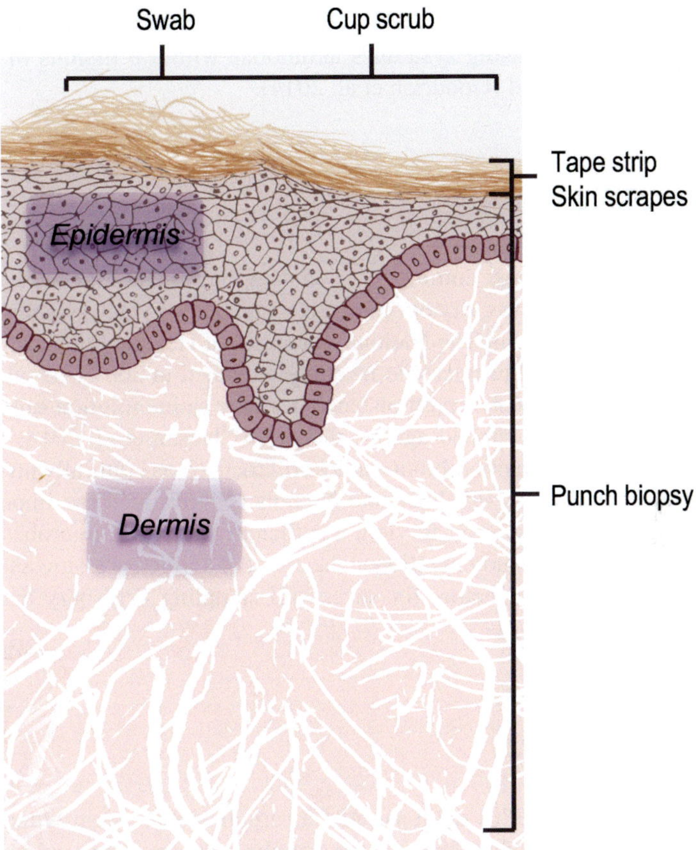

Fig. 3.1 Representation of sampling depth each sampling method can reach

according to our bathing and skin care habits as well as use of antibiotics (Byrd et al. 2018; Kong et al. 2017). These factors can override experimental variable - induced variation in the microbiota, thus, skin microbiome studies commonly intend to control such confounders (Kong et al. 2017).

The intraindividual variation between physiologically distinct skin sites can be greater than the interindividual variation between anatomically analogous skin sites (Costello et al. 2009; Oh et al. 2016). Therefore, a skin microbiota study needs to be exclusive with the anatomical sampling site across the study cohort. Moreover, in order to control lifestyle-induced fluctuations in the microbiota composition, such as skin hygiene and care, the study subjects are commonly given behavioral regulations (Kong et al. 2017). Typically, bathing and application of moisturizers is not allowed 24 h prior to sampling. Several studies have also instructed the participants to only use a non-antimicrobial soap for hygiene and to avoid using topical antiseptics for minimum 7 days before sampling (Fyhrquist et al. 2019; Grice et al. 2009; Oh et al.

2014). According to the greatly varying impact of antibiotics for microbes, study subjects who have been using systemics antibiotics within 6 months of sampling should always be excluded (Goodrich et al. 2014).

3.1.2 Swabbing

Swabbing is so far the most commonly used sampling method because it is non-invasive and fast and easy to carry out (Grogan et al. 2019). In fact, swabbing was the standard sampling method in The National Institutes of Health Human Microbiome Project, a large-scale human microbiome study launched in 2007 (Versalovic et al. 2010). Consistently, the swab is premoistened in sterile saline solution supplemented with 0.1% Tween20, and rubbed against the skin (Clausen et al. 2018; Gao et al. 2007). Early on, when skin microbiota studies still focused on culturally investigating the microbial composition, Pillsbury and Nichols (1946) noted the importance of premoistening the swab in order to yield a sufficient amount of microbes from the skin. Moreover, the same study mentioned the effect of applied pressure and duration of swabbing as important factors for successful sampling (Pillsbury and Nichols 1946).

3.1.3 Cup Scrubbing

Pillsbury and Nichols (1946) demonstrated a sampling method in which bacteria are rubbed from the skin while keeping the sampling site soaked in culturing broth, releasing the microbes from the skin directly into the broth. Later Williamson and Kligman (1965) changed the broth into surfactant, and demonstrated that 97% of all bacteria in the sampling site can be captured using this method. Williamson and Kligman's recommended surfactant solution is still being used today for the cup scrubbing method. A sterile cylinder 25 mm in diameter is pressed against the skin and filled with phosphate buffer saline (PBS) solution supplemented with 0.01% Triton X100. The surface of the skin inside the cylinder is then rubbed with an inoculating loop, swab, or any sterile blunt device for 1 min. The scrubbing releases microbes from the skin into the solution, which is collected (Chng et al. 2016; Williamson and Kligman 1965).

3.1.4 Tape Stripping

After its introduction in 1939, tape stripping was widely used in studies examining the structure of the human epidermis, and the regeneration of stratum corneum (Menton and Eisen 1971; Pinkus 1952). Two decades later, tape stripping was used for the quantification of microbes on the skin, as well as for diagnosing pathogen-associated skin disorders (Noble 1968; Updegraff 1964). To date, tape stripping is mostly used in the investigation of damage-induced skin transcriptomics and the protein and lipid composition of stratum corneum (Clausen et al. 2016; Kezic et al. 2009; Zeeuwen et al. 2012).

As the stripping method can be used for the removal of stratum corneum, it could potentially be used for complete sampling of microbes residing in the uppermost layer of the skin (Ogai et al. 2018; Updegraff 1964). A study by Chng et al. (2016) is one of the few that has used tape stripping in sampling the skin microbiota in combination with culture-independent identification methods. The skin was tape stripped up to 50 times using the same tape for every strip. The study proposes that tape stripping performs better than swabbing in capturing microbes from the skin (Chng et al. 2016). However, other studies show that swabbing recovers similar skin microbial composition as tape stripping (Ogai et al. 2018).

3.1.5   Skin Scraping

Skin scraping is another method for sampling microbes residing underneath the uppermost layers of dead skin (Grice et al. 2008). The method was introduced in 1929 by Jordin as a well-performing sampling method for culturing fungal organisms from the skin (Pillsbury and Nichols 1946). To date, skin scrapings are still widely used for fungal cultivations from the skin and in the diagnosis of fungal and parasitic skin diseases (Findley et al. 2013; Markle and Makhoul 2004). Grice and colleagues (2008) compared skin scraping to swabbing, and concluded that the dominant taxa are identified equally well with these two sampling methods. Skin scrapings are carried out by shaving the surface of the skin with few strokes using a fine blade, and collecting the released skin scrapings (Grice et al. 2008).

3.1.6   Punch Biopsies

A skin biopsy is used for sampling microbes jointly from the epidermis and dermis, offering a full-thickness profile of the human skin microbiota (Grice et al. 2008; Nakatsuji et al. 2013). Skin biopsies are commonly utilized in the investigation of skin transcriptomics, as well as in skin pathology (Sina et al. 2009; Zeeuwen et al. 2012). However, as research is revealing more about the possible interactions between the skin microbiota and the dermal cells, investigating the microbial composition in the subcutaneous compartments of the skin is becoming more important (Nakatsuji et al. 2013; Prast-Nielsen et al. 2019).

A skin punch biopsy is taken from locally anesthetized skin with a circular device, 4-mm in diameter reaching few millimeters deep in the skin (Grice et al. 2008; Nakatsuji et al. 2013; Prast-Nielsen et al. 2019). This sampling method is the most invasive option resulting in scarring of the sampling site, thus many study participants might refuse to give such sample (Grice et al. 2008; Kim et al. 2019). Grice and colleagues (2008) showed that the microbial composition in skin biopsies is comparable with what can be obtained using the non-invasive swabbing method. However, Prast-Nielsen et al. (2019) published results in contrary to what Grice et al. had reported, that is, skin swabs and biopsies capture different composition of microbes when the alpha-diversity and relative abundance of bacterial phyla are compared between the two sample types. Although punch biopsy is the most invasive of the established sampling methods, skin biopsies remain the only method that can reach the deepest compartments of the skin, thus revealing information that cannot be concluded from the surface of the skin (Nakatsuji et al. 2013).

3.2 DNA Extraction

Different approaches for cell lysis can create bias due to their effectiveness in lysing microbial cells with different cell wall properties, thus the choice of DNA extraction method can greatly influence the eventually observed sample-specific microbial composition (Goodrich et al. 2014). The presence of contaminating cells or DNA in extraction kits and laboratory reagents have been recognized early on, and becomes particularly problematic when processing samples with low microbial mass, for contaminating DNA can supersede the minute amount of sample-specific microbial DNA (Tanner et al. 1998; Weyrich et al. 2019).

3.2.1 The Effects of Extraction Method

The choice of DNA extraction method has a great impact on the compositional outcome of microbial samples due to the differences in the cell wall properties of microbial cells. Incomplete lysis of some of the cells in a sample would bias the observed community representation in the sample (Hugerth and Andersson 2017). Microbial cell walls can be lysed mechanically, thermally, chemically or enzymatically, with distinct methods changing in effectiveness against cells that bear structurally different cell wall (Shehadul Islam et al. 2017). For example, to extract DNA more effectively from gram-positive bacteria with thick peptidoglycan-comprised cell wall, mechanical lysis step should be part of the extraction protocol (Yuan et al. 2012). Including a mock community sample, that is, a sample containing a combination of specified microbial strains of defined quantity, in the DNA extraction step as a positive control will allow for quality-check on the choice of cell lysis method (Grogan et al. 2019).

With the use of a mock community, Brooks et al. (2015) demonstrated that any bias introduced to the microbial community composition can vary greatly depending on the use of different DNA extraction kits, due to utilization of different cell lysis methods. Walker and colleagues (2015) used fecal samples to compare two extraction methods, and concluded that the yield of bacterial DNA can be increased, and the bias in the bacterial profile decreased by mechanically lysing the cells with bead-beating. Furthermore, a combination of mechanical and enzymatic cell lysis have been shown to recover the most truthful representation of microbial composition in the samples (Yuan et al. 2012).

3.2.2 Laboratory Contamination is a Common Problem

Samples taken from the skin bear low yield of microbial DNA due to relatively low microbial mass on the skin. Introduction of contaminating microbial DNA is an inevitable problem in such samples, for the contaminating DNA can supersede the minute amount of sample-specific DNA (Hugerth and Andersson 2017). Contaminating organisms have been detected in DNA extraction kits, PCR reagents and ultrapure molecular biology grade water, and in the cleanest laboratory environment, that is, in ultraclean ancient DNA laboratory (Salter et al. 2014; Weyrich et al. 2019). Moreover, the composition of contaminating organisms in DNA samples have been shown to vary according to the season, the laboratory facility and the researchers working at the facility (Weyrich et al. 2019). Typically identified contaminating organisms include strains that are commonly found in soil and water, such as *Pseudomonas, Ralstonia, Burkholderia* and *Sphingomonas,* as well as members of the human skin and oral microbiota, such as *Cutibacterium, Corynebacterium* and *Streptococcus* (Salter et al. 2014).

Earlier in microbial ecology research, Tanner et al. (1998) reported that several microbes thought to be present in a broad range of extreme environments, such as the Antarctica or deep marine sediment, could also be cloned from samples lacking environmental template DNA, suggesting that the sample-specific DNA is derived from the laboratory reagents rather than the environmental sample itself. Similar findings have later been made by Lauder and colleagues (2016) who could not distinguish between the collection of microbes that were specific for placenta-derived samples and the composition observed in the negative DNA extraction controls. Furthermore, kit-specific contamination can account for the observation of temporal shifts in the microbiota composition in longitudinal studies, as described by Salter and colleagues (2014) who re-analyzed 16S rRNA gene sequencing data derived from nasopharyngeal swabs taken from a cohort of 20 children who were sampled monthly from birth to 24 months of age. DNA was extracted from the swabs in chronological order, eventually using four batches of one specific DNA extraction kit. Due to different combinations of contaminating microbes in each batch, the nasopharyngeal microbiota composition was thought to change by age, when essentially the composition changed according to each batch. If the contaminating taxa were removed from the sequencing data, the age-associated variation in the nasopharyngeal microbiota disappeared (Salter et al. 2014).

Several methods are used in elimination of contamination in laboratory reagents and equipment, including UV radiation and treatment with DNases, but there are several microbial taxa that can resist such treatment, not to mention that extracellular DNA released in the environment from rupturing microbial cells can be preserved in the environment long after the cell itself has died (Alexeyev 2013; Salter et al. 2014; Weyrich et al. 2019). Therefore, it is of extreme importance to collect negative controls and process them in parallel with the samples, as well as report for contaminated organisms. As the composition of contaminant organisms changes over time and according to different batches of reagents, the sampling of negative controls should be part of routine quality check in a DNA laboratory (Grogan et al. 2019; Weyrich et al. 2019).

3.3 Microbial DNA Sequencing

The two most widespread approaches to metagenomics are marker gene-based and whole-genome sequencing (also referred to as Whole-Genome Shotgun sequencing, WGS). As the cost of DNA sequencing is steadily dropping while the throughput and accuracy of instruments increases, both methods are becoming ubiquitous in molecular biology laboratories. Presently, the more cost-effective marker gene method is used in thousands of experiments, generating microbial sequence datasets on the order of millions yearly. WGS, on the other hand, offers superior detail and functional information with more complex analysis options, although at a higher cost. The main steps, differences and similarities between methods are illustrated in Fig. 3.2 and detailed in the paragraphs below.

3.3.1 Marker Gene Sequencing

Marker genes are highly conserved DNA sequences containing variable regions, suitable for the reconstruction of phylogenetic relationships between microbial taxa. In the case of prokaryotes, the gene encoding the 16S ribosomal RNA (component of the 30S small subunit of the prokaryotic ribosome) (Woese and Fox 1977) is used as marker. For fungi, the Internal Transcribed Spacer 1 (ITS1, located between the genes encoding the 18S and 5.8S rRNA subunits) serves this purpose most commonly.

Marker gene sequences are amplified using polymerase chain reaction (PCR) from isolated bacterial or fungal DNA, with the resulting product known as the amplicon. Amplicons are then characterized by DNA sequencing either by the traditional Sanger capillary method or high-throughput sequencing (also called "Next Generation Sequencing", NGS) (van Dijk et al. 2018). As the 2010s have seen a dramatic improvement in NGS technologies, 16S rRNA gene sequencing has become a standard and affordable method of microbiome analysis. Using NGS, relatively short fragments (100–300 bp) of DNA are characterized. As the 16S rRNA

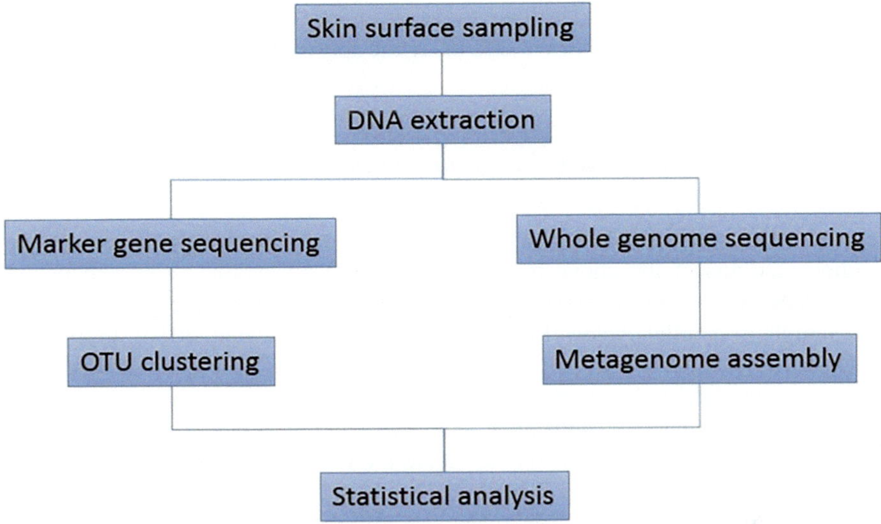

Fig. 3.2 Overview of the main steps of metagenomics workflow

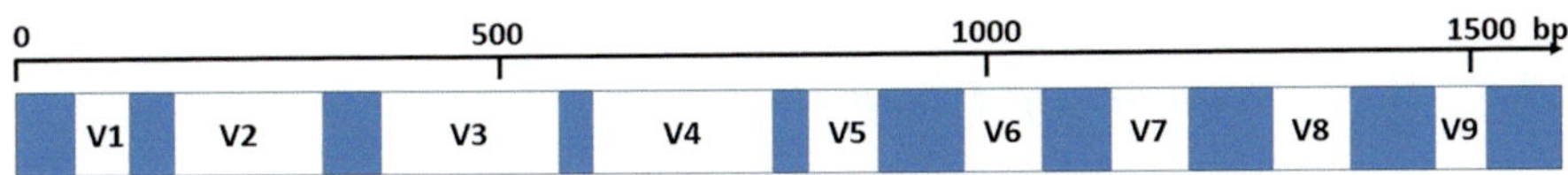

Fig. 3.3 Schematic structure of the bacterial 16S ribosomal RNA gene

gene stretches approx. 1,500 bp, only specific, informative regions are sequenced by NGS. The 16S rRNA contains 9 so-called "hypervariable regions" labelled V1–V9, anchored between highly conserved sequences, which enables the design of universal PCR primers binding to conserved regions across nearly all bacterial species, while creating amplicons spanning one or more of the evolutionarily informative hypervariable regions, thus referred to as V1-V3, V4-V5, V6-V8 primers (Fig. 3.3).

3.3.2 Alternative Marker Genes

While the 16S rRNA subunit is the most widely used marker gene in bacterial metagenomics, there exist a number of alternatives, which are mostly used in conventional culture-dependent settings, but also have utility in WGS metagenomic studies. Multi-Locus Sequence Typing (MLST) is used for the characterization of a pre-defined set of microbes, i.e. a specific genera or species, and uses conserved genes of a given genus to reconstruct evolutionary relationships. Usually 5 to 10 such genes are used; while the scope of MLST typing is narrower, the advantages include finer resolution for the targeted genus or species down to the strain level, and application to not only to bacteria but archaea, fungi or viruses, using the appropriate set of genetic markers.

3.3.3 Generation of Raw Sequence Data

The generated amplicon DNA is then subjected to high-throughput sequencing, yielding readouts of the above mentioned 100–300 bp length, called sequencing reads. Depending on experimental design, several million reads are generated from each sample in parallel cycles of automated reactions (Liu et al. 2012). In the most widely used sequencing-by-synthesis approach, fragments of single-stranded DNA are used as templates to incorporate fluorescently labelled nucleotides during a series of hybridization reactions, with each new cycle adding a new base for 100–300 cycles. The fluorescent signal is recorded and the resulting microscopic images are analyzed computationally to reconstruct the nucleotide sequence of each DNA fragment. Other, more specialized instruments use pH or electric resistance of individual nucleotides instead of fluorescence detection.

3.3.4 Basic Sequencing Parameters

A crucially important experimental design question is the quantity of reads to be generated: the higher the number of reads (the sequencing depth), the greater the resolution of the experiment; thus, chances are better for identifying rare species that represent a low percentage of DNA in the given microbiome sample. Most commonly it is expressed in millions of reads sequenced, with certain studies generating reads on the order of 100 M per sample. The next key factor, read length is dependent on the sequencing instrument and is expressed in base pairs: as mentioned earlier, 100–300 bp reads are used most commonly, while specialized instruments offer read lengths of up to 150,000 bp at the cost of accuracy and increased complexity. In genomic studies, sequencing depth and read length are usually used to calculate the expected coverage, e.g. if a DNA sample of human blood is sequenced using a read length of 300 bp and a depth of 20 million reads, knowing that the haploid human genome is ~ 1.8 billion bp long, we can expect an average of 300*20 M/1800 M = 3.3 reads covering each genomic base. In the case of microbial samples often made up of hundreds of different species, however, there is no prior knowledge of either the total length of all microbial genomes (or equivalently, all marker genes), or the ratio at which a species is present and "takes up" sequencing depth. However, as with all quantitative or semi-quantitative nucleotide sequencing methods, count data, i.e. how many reads represent a bacterial species in a sample, and in the complete study population, form the basis for all subsequent analyses.

3.3.5 Data Characteristics

As a consequence, metagenomic sequencing data is highly *compositional*, posing analytical challenges detailed in further sections. The expected coverage can only be estimated based on previous studies of a similar environment, making the identification of novel species and microbial communities highly sensitive to the pre-determined sequencing depth. Another fundamental property of metagenomics datasets is *sparsity*. As each read is assigned to a specific species, the counts of how many reads represent a species are stored in a tabular format (the OTU table, detailed below). Since many bacterial species are observed in only one or few subjects due to the high inter-individual variability of the microbiome, the resulting table contains many zeros, which poses difficulties for most statistical methods (Calle 2019).

3.4 Data Analysis

The generated sequence data is pre-processed, subjected to initial quality control and stored in a format suitable for further computational analysis. Reads are stored in files of the *.fastq* format, storing not only DNA sequence data, but critically important information on the quality of readout and technical information of the sequencing instrument. This highly uniform file format is then used as the basis for further analysis, and also frequently deposited in public databases for future use by the scientific community. The practice of sharing raw experimental data, made ubiquitous during the recent decade, not only makes the conduct of studies more transparent, but enables reanalysis of past results using more up-to-date data analysis methods, and the ongoing integration of past and current knowledge. The most prominent deposits for microbial sequencing data are the NCBI Sequence Read Archive (US), the EBI-EMBL Metagenomics database (EU) and DDBJ (Japan).

3.4.1 Normalization

A specific drawback of NGS methods is the great variance in the number of reads obtained from different samples of the same population. In metagenomics, it is difficult to estimate the amount of DNA sampled from a given body site- e.g. heavily infected skin in certain diseases might yield a significantly higher biomass than the matching skin area of healthy controls, but there might be similar differences between normal skin samples as well, due to natural variations in microbial content and skin structure. Direct comparison of the abundance of microbes is hindered by this phenomenon, and a multitude of normalization measures were developed to circumvent the problem (Weiss et al. 2017). Widely used approaches include *rarefaction,* or drawing without replacement, where samples containing above-average read counts are "rarefied", i.e. reads are randomly discarded. Samples with less reads than the average or an arbitrarily defined limit need to be excluded completely, thus data loss might be unacceptably high when rarefaction parameters are not considered carefully (McMurdie et al. 2014). To avoid data loss, *scaling* might be applied, where samples might be scaled e.g. according to a pre-defined quantile of their read counts. However, scaling does not take into account sequencing depth and the fact that samples with more reads have a higher chance of detecting rare species, thus, when the depth of sequencing is highly variable among samples, scaling is also not a favorable approach (Weiss et al. 2017). *Aitchinson's log-ratio* transformation is also a widely applied normalization method, where the sparsity of microbiome data is handled by adding a small pseudocount to all observations, thus eliminating zeros in the dataset.

3.4.2 Taxonomic Classification

The most commonly used NGS platforms provide DNA sequence readout (i.e. base calling) at > 99.9% accuracy (Ledergerber and Dessimo 2011). Nonetheless, strict quality-based filtering is applied to.*fastq* files and identical amplicon sequences are grouped together, with statistical methods used to determine the likelihood of a specific amplicon representing true biological signal or residual artefacts of sample preparation and sequencing. Amplicon sequences are then used to determine taxonomic groups present in the sample, by classification according to similarity. Two major avenues of taxonomic analysis are available: Operational Taxonomic Unit (OTU) picking, and Amplicon Sequence Variant (ASV) classification.

3.4.2.1 Operational Taxonomic Unit-Based Methods

OTUs traditionally refer to groups of individuals displaying a predetermined degree of similarity (Sokal and Sneath 1963). In the context of the microbiome, OTUs represent bacterial or fungal DNA isolates with a certain percentage of sequence similarity in the 16S rRNA gene. OTUs are most often clustered using hierarchical clustering algorithms or heuristic approximations thereof (Schmidt et al. 2014). An arbitrary similarity threshold is then used to define clusters; while 97% similarity is used most commonly, this can vary based on study design.

During so-called *"closed-reference"* OTU picking, a pre-existing rRNA database is used as reference, where each marker gene sequence has been assigned its proper taxonomic classification. Sequencing reads from our experiments are then assigned to an OTU based on the percentage similarity to the reference database sequences. While this approach enables direct identification of species and is computationally efficient, only already known bacteria can be characterized in the sample, as all 16S rRNA sequences that do not match the reference database above a pre-defined similarity threshold are discarded.

Using a de novo OTU picking method, novel species can be characterized at the cost of higher computational complexity. All sequenced 16S rRNA information is used, and OTUs are assigned regardless of pre-existing taxonomic data, based on the pairwise similarity of each read in the sample to one another. Reads sharing a similarity higher than a threshold (usually 97%) are clustered together, and the cluster of reads is represented by the most common shared nucleotide sequence, resulting in a de novo OTU. The most commonly used algorithm is hierarchical or heuristic clustering.

A hybrid of the two previous methods is *open-reference* OTU picking, where classification based on a taxonomic database is carried out when possible, however novel sequences are not discarded, but subjected to de novo OTU picking. While the latter method holds many advantages, certain study design and technical parameters limit its application. As most species of the human skin microbiome have been characterized, the use of closed-reference OTU picking offers the greatest efficiency coupled with negligible loss of novel information.

3.4.2.2 Amplicon Sequence Variant-Based Classification

As a recently emerged and dynamically growing field, metagenomic analysis techniques are constantly evolving. During recent years, Amplicon Sequence Variant-based classification has been increasingly used as an alternative to OTU-based taxonomies (Callahan et al. 2016). Despite high sequencing accuracy and subsequent quality control of data, sequencing errors and artefacts introduced during the generation of amplicons by PCR may remain, biasing downstream results. For this reason, during ASV picking, each sequencing read is used in the construction of a specific error model that is customized to fit the set of samples sequenced in the experiment. In the process of denoising, true biological variation is distinguished from random errors using this model, and the original sequence content is inferred (Callahan et al. 2016; McMurdie et al. 2014). The resulting ASVs may provide single-nucleotide level discrimination of sequences instead of clustering based on a pre-determined similarity threshold, as in the case of OTUs. This increased resolution results in a more accurate identification at the species, or in some cases, the strain level. As ASVs are not dependent on a reference database, such as closed-reference OTUs, and represent exact DNA sequences instead of clusters of sufficiently similar ones, such as de novo OTUs, this method provides favorable results and is increasingly utilized in metagenomics.

3.4.3 *Phylogenetic Tree Construction*

A phylogenetic or evolutionary tree is a structure representing evolutionary relationships between biological species, or other taxonomic ranks. These relationships are called the phylogeny of the species and are based upon differences or similarities in their physical or genetic characteristics. Trees represent taxonomic groups at the tips or leaves, with branches indicating inferred evolutionary relationships between them. Groups are organized by derived traits, with branching points, or internal nodes, representing evolutionary divergence. The reconstruction of the Tree of Life, an evolutionary tree spanning all known organisms and organized by the pairwise similarity of their DNA sequences is one of the most complex undertakings of molecular biology (Delsuc et al. 2005). A particular challenge in phylogenetics is posed by homoplasy, the gain or loss of a trait occurring independently across multiple lineages during the course of evolution. Examples of homoplasy are convergent, parallel and reverse evolution. While constructing trees based on phenotype leads to several biases due to the effects of e.g. convergent evolution, molecular phylogeny also poses technical limitations. When constructing a phylogeny based on pre-defined markers such as the 16S rRNA gene, the biases introduced by e.g. horizontal gene transfer are minimized due to the high level of conservation, however, in certain cases, the 16S rRNA marker is not sufficient to distinguish e.g. closely related species. This limitation is further emphasized in the case of low-coverage or low-quality sequencing data. Approaches to phylogenetic tree construction include:

Maximum parsimony- while building a phylogenetic tree, unknown evolutionary events need to be reconstructed from limited information, i.e. the nucleotide sequences of OTUs, ASVs or selected marker genes in the case of WGS. As the process requires a set of assumptions, given sample sequences give rise to a multitude of possible phylogenetic tree versions, of which one is selected which represents the actual relationships with the highest probability. To ensure the correctness of this inference, different methods use different sets of *optimality criteria*, conditions that must be satisfied at a function's minimum point. Maximum parsimony is used to infer a phylogenetic tree through minimizing the total number of evolutionary steps required to explain the relationships of OTUs in a given sample—in other words, usage of the simplest available hypothesis, a general principle in all scientific fields.

Neighbor joining trees apply an agglomerative clustering method, where pairs of OTUs are selected in each stage of tree construction which minimize the total branch length of the tree, thus creating a parsimonious tree.

Maximum likelihood trees apply an underlying nucleotide substitution model in order to reconstruct evolutionary events, assigning probabilities to mutation events. Although computationally demanding, recently ML methods have become the standard for 16S marker-gene based phylogenetics.

Markov Chain Monte Carlo (MCMC)-Bayesian approaches, introduced in the 1990s, aim to find the most likely phylogenetic tree for the given data using a likelihood function with suitable evolutionary models. MCMC provides a simulation-based estimation of the posterior probability used in Bayesian inference. With advances in computing capacity and simulation algorithms, MCMC has become a valuable tool in phylogenetic tree construction. (Nascimento et al. 2017).

3.4.4 Measurements of Microbial Richness

Microbial richness, the breadth of different microbial taxa found in a given sample, is characterized using two key measures: within-sample, or *alpha diversity* and between-sample, or *beta diversity*, which are summarized for the overall population by *gamma diversity*. These terms originate from ecology, introduced by R.H. Whittaker in 1972 (Whittaker 1972), and refer to the richness of species in a habitat and the ratio of species counts between habitats. While the exact level of organization at which alpha diversity is measured is not defined strictly, considering human subjects, it is important to establish that different body sites harbor markedly different microbial communities, thus representing distinct habitats. However, traditionally alpha- and beta diversity refer to intra-individual and inter-individual measures in human studies, and consequently are used for the characterization of the microbiome composition of a single subject (alpha diversity) versus the differences between microbiomes of all study subjects (beta diversity). In its simplest form, alpha diversity refers to the number of taxa found in an individual sample. Beta diversity, while also succeeded by more complex formulas, originally indicates the ratio of species observed in individual samples versus the complete species diversity of the population, which is termed *gamma diversity*. As mentioned, the original metrics proposed by Whittaker were followed by several different calculations of species diversity, evenness, or the ubiquity of given species in a population, or missingness, the estimation of what percentage of data might be missed in the sample due to the technical constraints of sampling and DNA sequencing (detailed below). While these novel measures are often referred to as alpha or beta diversity collectively, in scientific practice it is common to refer to them by exact names in order to avoid misinterpretation. It is important to note that most diversity measures do not include a notion of space, i.e. if there are differences in the sampled area, these need to be adjusted for beforehand. Also, a specific drawback of sequencing, the variable number of sequencing reads obtained from each sample, needs to be addressed through normalization (McMurdie et al. 2014) before diversity measures and further statistical analyses can be applied.

3.4.5 Abundance Measures

As previously mentioned, metagenomic studies -either marker gene-based or WGS- offer information on the quantities of microbial taxa in each sample. However, metagenomic sequencing yields compositional data, where the sequencing depth defines the chance with which low-abundance species can be detected. For example, a relatively rare species usually present in minor quantities on the skin, *Halomonas phoceae* may not be detected in a sample sequenced using 1 million reads, while a common skin bacterium, *Acinetobacter johnsonii* might be detected in the same sample with a sequencing depth of only 250,000 reads. Since absolute quantification of bacteria is not achievable, *relative abundance* is calculated, based on the normalized counts of reads representing each taxon.

3.4.6 *Additional Commonly Used Indices*

The *Shannon diversity index* or Shannon's H is an alpha diversity measure, however it also indicates how evenly the taxa are distributed in a sample, i.e. whether one or more species are overgrowing others, and thus takes into account abundance information. The proportion of species *i* relative to the total number of species (*pi*) is taken and multiplied by the natural logarithm of this proportion (ln*pi*). The product is summed across species, and the reciprocal is taken:

$$H = -\sum_{i=1}^{S} p_i \ln p_i$$

where H is Shannon's diversity index, S is the total number of species in the community, p_i is the proportion of S made up of the *i*th species (Shannon 1948).

Simpson diversity is another commonly used measure, indicating species evenness similarly to Shannon's H, where the proportion of species *i* relative to the total number of species (*pi*) is calculated and squared. The squared proportions for all the species are summed, and the reciprocal is taken:

$$D = \frac{1}{\sum_{i=1}^{S} p_i^2}$$

where D represents the Simpson diversity index, while S is the total number of species in the community, p_i is the proportion of S made up of the *i*th species. Although Shannon's and Simpson's diversity measures are quite similar, the former places more weight on species richness, while the latter weighs species evenness more, and the two may be used jointly during exploratory data analysis.

A more abstract approach to diversity estimation, the *Abundance-based Coverage Estimator (ACE)* was introduced by Anne Chao and is a non-parametric diversity measure for estimating species richness based on the observed OTUs (Chao and Lee 1992). The observed frequencies of OTUs are divided into abundant and rare groups based on presence/absence information, and quantities of abundant species are not considered directly (Kim et al. 2017). This formula makes use of the observation of singleton species, rare species (or OTUs) that appear in only a single sample of the complete dataset. Their frequency is then used to estimate how many species are likely to be missed in the dataset due to the above-mentioned limitations of DNA sequencing, thus species missingness is considered:

$$S_{ACE} = S_{abund} + \frac{S_{rare}}{C_{ACE}} + \frac{F_1}{C_{ACE}}\gamma_{ACE}^2$$

where S_{abund} and S_{rare} are the number of abundant and rare OTUs, respectively, C_{ACE} is the sample coverage estimation, F_1 is the frequency of singletons and γ_{ACE}^2 is the estimated coefficient of variation for rare OTUs.

The *Jaccard index* (Jaccard 1912), also known as Intersection over Union or Jaccard similarity coefficient is a simple similarity measure used across all scientific disciplines, and suitable for beta diversity analysis. Only presence/absence status of species is considered, where the index specifies the size of the intersection divided by the size of the union of two sets of samples:

$$J(A, B) = \frac{|A \cap B|}{|A \cup B|}$$

where J is the Jaccard index and A and B are different samples or sets of samples. It is easily converted into a dissimilarity metric between samples by subtracting from 1:

$$d_J(A, B) = 1 - J(A, B)$$

Bray–Curtis dissimilarity (Bray and Curtis 1957) takes into account the difference of microbial abundances between sets of samples, opposed to the presence/absence information of the Jaccard index:

$$BC_{ij} = \frac{2C_{ij}}{S_i + S_j}$$

where S_i and S_j are the total number of species counted in each sample, while C_{ij} is the sum of species present in both samples taking only the lesser count. (e.g. if *Propionibacterium acnes* is represented by 100 reads in sample A and 500 reads in sample B, while *Acinetobacter johnsonii* is present with 120 and 300 reads in A and B respectively, $C_{ij} = 100 + 120 = 220$).

3.4.7 Ordination

Ordination is used as an important exploratory data analysis tool. Multidimensional Scaling (MDS) represents pairwise distances among the samples of a study population, thus providing information on their similarity. When studying populations harboring markedly different microbiota, MDS methods represent these as distinct clusters. *Principal Coordintate Analysis* applies variance-maximizing data transformation, and is usually applied to one of the above-mentioned dissimilarity metrics, e.g. the Jaccard dissimilarity. The results are usually presented on a two-dimensional plot indicating samples along the two main axes of variation found in the data, where distinct sample clusters may be observed.

3.4.8 Differential Abundance

While diversity measures provide information on the richness and evenness of the microbiome in a population, the quantification of microbial species also enables the comparison of communities between different sets of samples. The most common application to the skin microbiome might be the comparison between different body sites of a study population, or that of control and diseased individuals. The most widespread applications apply generalized linear models which assume a particular data distribution, e.g. negative binomial distribution (Robinson et al. 2010; Love et al. 2014), or apply zero-inflated Gaussian or lognormal models (Weiss et al. 2017). While all of these methods have unique benefits and drawbacks, statistical testing of microbial community differences is not straightforward due to the compositional nature of the data. However, such measurements are of key importance to future clinical applications of metagenomics, and are thus an area of active methodological research.

3.4.9 Co-occurence Network Construction

Co-occurrence refers to species or OTUs in a study population which appear in the same samples at a given frequency, thus is a tool for identifying microbial communities. Determining which species occur together frequently could be achieved by measuring their Pearson or Spearman correlation coefficients, however the relative nature, and most importantly the sparsity of microbiome data again raise complications for these methods (Hirano and Takemoto 2019). As a consequence, several alternatives have been proposed, such as SparCC, CCLasso or SPIEC-EASI, algorithms optimized for sparse data. The resulting networks represent bacteria or OTUs as nodes, with connecting lines (edges) showing negative or positive correlations between them.

3.5 Whole-Genome Sequencing

So far we have examined examples of data analysis related to 16S marker gene sequencing, however, most of the above methodologies apply to WGS metagenomics as well. While more costly and complex, a great advantage of WGS over 16S rRNA sequencing is that the actual genome content and precise gene sequences of the microbiota are identified. Functions of unknown bacterial genes may be inferred by sequence homology, while clustering and network construction approaches can be used to compare the metabolic capacity between different study populations, reflecting e.g. antibiotic resistance or the secretion of toxins or proteases. Not restricted by the 16S subunit, viruses and fungi are also present in the samples, however, for the routine detection of non-prokaryotes, the reference databases for these organisms need considerable improvement.

3.6 Outlook

Metagenomics is among the most dynamically evolving research fields of the decade, holding the promise to answer crucial questions on the structure of the human and environmental microbiota, host-microbe interplay and the homeostatic microflora, clinical treatment options and much more. As mentioned previously, microbial DNA sequencing approaches cannot distinguish between living or dead microbes in the sample; however, sequencing of microbial RNA, subsequent gene expression profiling and metabolite screening are rapidly developing. Novel sequencing technologies enable the reconstruction of microbial genomes with unprecedented precision, with handheld, portable devices being capable of microbiome profiling on-site in certain scenarios. Computational methods adapted from different fields of science are also tailored to suit microbial analyses and provide higher precision at reduced computational requirements, altogether making metagenomics more accessible and applicable to current clinical and research challenges.

References

Aitchison J. The statistical analysis of compositional data. J Roy Stat Soc B Met. 1982;44(2):139–77.

Alexeyev OA. Bacterial landscape of human skin: seeing the forest for the trees. Exp Dermatol. 2013;22:443–6. https://doi.org/10.1111/exd.12160.

Beals M, Gross L, Harrell S. Diversity Indices: Simpson's D and E 1999. http://www.tiem.utk.edu/~gross/bioed/bealsmodules/simpsonDI.html.

Bray JR, Curtis JT. An ordination of upland forest communities of southern Wisconsin. Ecol Monogr. 1957;27:325–49.

Brooks JP, Edwards DJ, Harwich MD, Rivera MC, Fettweis JM, Serrano MG, Reris RA, Sheth NU, Huang B, Girerd P. Vaginal microbiome consortium (additional members). In: Strauss JF, Jefferson KK, Buck GA, editors. The truth about metagenomics: quantifying and counteracting bias in 16S rRNA studies. BMC Microbiol. 2015;15:66. https://doi.org/10.1186/s12866-015-0351-6.

Byrd AL, Belkaid Y, Segre JA. The human skin microbiome. Nat Rev Micro. 2018;16:143–55. https://doi.org/10.1038/nrmicro.2017.157.

Callahan BJ, McMurdie PJ, Holmes SP. Exact sequence variants should replace operational taxonomic units in marker-gene data analysis. ISME J. 2017;11(12):2639–43. https://doi.org/10.1038/ismej.2017.119.

Callahan B, McMurdie P, Rosen M. DADA2: High-resolution sample inference from Illumina amplicon data. Nat Methods. 2016;13:581–583. https://doi.org/10.1038/nmeth.3869.

Calle ML. Statistical analysis of metagenomics data. Genomics Inform. 2019;17(1):e6. https://doi. org/10.5808/GI.2019.17.1.e6.

Chao A, Chun-Huo C, Lou J. Phylogenetic diversity measures and their decomposition: a framework based on hill numbers. Biodiversity Conservation and Phylogenetic Systematics. 2016, p. 141–172.

Chao A, Lee SM. Estimating the number of classes via sample coverage. J Am Stat Assoc. 1992;87(417):210–217. https://doi.org/10.1080/01621459.1992.10475194.

Chng KR, Tay ASL, Li C, Ng AHQ, Wang J, Suri BK, Matta SA, McGovern N, Janela B, Wong XFCC, Sio YY, Au BV, Wilm A, De Sessions PF, Lim TC, Tang MBY, Ginhoux F, Connolly JE, Lane EB, Chew FT, Common JEA, Nagarajan N. Whole metagenome profiling reveals skin microbiome-dependent susceptibility to atopic dermatitis flare. Nat Microbiol. 2016;1:16106. https://doi.org/10.1038/nmicrobiol.2016.106.

Clausen M-L, Slotved H-C, Krogfelt KA, Agner T. Tape stripping technique for stratum Corneum protein analysis. Sci Rep. 2016;6:19918. https://doi.org/10.1038/srep19918.

Clausen M-L, Agner T, Lilje B, Edslev SM, Johannesen TB, Andersen PS. Association of disease severity with skin microbiome and Filaggrin gene mutations in adult atopic dermatitis. JAMA Dermatol. 2018;154:293. https://doi.org/10.1001/jamadermatol.2017.5440.

Costello EK, Lauber CL, Hamady M, Fierer N, Gordon JI, Knight R. Bacterial community variation in human body habitats across space and time. Science. 2009;326:1694–7. https://doi.org/10. 1126/science.1177486.

Delsuc F, Brinkmann H, Philippe H. Phylogenomics and the reconstruction of the tree of life. Nat Rev Genet. 2005;6:361–375. https://doi.org/10.1038/nrg1603.

Evans CA, Smith WM, Johnston EA, Giblett ER. Bacterial flora of the normal human skin*. J Investig Dermatol. 1950;15:305–24. https://doi.org/10.1038/jid.1950.105.

Findley K, Oh J, Yang J, Conlan S, Deming C, Meyer JA, Schoenfeld D, Nomicos E, Park M, Intramural Sequencing Center Comparative Sequencing Program NIH, Kong HH, Segre JA. Topographic diversity of fungal and bacterial communities in human skin. Nature. 2013;498:367–70. https://doi.org/10.1038/nature12171.

Fitch WM. Toward defining the course of evolution: minimum change for a specified tree topology. Syst Zool. 1971;20(4):406–16. https://doi.org/10.2307/2412116.

Fyhrquist N, Muirhead G, Prast-Nielsen S, Jeanmougin M, Olah P, Skoog T, Jules-Clement G, Feld M, Barrientos-Somarribas M, Sinkko H, van den Bogaard EH, Zeeuwen PLJM, Rikken G, Schalkwijk J, Niehues H, Däubener W, Eller SK, Alexander H, Pennino D, Suomela S, Tessas I, Lybeck E, Baran AM, Darban H, Gangwar RS, Gerstel U, Jahn K, Karisola P, Yan L, Hansmann B, Katayama S, Meller S, Bylesjö M, Hupé P, Levi-Schaffer F, Greco D, Ranki A, Schröder JM, Barker J, Kere J, Tsoka S, Lauerma A, Soumelis V, Nestle FO, Homey B, Andersson B, Alenius H. Microbe-host interplay in atopic dermatitis and psoriasis. Nat Commun. 2019;10:4703. https://doi.org/10.1038/s41467-019-12253-y.

Gao Z, Tseng C, Pei Z, Blaser MJ. Molecular analysis of human forearm superficial skin bacterial biota. PNAS. 2007;104:2927–32. https://doi.org/10.1073/pnas.0607077104.

Goodrich JK, Di Rienzi SC, Poole AC, Koren O, Walters WA, Caporaso JG, Knight R, Ley RE. Conducting a microbiome study. Cell. 2014;158:250–62. https://doi.org/10.1016/j.cell.2014. 06.037.

Grice EA, Kong HH, Renaud G, Young AC, Comparative Sequencing Program NISC, Bouffard GG, Blakesley RW, Wolfsberg TG, Turner ML, Segre JA. A diversity profile of the human skin microbiota. Genome Res. 2008;18:1043–50. https://doi.org/10.1101/gr.075549.107.

Grice EA, Kong HH, Conlan S, Deming CB, Davis J, Young AC, Comparative Sequencing Program NISC, Bouffard GG, Blakesley RW, Murray PR, Green ED, Turner ML, Segre JA. Topographical and temporal diversity of the human skin microbiome. Science. 2009;324:1190–2. https://doi. org/10.1126/science.1171700.

Grogan MD, Bartow-McKenney C, Flowers L, Knight SAB, Uberoi A, Grice EA. Research techniques made simple: profiling the skin microbiota. J Investig Dermatol. 2019;139:747–752.e1. https://doi.org/10.1016/j.jid.2019.01.024.

Heather JM, Chain B. The sequence of sequencers: the history of sequencing DNA. Genomics. 2016;107:1–8. https://doi.org/10.1016/j.ygeno.2015.11.003.

Hirano H, Takemoto K. Difficulty in inferring microbial community structure based on co-occurrence network approaches. BMC Bioinform. 2019;20:329. https://doi.org/10.1186/s12 859-019-2915-1.

Hugerth LW, Andersson AF. Analysing microbial community composition through amplicon sequencing: from sampling to hypothesis testing. Front Microbiol. 2017;8:1561. https://doi.org/10.3389/fmicb.2017.01561.

Jaccard P. The distribution of the flora in the alpine zone. New Phytol. 1912;11:37–50. https://doi.org/10.1111/j.1469-8137.1912.tb05611.x.

Kezic S, Kammeyer A, Calkoen F, Fluhr JW, Bos JD. Natural moisturizing factor components in the stratum corneum as biomarkers of filaggrin genotype: evaluation of minimally invasive methods. Br J Dermatol. 2009;161:1098–104. https://doi.org/10.1111/j.1365-2133.2009.09342.x.

Kim BR, Shin J, Guevarra RB, Lee JH, Kim DW, Seol KH, Lee J, Kim HB, Isaacson RE. Deciphering diversity indices for a better understanding of microbial communities. J Microbiol Biotechnol. 2017;27(12):2089–93.

Kim BE, Goleva E, Kim PS, Norquest K, Bronchick C, Taylor P, Leung DYM. Side-by-side comparison of skin biopsies and skin tape stripping highlights abnormal stratum Corneum in atopic dermatitis. J Investig Dermatol. 2019;139:2387-2389.e1. https://doi.org/10.1016/j.jid.2019.03.1160.

Kong HH, Segre JA. Skin microbiome: looking back to move forward. J Investig Dermatol. 2012;132:933–9. https://doi.org/10.1038/jid.2011.417.

Kong HH, Andersson B, Clavel T, Common JE, Jackson SA, Olson ND, Segre JA, Traidl-Hoffmann C. Performing skin microbiome research: a method to the madness. J Investig Dermatol. 2017;137:561–8. https://doi.org/10.1016/j.jid.2016.10.033.

Lauder AP, Roche AM, Sherrill-Mix S, Bailey A, Laughlin AL, Bittinger K, Leite R, Elovitz MA, Parry S, Bushman FD. Comparison of placenta samples with contamination controls does not provide evidence for a distinct placenta microbiota. Microbiome. 2016;4:29. https://doi.org/10.1186/s40168-016-0172-3.

Ledergerber C, Dessimoz C. Base-calling for next-generation sequencing platforms. Brief Bioinform. 2011;12:489–497. https://doi.org/10.1093/bib/bbq077.

Liu L, Li Y, Li S, et al. Comparison of next-generation sequencing systems. J Biomed Biotechnol. 2012;2012: 251364. https://doi.org/10.1155/2012/251364.

Love MI, Huber W, Anders S. Moderated estimation of fold change and dispersion for RNA-seq data with DESeq2. Genome Biol. 2014;15(12):550. https://doi.org/10.1186/s13059-014-0550-8.

Markle WH, Makhoul K. Cutaneous leishmaniasis recognition and treatment. AFP. 2004;69:1455–1460.

Marples MJ. The normal flora of the human skin†. Br J Dermatol. 1969;81:2–13. https://doi.org/10.1111/j.1365-2133.1969.tb12827.x.

McMurdie PJ, Holmes S. Waste not, want not: why rarefying microbiome data is inadmissible. PLOS Comput Biol. 2014;10(4):e1003531. https://doi.org/10.1371/journal.pcbi.1003531.

Menton DN, Eisen AZ. Structure and organization of mammalian stratum corneum. J Ultrastruct Res. 1971;35:247–64. https://doi.org/10.1016/S0022-5320(71)80155-7.

Nakatsuji T, Chiang H-I, Jiang SB, Nagarajan H, Zengler K, Gallo RL. The microbiome extends to subepidermal compartments of normal skin. Nat Commun. 2013;4:1431. https://doi.org/10.1038/ncomms2441.

Nascimento FF, Reis MD, Yang Z. A biologist's guide to Bayesian phylogenetic analysis. Nature Ecol Evol. 2017;1(10):1446–54. https://doi.org/10.1038/s41559-017-0280-x.

Noble WC. Observations on the surface flora of the skin and on the skin pH. Br J Dermatol. 1968;80:279–81. https://doi.org/10.1111/j.1365-2133.1968.tb12299.x.

Ogai K, Nagase S, Mukai K, Iuchi T, Mori Y, Matsue M, Sugitani K, Sugama J, Okamoto S. A comparison of techniques for collecting skin microbiome samples: swabbing versus tape-stripping. Front Microbiol. 2018;9:2362. https://doi.org/10.3389/fmicb.2018.02362.

Oh J, Byrd AL, Park M, Kong HH, Segre JA. Temporal stability of the human skin microbiome. Cell. 2016;165:854–66. https://doi.org/10.1016/j.cell.2016.04.008.

Oh J, Byrd AL, Deming C, Conlan S, Kong HH, Segre JA. NISC comparative sequencing program, fifth, 2014. Biogeography and individuality shape function in the human skin metagenome. Nature. 2014;514:, 59–64. https://doi.org/10.1038/nature13786.

Pillsbury DM, Nichols AC. Bacterial flora of the normal and infected skin: an evaluation of various methods of performing skin cultures1. J Investig Dermatol. 1946;7:365–73. https://doi.org/10.1038/jid.1946.43.

Pinkus H. Examination of the epidermis by the strip method: II. Biometric data on regeneration of the human epidermis1. J Investig Dermatol. 1952;19:431–47. https://doi.org/10.1038/jid.1952.119.

Prast-Nielsen S, Tobin A-M, Adamzik K, Powles A, Hugerth LW, Sweeney C, Kirby B, Engstrand L, Fry L. Investigation of the skin microbiome: swabs vs. biopsies. Br J Dermatol. 2019;181:572–9. https://doi.org/10.1111/bjd.17691.

Robinson MD, McCarthy DJ, Smyth GK. EdgeR: a bioconductor package for differential expression analysis of digital gene expression data. Bioinform (Oxford, England). 2010;26(1):139–40. https://doi.org/10.1093/bioinformatics/btp616.

Saitou N, Nei M. The neighbor-joining method: a new method for reconstructing phylogenetic trees. Mol Biol Evol. 1987;4(4):406–25. https://doi.org/10.1093/oxfordjournals.molbev.a040454.

Salter SJ, Cox MJ, Turek EM, Calus ST, Cookson WO, Moffatt MF, Turner P, Parkhill J, Loman NJ, Walker AW. Reagent and laboratory contamination can critically impact sequence-based microbiome analyses. BMC Biol. 2014;12:87. https://doi.org/10.1186/s12915-014-0087-z.

Schmidt TSB, Matias Rodrigues JF, von Mering C. Ecological consistency of SSU rRNA-Based operational taxonomic units at a global scale. PLOS Comput Biol. 2014;10(4):e1003594. https://doi.org/10.1371/journal.pcbi.1003594.

Shannon CE. A mathematical theory of communication. Bell Syst Tech J. 1948;27:379–423.

Shehadul Islam M, Aryasomayajula A, Selvaganapathy P. A review on macroscale and microscale cell lysis methods. Micromachines. 2017;8:83. https://doi.org/10.3390/mi8030083.

Simpson EH. Measurement of diversity. Nature. 1949;163:688. https://doi.org/10.1038/163688a0.

Sina B, Kao GF, Deng AC, Gaspari AA. Skin biopsy for inflammatory and common neoplastic skin diseases: optimum time, best location and preferred techniques. a critical review. J Cutan Pathol. 2009;36:505–10. https://doi.org/10.1111/j.1600-0560.2008.01175.x.

Sokal RR, Sneath PHA. English, miscellaneous, principles of numerical taxonomy. W. H. Freeman and Co., San Francisco and London; 1963.p.359. 19650300280.

Tanner MA, Goebel BM, Dojka MA, Pace NR. Specific ribosomal DNA sequences from diverse environmental settings correlate with experimental contaminants. Appl Environ Microbiol. 1998;64:3110–3.

Updegraff DM. A cultural method of quantitatively studying the microorganisms in the skin**from the central research laboratories, minnesota mining and manufacturing company, Saint Paul, Minnesota. J Investig Dermatol. 1964;43:129–37. https://doi.org/10.1038/jid.1964.130.

Van Dijk EL, Jaszczyszyn Y, Naquin D, Thermes C. The third revolution in sequencing technology. Trends Genet. 2018;34(9):666–681. https://doi.org/10.1016/j.tig.2018.05.008.

Versalovic J, Keitel W, Petrosino J. Coordinating Investigator and Study Chair 2010;67.

Walker AW, Martin JC, Scott P, Parkhill J, Flint HJ, Scott KP. 16S rRNA gene-based profiling of the human infant gut microbiota is strongly influenced by sample processing and PCR primer choice. Microbiome. 2015;3:26. https://doi.org/10.1186/s40168-015-0087-4.

Weiss S, Xu ZZ, Peddada S, Amir A, Bittinger K, Gonzalez A, Knight R. Normalization and microbial differential abundance strategies depend upon data characteristics. Microbiome. 2017;5(1):27. https://doi.org/10.1186/s40168-017-0237-y.

Weyrich LS, Farrer AG, Eisenhofer R, Arriola LA, Young J, Selway CA, Handsley-Davis M, Adler CJ, Breen J, Cooper A. Laboratory contamination over time during low-biomass sample analysis. Mol Ecol Resour. 2019;19:982–96. https://doi.org/10.1111/1755-0998.13011.

Whittaker RH. Evolution and measurement of species diversity. Taxon. 1972;21(2/3):213–51. https://doi.org/10.2307/1218190.

Williamson P, Kligman AM. A new method for the quantitative investigation of cutaneous bacteria*. J Investig Dermatol. 1965;45:498–503. https://doi.org/10.1038/jid.1965.164.

Woese CR, Fox GE. Phylogenetic structure of the prokaryotic domain: the primary kingdoms. Proc Natl Acad Sci USA. 1977;74:5088–90. https://doi.org/10.1073/pnas.74.11.5088.

Yuan S, Cohen DB, Ravel J, Abdo Z, Forney LJ. Evaluation of methods for the extraction and purification of DNA from the human microbiome. PLoS ONE. 2012;7: e33865. https://doi.org/10.1371/journal.pone.0033865.

Zeeuwen PL, Boekhorst J, van den Bogaard EH, de Koning HD, van de Kerkhof PM, Saulnier DM, van Swam II, van Hijum SA, Kleerebezem M, Schalkwijk J, Timmerman HM. Microbiome dynamics of human epidermis following skin barrier disruption. Genome Biol. 2012;13:R101. https://doi.org/10.1186/gb-2012-13-11-r101.

Chapter 4
Skin Microbiota—Host Interactions in Health and Disease

Antti Lauerma

Abstract Human skin microbiota has been studied intensively for over 10 years. Several important findings have been made, but also gaps in knowledge are wide. The structure and interaction of microbiota and skin immunity has been shown to be significant in many skin conditions. Interaction depends on skin site, age, overall health and anatomical location in skin area. Of particular importance are antimicrobial peptides. Microbiota acts as natural adjuvant in skin and aids innate responses. Skin-infiltrating T lymphocytes interact directly with cutaneous microbiota. An emerging area is the effect of commensals on immune imprinting early in life, with unconventional T cells and dendritic cells playing a key role. Interactions with the host during bacterial, fungal and viral infections have been shown. Other areas include effects on maturation of mast cells, skin barrier and wound healing, as well as neoplastic transformation.

Keywords Microbiome · Microbiota · Immunity · Skin · Barrier · Commensal · Pathogen · Cancer

4.1   Introduction

Microbiome has been well known since advent of next generation techniques (Byrd et al. 2018). A nomenclature group suggests that microbiome and microbiota are used synonymously as microbiome has become a word in lay language. The importance of interaction between immune system and microbiota is apparent because microbes are controlled by immune systems. In non-vertebrates innate immunity is the main function, whereas in vertebrates there are also "learned/educated" immune responses, adaptive immunity. The emergence of information for microbiome-immune-interactions has been enormous during last 15 years. However, significant gaps in our knowledge still remain. This chapter will describe the latest findings and status of these interactions.

A. Lauerma (✉)
Department of Dermatology, University of Helsinki, Helsinki, Finland
e-mail: antti.lauerma@helsinki.fi

© The Author(s), under exclusive license to Springer Nature Switzerland AG 2025
A. Lauerma et al. (eds.), *The Skin Microbiome Manual*,
https://doi.org/10.1007/978-3-031-82689-4_4

4.2 Skin, Microbiota and Immunity

Skin differs greatly from other barrier sites of the body, i.e. mucosal membranes, as it is dry, cool, and has hairs (pilosebaceous units). Biochemically skin is acidic as opposed to neutral other barriers. Skin has also plethora of lipids, such as fatty acids, ceramides and cholesterol, that are result of keratinocyte differentiation where keratoinocyte transform to lipid-rich corneocytes. The high lipid content in corneocytes acts also as barrier to water loss from body and entry of hydrophilic materials, including DNA, RNA, proteins as well as viruses and bacteria (Zhang et al. 2022).

Additionally, skin is in an environment rich in oxygen, a potent toxic substance, as opposed to mucosal membranes. The exception is skin appendages including eccrine and apocrine sweat glands and sebaceous glands. A shift to anaerobic conditions favors growth of *Cutibacterium acnes*, a bacterium prevalent especially in sebaceous glands. This growth results in excretion of short chain fatty acids (SCFAs) that are highly immunomodulatory. This has dual results, increased immune protection and on other hand increased non-specific inflammation, as seen in acne vulgaris (Chinappan and Haris-Tryon 2021).

While digestive tract has highest number of bacteria, skin comes in second. There are up to one million bacteria per square centimeter in skin (Selwvn 1980). Skin microbiota acts as natural cutaneous adjuvant. Skin commensals give continuous information to immune system to maintain skin homeostasis. Commensal bacteria contribute to cutaneous defense also by producing antimicrobial peptides (AMPs) and directing microbiota to produce its own AMPs. The composition of bacteria differs between skin sites, where lipophilic *Cutibacteria* dominate sebaceous sites and *Staphylococcae* and *Corynebacteriae* more humid areas. Skin keratinocytes and sebocytes carry toll-like receptors (TLRs) and NOD-like receptors (NLRs). TLR2, TLR6 and NOD2 are important in response to commensal *Staphylococcus* and *Streptococcus* species. For herpesviruses, poxviruses and papillomaviruses TLRs 2, 3, 7, 8 and 9 are, on the other hand, important. Additionally bacterial sensing induces an interleukin-1 family cytokine cascades that leads to inflammasome activation via its own sensors such as NLRP3 (Lai et al. 2010; Sun et al. 2019).

In addition to innate responses, skin is rich in skin-homing (CLA+) T lymphocytes. Most of these cells are not in blood circulation, but reside in skin sites, thus providing immediate adaptive responses to pathogens and other immunologically active antigens, such as allergens (Clark et al. 2006).

4.3 Commensals, Unconventional T Cells and New Dendritic Cells

In addition to CLA+ T lymphocytes, skin and other organs hosts also unconventional T cells, out of which many are involved in specific adaptive responses. The unconventional T cells with T cell receptors include gamma-delta-17 T cells, gamma-delta-intraepithelial T cells, invariant natural killer T (iNKT) cells and mucosal-associated invariant T (MAIT) cells. Out of skin T cells, approximately 11% are unconventional T cells (Constantinides and Belkai 2021).

iNKT cells are modulated during first 2 weeks of life by skin commensals, resulting in immune imprinting (Constantinides et al. 2019) of note is the role of MAIT cells. Most bacteria and fungi produce riboflavin (vitamin B2) and MAIT cells recognize it. In animal experiments it has been shown that if mice are not exposed to riboflavin, or lack MAIT cells, during first two weeks after birth, it is not possible to mount the response later in life (Constantinides et al. 2019). Thus, early exposure is critical period to develop healthy immune responses, and if time window closes, it may not open again.

Unconventional T cells also compete for niches of tissue and immune responses between each other, filling the gaps left out. In addition to inflammation responses, unconventional T cells are also important in tissue repair. Especially MALT cells that reside conveniently under basement membrane in skin, are of importance in barrier and tissue repair (Constantinides and Belkaid 2021).

Dendritic cells that present antigens are central in immune responses. Recently, a new specialized subset of antigen presenting dendritic cells was found, that is important also in in neonatal skin, such as with unconventional T cells (Weckel et al. 2023).CD301b+ type 2 dendritic cells were found to be specifically capable of uptake and presentation of commensal bacteria to regulatory T cells, creating tolerance, instead of inflammation response, to these. This interaction seems to be decisive in inducing healthy tolerogenic responses to commensals, that are important to health (Weckel et al. 2023).

4.4 Microbiome and Maturation of Immune Cells

Immune cell maturation has been shown to be modulated by commensals early in life, leading to maturation of regulatory T cells among others. It has also been shown that skin microbiome is important in maturation of mast cells, a leukocyte subset that is involved not only in allergic and anti-helminth responses, but that is also major producer of cytokines, chemokines, tryptase and other immune-activating mediators. When mice were grown in germ-free conditions, their maturation was incomplete, they lacked the important stem cell factor for maturation, and were largely undifferentiated. However, when environment was supplemented with bacterial factors such as TLR2-activating staphylococcal LTA, the maturation was restored (Wang et al. 2017).

4.5 Microbiome and Tissue Repair

The epidermis is a major barrier between body and environment. The proper development of this barrier depends on skin microbiome early in life. The barrier is a necessity for terrestrial life. It was shown that if early in life there was no proper microbiota, the barrier failed to develop fully. Also, repair processes were compromised. The signaling acts via aryl hydrocarbon receptor, representing a key sensor/communication hub between commensals and barrier development and repair. These findings may have important consequences to many skin diseases that include barrier defects and delayed repair (Uberoi et al. 2021).

4.6 Protection from Infections and Skin Cancer by Skin Commensal Microbiome

Staphylococcus hominis is common commensal in human skin. It is closely related to *Staphylococcus aureus*, an infective strain. *Staphylococcus hominis* counteracts *Staphylococcus aureus* by producing six autoinducing peptides (AIPs) that inhibit the major virulence factor accessory gene regulator (agr) sensing system of *Staphylococcus aureus*. Such results have also been shown earlier with *Staphylococcus epidermis*. It is now well established that commensals regulate infectious bacteria and maintain skin health (Severn et al. 2022).

Staphylococcus epidermidis produces 6-N-hydroxyaminepurine (6-HAP) that suppresses DNA polymerase activity. Injections of 6-HAP in mice inhibited growth of malignant melanoma with no adverse effects. 6-HAP prevented the development of new skin cancers in a model of UV-inducible skin neoplasia. Skin commensals such as *Staphylococcus epidermidis* may protect against skin cancer (Nakatsuji et al. 2018).

4.7 Conclusions

Overwhelming evidence is gathering on the importance of microbiome-immune-interaction in skin health. Skin commensals act in concert with the host to maintain skin homeostasis. These emerging results underline the need for further investigations, and, already, avoidance of unnecessary antibacterial interventions especially early in life.

References

Byrd AL, Belkaid Y, Segre JA. The human skin microbiome. Nat Rev Microbiol. 2018;16(3):143–55.

Chinnappan M, Harris-Tryon TA. Novel mechanisms of microbial crosstalk with skin innate immunity. Exp Dermatol. 2021;30(10):1484–95.

Clark RA, Chong B, Mirchandani N, Brinster NK, Yamanaka K, Dowgiert RK, Kupper TS. The vast majority of CLA+ T cells are resident in normal skin. J Immunol. 2006;176(7):4431–9.

Constantinides MG, Belkaid Y. Early-life imprinting of unconventional T cells and tissue homeostasis. Science. 2021 Dec 10;374(6573):eabf0095.

Constantinides MG, Link VM, Tamoutounour S, Wong AC, Perez-Chaparro PJ, Han SJ, Chen YE, Li K, Farhat S, Weckel A, Krishnamurthy SR, Vujkovic-Cvijin I, Linehan JL, Bouladoux N, Merrill ED, Roy S, Cua DJ, Adams EJ, Bhandoola A, Scharschmidt TC, Aubé J, Fischbach MA, Belkaid Y. MAIT cells are imprinted by the microbiota in early life and promote tissue repair. Science. 2019 Oct 25;366(6464).

Lai Y, Cogen AL, Radek KA, Park HJ, Macleod DT, Leichtle A, Ryan AF, Di Nardo A, Gallo RL. Activation of TLR2 by a small molecule produced by Staphylococcus epidermidis increases antimicrobial defense against bacterial skin infections. J Invest Dermatol. 2010;130(9):2211–21.

Nakatsuji T, Chen TH, Butcher AM, Trzoss LL, Nam SJ, Shirakawa KT, Zhou W, Oh J, Otto M, Fenical W, Gallo RL. A commensal strain of Staphylococcus epidermidis protects against skin neoplasia. Sci Adv. 2018 Feb 28;4(2):eaao4502.

Selvan S. Microbiology and ecology of human skin. Practitioner. 1980;224:1059–62.

Severn MM, Williams MR, Shahbandi A, Bunch ZL, Lyon LM, Nguyen A, Zaramela LS, Todd DA, Zengler K, Cech NB, Gallo RL, Horswill AR. The ubiquitous human skin commensal staphylococcus hominis protects against opportunistic pathogens. mBio. 2022 Jun 28;13(3):e0093022.

Sun L, Liu W, Zhang LJ. The role of toll-like receptors in skin host defense, psoriasis, and atopic dermatitis. J Immunol Res. 2019;14(2019):1824624.

Uberoi A, Bartow-McKenney C, Zheng Q, Flowers L, Campbell A, Knight SAB, Chan N, Wei M, Lovins V, Bugayev J, Horwinski J, Bradley C, Meyer J, Crumrine D, Sutter CH, Elias P, Mauldin E, Sutter TR, Grice EA. Commensal microbiota regulates skin barrier function and repair via signaling through the aryl hydrocarbon receptor. Cell Host Microbe. 2021;29(8):1235-1248.e8.

Wang Z, Mascarenhas N, Eckmann L, Miyamoto Y, Sun X, Kawakami T, Di Nardo A. Skin microbiome promotes mast cell maturation by triggering stem cell factor production in keratinocytes. J Allergy Clin Immunol. 2017;139(4):1205–16.

Weckel A, Dhariwala MO, Ly K, Tran VM, Ojewumi OT, Riggs JB, Gonzalez JR, Dwyer LR, Okoro JN, Leech JM, Bacino MS, Cho GD, Merana G, Anandasabapathy N, Kumamoto Y, Scharschmidt TC. Long-term tolerance to skin commensals is established neonatally through a specialized dendritic cell subgroup. Immunity. 2023;56(6):1239-1254.e7.

Zhang C, Merana GR, Harris-Tryon T, Scharschmidt TC. Skin immunity: dissecting the complex biology of our body's outer barrier. Mucosal Immunol. 2022;15(4):551–61.

Chapter 5
Biodiversity Hypothesis: The Role of Environmental Microbial Exposures in Non-communicable Diseases

Jenni Lehtimäki

Abstract Biodiversity hypothesis suggests that two global megatrends, increasing global burden of chronic, non-communicable diseases and declining biological diversity on Earth are connected. The link between the two is hypothesized to be a decreasing exposure to beneficial environmental microbes that support development and function of immune system. Skin is open for microbial colonization from the environment, and a large proportion of skin microbes are transient. Skin and its microbiome are active both in local and systemic immune responses. These features make skin microbiome a potential link between living environment and human health. Urban environments provide homogenous microbial exposures enriched with common human skin bacteria, while rural and farming environments provide heterogenous microbial exposures. Active contact with soil or other natural elements shapes composition of skin microbiome relatively fast and living in greener environment impacts on microbial taxa found on human skin. These findings support the notion that surrounding nature and contact with it are influencing microbial communities on skin. Importantly, skin microbes originating from nature have been associated with immunoregulatory pathways and decreased risk on asthma and atopic diseases. Therefore, ongoing biodiversity decline and inadequate green areas in residential environments can limit human exposure to beneficial microbes. This chapter describes the history and current evidence of the biodiversity hypothesis, and represents related concepts including hygiene hypothesis, exposome and planetary health.

Keywords Environmental health · Asthma · Atopic diseases · Immunology · Children · Farming · Rural · Urban · Inflammatory diseases · Autoimmune diseases · Microbiome · Hygiene hypothesis · Old friends hypothesis · The developmental origins of health and disease · Exposome · Planetary health

J. Lehtimäki (✉)
Finnish Environment Institute, Helsinki, Finland
e-mail: jenni.lehtimaki@syke.fi

5.1 Introduction

Non-communicable diseases, such as cardiovascular diseases, cancers, autoimmune and allergic diseases, have passed infectious diseases as a main cause of global mortality (Collaborators et al. 2017). Many non-communicable diseases are more prevalent in high-income countries than in low-income countries. Therefore, non-communicable diseases are also known as lifestyle diseases, or diseases of affluence. However, some noncommunicable diseases, e.g., cardiovascular diseases, have recently became common around the globe. Adaptation of western diet, tobacco smoking, air pollution exposure, sedentary lifestyle, aging population, and urbanized living environment associate with their global spread. These adverse lifestyles and exposures are suggested to cause a prolonged low-level inflammation and disturbed immune function, which may be common explanators of these various diseases. Some scientists call them inflammatory diseases to emphasize the importance of chronic inflammation in disease etiology ('causes of disease').

Microbiome has been recognized to be disturbed in people with non-communicable diseases (Blaser 2014), which explains the motivation for intensive research of human microbiomes during recent decades. This chapter focus the factors that are beneficial for human microbiome. The main emphasis is placed on biodiversity hypothesis suggested by ecologist Ilkka Hanski and allergologist Tari Haahtela at 2011 (Hertzen et al. 2011). They proposed that increasing prevalence of non-communicable diseases is tightly linked to other global megatrend, decreasing biological diversity. They reasoned that diverse natural environments support beneficial environmental microbial exposures, which further maintain healthy human microbiome composition and, by stimulating immune function, prevent non-communicable diseases. In this chapter, components of biodiversity hypothesis are discussed, the research around hypothesis is reviewed, the potential role of skin microbiome is covered, and, finally, microbiome is considered as an important part of the health of the whole planet.

5.2 Declining Biological Diversity and Human Wellbeing

Biological diversity i.e., biodiversity, means a total variety of life in all its levels from genes to species and finally to ecosystems. Diversity of species in terrestrial and aquatic ecosystems has been consistently shown to be an important determinant of ecosystem productivity, stability, nutrient dynamics, and ability to resist invasion by exotic species or by pathogens (Tilman et al. 2014). The root reason for importance of biodiversity is less clear, but some ideas have extensive scientific support. For example, a large number of functional groups (=groups of organisms having partly overlapping roles within a habitat) increases productivity and resource use in natural ecosystems, but also prevents overuse of limited resources (Tilman et al. 2014). It has been estimated that more species are needed for maintaining ecosystem processes than can be directly linked to those processes. Thus, numerous direct and indirect interactions take place between organisms and are not fully described. Besides of "visible" ecosystems, complex dynamics between organisms take place in human microbiomes, which are part of all biodiversity and one kind of natural habitats.

Biodiversity is currently decreasing in unprecedented rates. The speed of species loss is even a thousand times faster than compared to historical extinction rates (Pimm et al. 2014) and we are seeing extensive decreases in the population and range sizes of even many common species that increases their extinction risk. Alarming decline is explained by human actions as growing human population has transformed the land use around the planet, overused natural resources and driven major shifts in global climate. These changes decrease the land available for species, destroy sensitive and unique ecosystems and change natural dynamics within ecosystems and between species. It is less clear what is happening for microbial diversity as baseline understanding on their numbers as well as long-term monitoring is missing (Cavicchioli et al. 2019). It is reasonable to assume that microscopic taxa are facing similar decline as macroscopic species as they partly depend on the same ecosystems. For example, diversity of plant species associates with diversity of soil microbes (Prober et al. 2015). Yet, global analysis showed that microscopic biodiversity does not follow the occurrence patterns of macroscopic biodiversity in one-third of the comparisons (Cameron et al. 2019). Therefore, the current understanding of microscopic biodiversity and trends in their species and population numbers are inadequately described.

The decline of biodiversity raises worries about the future of ecosystem services which support human wellbeing. For example, cycle of nutrients and water, pollination and infectious disease regulation are maintained by healthy ecosystems. In most ecosystem services, microbes have essential roles (Cavicchioli et al. 2019). Thus, decline of both macroscopic and microscopic biodiversity threats the stability of ecosystems, consequently threatening human wellbeing. For example, declining food security due to disturbed ecosystem services can cause lack of nutrients and energy and thus harm human health. Further, biodiverse environments control spread of pathogens and decrease emergence of new zoonoses (Tilman et al. 2014). Besides these examples, declining biodiversity can also have more *direct* influence on human wellbeing as suggested by biodiversity hypothesis.

5.3 Environment and Lifestyle Associate with the Risk of Non-communicable Diseases

The biodiversity hypothesis builds on scientific discoveries made around 1990's. At that time, several studies showed large disparities in the risk of asthma and atopic diseases between East and West at European continent. Erika von Mutius investigated child health disparities between East- and West-Germany after the German reunification. They assumed that as children in deprived East-Germany were heavily exposed to industrial air pollution, they would have more asthma and atopic diseases than children living in wealthier West-Germany. However, they discover exactly the opposite. Children from affluent West-Germany had higher prevalence of these diseases (von Mutius et al. 1994). Similar discoveries were made in comparisons between people living at opposite sides of Finnish and Russian border. Wealthier Finnish population had substantially higher prevalence of self-reported allergic symptoms and allergic sensitization (i.e. over-representation immunoglobulin E against non-harmful allergens) than Russian population (Vartiainen et al. 2002). These disparities were explained by differences in lifestyle. Eastern populations had not adopted western standards of living, and were, e.g., more commonly cultivating their own food. Disparities between East and West were reported across Europe: Eastern counties were consistently less likely to have as high prevalence of allergic diseases than wealthier Western countries (Matricardi 2001).

Asthma and atopic diseases are very common in (western) populations, which eases research on their potential root causes. Nowadays, in many westernized countries between a quarter and a third of adults suffer from asthma or atopic disease. Already decades ago, living environment and lifestyle were among top candidates as causes to these diseases. In the context of this chapter, it is interesting that green living environment is associated to lower risk of asthma and atopic diseases. However, there is also contradictory findings (Konijnendijk et al. n.d.) suggesting that the relation between living environment and risk of asthma and atopic diseases is complex. The various findings have been explained, e.g., by lack of longitudinal studies and differing methods to define greenness of living environment and disease outcomes. The biodiversity hypothesis suggests that as long as microbial exposures linking the environment and risk of these diseases is not included into the research approaches, the understanding remains partial.

Even though this chapter mainly focus on the asthma and atopic diseases (as current research around biodiversity hypothesis is based on these diseases), there is a plenty of evidence that green residential environment associates with numerous other health benefits. The most coherent evidence comes from beneficial effect of visiting in nature or living close to nature and mental health. Visits in nature are known to reduce blood pressure as well as stress levels rather immediately, which has led some doctors to guide their patients to visit in forests and parks. Living in greener environments also reduces rates of depression and anxiety (Konijnendijk et al. n.d.). Spending two hours in green areas a week supports mental health in adults (White et al. 2019). Further, green areas in childhood living environment decreased the risk of ADHD (Donovan et al. 2019). Green living environment has also been associated with physical health. For example, in meta-analysis including nearly eight million subjects, green living environment reduced all-cause, non-accidental mortality (Rojas-Rueda et al. 2019). Also cardiovascular diseases, which are the leading cause of global mortality, have inverse relationship with greenness in living environment in several studies around the world (Liu et al. 2022), and also in urban areas (Bianconi et al. 2023).

Underlining reasons for the health benefits of nature can be several. Green environments provide places for exercise and other leisure activities, they reduce the exposure to air pollution and noise, and can provide a sensory environment that is beneficial for people. In green spaces humans get exposed directly to various natural elements by breathing in, touching or sometimes by eating (such as berries). For example, trees produce volatile organic compounds, which can be sensed as smells, and experimental studies on animal models suggest these can provide health benefits (Antonelli et al. 2020). Natural environments are also rich in microbial species. In following sections, the microbes in our living environments and their association to skin microbiome are described.

5.4 Environmental Microbiomes in Our Daily Environments

If biodiversity hypothesis holds, then dissimilar environments should harbor contrasting environmental microbiomes. Indeed, differences in the environmental microbes between rural and urban areas, between geographical gradients and even within a single plant have been described. In a pioneering study, Albert Barberán (Barberán et al. 2015) showed with more than thousand samples that microbial communities in outdoor air were highly variable across the North American continent. Climatic and soil-related factors were important determinants of microbial communities. Authors made discovery with potential relevance for human health: Urban airborne microbiome was not less diverse than rural microbiome as commonly believed. Instead, urban microbial communities tended to be more *homogenous,* i.e., variability between samples was small. In other words, a person walking around in a city confronts similar microbial exposures everywhere while hiker in a rural area confronts constantly new types of microbial exposures.

Considering human health, it is interesting which type of environmental microbes are in our daily environments. Most people live in urbanized areas and hence the differences between built and green land cover types as well as between different types of green areas are potentially important. Interestingly, environmental microbes in green areas do not seem to colonize efficiently nearby built environments. Environmental microbes were studied in urban parks and in parking lots next to them. Microbial communities in parking lots were similar to each other while parks differed from each other. Parking lot microbiomes did not resemble microbiomes of parks next to them (Mhuireach et al. 2016). The homogenization of urban microbiomes can be caused by materials, such as asphalt, not supporting all microbial life, but also by citizens. In urban areas, human skin related microbes are enriched, particularly in public transportation.

Different types of urban green spaces such as open sport yards, managed parks and natural forests harbor different soil microbial communities (Baruch et al. 2020). Soil microbes are probably important determinants of microbial communities on air. Microbial communities on air in green areas depend on distance from soil as well as the canopy coverage in the green space (Robinson et al. 2021). Together these studies suggest that a baby crawling in the ground of urban forest with closed canopy is breathing in highly diverse microbial communities while adult person walking in an open green space such as lawn field is breathing in much less diverse microbial communities.

As people spend most of their time indoors, microbial communities there may form a large majority of our total microbial exposures. Indoor microbiomes have been intensively studied due to their potential importance for health. Studies have described that inhabitants have a large influence on indoor microbiome (Adams et al. 2016). Not surprisingly, common human skin microbes are enriched indoors. Microbiome indoors rapidly starts to resemble the skin microbiome of new residents and thus its composition can be individualized in each household. Arrival of pet also changes microbiome in homes. Dogs do not just bring common dog skin microbes to indoors, but also environmental microbiomes. For example, in rural and urban areas dogs carry dissimilar microbes indoors (Parajuli et al. 2018). Depending on the ventilation system of the building, indoor spaces are not completely independent of outdoor spaces, especially if the air flow is based on air pressure instead of mechanical ventilation (Adams et al. 2016). Surrounding environment also modifies indoor microbiomes. Indoor microbiome differs between rural and urban areas (Gupta et al. 2020) and farmers' homes tend to have own microbial signatures (Kirjavainen et al. 2019).

5.5 Environmental Microbes on Human Skin

The composition of human microbiomes is defined by numerous factors. Microbes inherited from mother, human genetics, chronological age and physiology can pose selection to microbial communities. Components of our diet both bring microbes, but also select them, and contacts with other people and animals can shape human microbiomes. Besides these, surrounding environment can shape microbiome, especially skin and airway microbiomes, because they are more open for the colonization by transient microbes than selective gut environment. Many studies have shown that gut, skin and airway microbiomes are dissimilar between populations living in traditional ways (such as hunter-gatherers, rain forest tribes and migrating shepherds) and westernized populations (Sonnenburg and Sonnenburg 2019). These differences could be explained with other than environmental factors, such as genetic background and diet, but accumulating evidence suggest that also living environment is important in these differences. For example, across gradient from a Peruvian Amerindian village in rainforest to the large Brazilian city of Manaus, the exposure to outdoor microbes decreases (McCall et al. 2019). The influence of the living environment to human skin microbiome is probably related with the amount of direct contact with outdoor environments. In age-gradient from newborns to teenagers, the difference in the skin microbiome composition between rural and urban children was largest in toddlers who probably actively touch their environment during outdoor plays. Interestingly, already newborns had dissimilar skin microbiome between rural and urban areas (Lehtimäki et al. 2017).

Direct contact with soil can impact on skin microbiota composition. Contact with soil immediately shapes the skin microbiota composition and diversifies it (Grönroos et al. 2019). Visit in urban green spaces can also influence on the composition of skin and nasal microbiomes. Comparisons of samples taken before and after the visits to various green spaces revealed that richness and diversity of microbial communities in skin and nasal samples increased after the visits. Moreover, skin started to resemble the soil microbiota while nasal samples become similar to the air samples collected from the visited parks (Selway et al. 2020). However, subjects were in active contact with the ground during the park visits. Hence, it remains unknown if such fast and large changes in skin microbiome compositions can be seen if a person just walks through a park. Moreover, changes in the skin microbiota do not remain long, probably just a day (Bateman 2017). Hence, very regular contact would be needed for such a large change to remain on skin. However, the differences in the skin microbiota between populations (as explained in previous paragraph) suggest that type of living environment can influence on skin microbes. It is speculated, that humans in westernized countries harbor microbiome which is not compatible with our biology (Rook 2013; Sonnenburg and Sonnenburg 2019). Evidence for this idea is discussed in the following sections.

5.6   Extending Hygiene Hypothesis

The importance of environmental microbial exposures, including pathogens, in human health has been speculated for decades. In 1989, David Strachan discovered an inverse relation between the number of siblings and the risk of hay fever in a sample of 17,000 British children. Especially older siblings associated with reduced risk of hay fever. Strachan explained his finding by decreasing exposure to childhood infections in families with fewer children as siblings are likely to transmit infections between each other in 'unhygienic contacts' (Strachan 1989). This idea was rather revolutionary at the time when common belief was that allergic diseases can be prevented by avoidance strategy and hygienic behavior. Strachan developed his findings into hygiene hypothesis, which originally stated that elimination of childhood infections in modern societies is causing increasing prevalence of allergic diseases. However, infections did not seem to coherently explain the lower risk of allergic diseases in families with many children (Strachan 2000). At same time, other protective factors correlating with family size were considered such as farming lifestyle and pet ownership. During the past decades, hygiene hypothesis has gradually generalized to the form it is usually nowadays understood. Too hygienic lifestyle associates with increasing risk of allergic and some other diseases, not just due to limited pathogen, but all microbe, exposures.

The hygiene hypothesis was further developed by Graham Rook. He placed hygiene hypothesis into evolutionary context and compared human life in the past and modern human societies. In both cases, humans are 'living in a microbial world', i.e., surrounded by extensive microbial diversity, but these microbial worlds are different. His ideas progressed into 'Old friends mechanism or hypothesis' which suggests that in modern societies people have lost the contact with those microscopic organisms that used to be present throughout human evolutionary history. According to Rook, humans have evolved dependency to some of these organisms, which are essential for our physiology and immunology (Rook et al. 2017). Rook parallels human immune system to the computer in order to explain the mechanism: hardware and software present (adaptive) immune system, but the computer is not functional without external data meaning microbial exposures (Rook 2013). Old friends hypothesis is hard to directly test due to evolutionary timescales. Yet, comparisons between human populations provide partial support (discussed later).

Biodiversity hypothesis closely relates to both hygiene hypothesis and Old friends hypothesis. Hypothesis warns that decline of biodiversity due to human actions pose a serious threat to human health by increasing the risk of non-communicable diseases (Hertzen et al. 2011). Macroscopic biological diversity is assumed to maintain those microbial species which are important for human health. Thus, declining biodiversity or urbanized living environments lacking natural environments may limit human exposure to microbial species providing health-supporting immune stimulation. Regardless of its name, hypothesis does not necessary assume that higher microbial diversity *in human bodies* is key for health but rather that surrounding biodiversity is needed for maintaining beneficial, environmental microbial communities.

Presented hypotheses are partly overlapping. They all assume that the lack of sufficient microbial exposure can disturb immune function or development that can be a root-cause of high prevalence of inflammatory, non-communicable diseases in modern societies. However, Hygiene hypothesis, Old friends hypothesis and Biodiversity hypothesis consider this phenomenon from different angles: focusing either on hygiene, evolutionary background, or global and local decline of biodiversity, respectively.

5.7 Interlinkages Between Microbial Exposures, Immune Function and Health

The starting point of research linking microbial exposures and asthma and atopic diseases was measurement of endotoxin, i.e., cell-wall structure of gram-negative bacteria, from indoor environments. Higher indoor endotoxin was discovered to be inversely associated with the risk of asthma in children across countries (Gehring et al. 2008). High endotoxin amount indoors was believed to indicate the total bacterial load people are exposed to. Importance of endotoxin exposure was also confirmed with experimental studies utilizing mice models (Schuijs et al. 2015). The development of next-generation sequencing, and marker-gene based sequencing techniques revealed that not just gram-negative bacteria, but other bacteria and also fungi indoors associate with reduced risk of atopic diseases.

Farming environments have been central in research of the associations between microbial exposures and asthma and atopic diseases. Farming have been linked to increasing microbial exposures indoors. Several qualified studies have discovered an inverse relation between farming related microbes and risk of asthma and atopic diseases. In two large birth cohorts, diversity of indoor microbiomes was higher in the homes of farmers and their children had reduced risk of asthma (Ege et al. 2011). Interestingly, if microbial community in non-farming home was similar to that of farming home, a child had reduced risk of asthma (Kirjavainen et al. 2019). This finding suggests that microbial exposures instead of some other farming related features are probably explaining the inverse relation between farming and asthma. Indoor microbial exposures can vary between farming homes depending on farming methods used. Both Amish and Hutterite populations in United States still have nineteenth century lifestyle. However, Hutterites have adopted modern agricultural methods while Amish utilize traditional nineteenth century farming. Amish population had richer indoor microbiota than Hutterite population and their children had significantly lower risk of asthma (Stein et al. 2016).

Besides contrasting risk of asthma between farm and non-farm homes, similar disparity has been described between rural and urban areas. In pioneering study testing biodiversity hypothesis, the skin microbiome and allergic sensitization were compared between teenagers living in various environments. Teenagers living in rural environments had more proteobacteria, especially gammaproteobacteria, on their skin, which were also higher on the skin of healthy than sensitized individuals. Authors concluded that there is interlinkages between living environment, skin microbiota composition and the risk of atopic diseases (Hanski et al. 2012; Ruokolainen et al. 2015). The study placed special focus on one type of gammaproteobacterial, Acinetobacter, which is environmental pathogen. It was associated with interleukin (IL)-10 that is an anti-inflammatory cytokine guiding immune system to regulate excessive inflammation. The association between Acinetobacter and IL-10 was dissimilar between sensitized and healthy individuals (Hanski et al. 2012) indicating disturbed cross-talk between skin microbiome and immune system in sensitized individuals.

The linkage between living environment, or related microbes, and immune function has been also described in other studies. For example, the expression of IL-10 increased in Ghanaian children along gradient from urban to rural families (Amoah et al. 2014). In farming studies presented earlier, also linkages to immune function were described. When laboratory mice were exposed to dust collected from the homes of Amish children, the responsiveness of airway epithelia was lower than if mice were exposed to dust collected from Hutterite homes (Stein et al. 2016). This indicates that microbes, or something else in the dust of Amish homes, guides the immune system to regulate its responsiveness better than that of Hutterite homes. Similar immunoregulatory potential was described in a study focusing on the effects of farm-like microbial exposures in non-farm homes (Kirjavainen et al. 2019). The molecular mechanisms behind these associations are not fully understood. However, some evidence suggests that microbial components can influence on epithelial layers. In experimental study, endotoxin as well as farming dust protected mice from allergic symptoms by modifying the communication between barrier epithelial cells in lungs and dendritic cells in epithelium of lungs. This required activation of A20, which is ubiquitin-modifying enzyme that decreases inflammatory reactions in epithelial layers (Schuijs et al. 2015).

Experimental approach has also been used to study the effect of other environmental bacteria. Mice that grew up in gazes including organic soil were compared to mice exposed to hygienic laboratory conditions. Both the gut microbiome and immune responsiveness differed between groups. Part of the mice were artificially turned to asthmatic, which showed that growing up with soil material protected individuals from excessive lung inflammation (Ottman et al. 2019). This interesting discovery indicates that soil exposure may not just prevent disease development, but may also control the severity of disease. In other experimental study, mice were exposed to home dust from the homes either having or not having a dog. Groups had dissimilar gut microbiota as well as differing immune responsiveness. Exposure to dust collected from the homes of dog reduced cytokine production in mice, which associated with hyperreactivity (Fujimura et al. 2014). Thus, experimental evidence supports that enriched microbial exposures can be behind a reduced risk of asthma and atopic diseases in rural and farming children. Yet, the benefits of rich microbial exposures can go beyond these diseases. Mice were exposed to diverse soil bacteria by breathing as authors wanted to control the effect coming from eating the material. Interestingly, high-diversity soil influenced the gut microbiota composition while low-diversity soil only produced comparable results to clean control material. High-diversity soil included environmental butyrate-producing bacteria, which also associated with decreased anxiety-like behavior in mice (Liddicoat et al. 2016). Butyrate is a type of short-chain fatty acid, which are produced by gut bacteria and have been found important in numerous physiological processes. Finding suggested that environmental bacteria, but only if highly diverse, can provide also mental health benefits.

5.8 Bacteria from Environment May Be Essential for Immune System Development

Early childhood is potentially efficient target for preventative approaches for many chronic diseases as some of them are known to have roots in early development and events (Renz et al. 2017). Based on 'Developmental origins of health and disease-hypothesis', there is a sensitive developmental window during first two or three year of life, particularly for immune system and other systems which are immature at the time of the birth. Development during this sensitive period can dictate the health later in life because it sets a baseline for some bodily responses. For example, both low birth weight and preterm birth has been associated with increasing risk for numerous non-communicable diseases (Gluckman et al. 2008). Preterm infants have been shown to have different gut microbiota development when compared to term infants (Healy et al. 2022), and, e.g., asthma risk is higher in children with disturbed gut microbiota maturation (Stokholm et al. 2018).

Current evidence suggests that exposure to environmental microbes can be especially important for developing infants. In Danish study, parents of six-months old infants were asked to vacuum beds of their children and use special filter to collect all dust form the beds. A decade later, this material was sequenced. It was discovered that bacteria in the beds originating from rural living environments associated with reduced risk of allergic rhinitis and asthma later in life (Lehtimäki et al. 2023). In the same cohort, bacteria in the airways of infants, which associated with rural environment, associated with largely distinct immune responsiveness in the airways when compared to urban-associated bacteria (Lehtimäki et al. 2020b). Yet, the composition of bacterial community in the beds and airways of infants were not corresponding (Gupta et al. 2020), which might indicate that environmental bacteria can impact human immune system and health through multiple routes and that environmental bacteria and those in human bodies can both be important for immune system development (Lee-Sarwar 2021).

Recent interventional research supports the hypothesis that environmental microbes can influence on immune function. Greening of daycare yards by adding forest floor and sod associated with increasing diversity of gammaproteobacteria on skin and enhanced immunoregulatory pathways in three to five years old children (Roslund et al. 2020). In another intervention, sand in the sandboxes used for playing was enriched with microbiologically rich forest material. Active and regular playing with enriched sand produced similar changes in children's skin and immune responsiveness as yard greening (Roslund et al. 2022). As sand material was not green, researchers concluded that seeing the green was not source the benefits for immune systems but instead the forest microbes. In coherence with these interventions, children participating to outdoor daycares, in which many hours a day is spent out in natural environments, even sleeping and eating, skin microbiome is remarkably more diverse when compared to children participating to average daycares (Lehtimäki et al. 2018a). These studies provide promising evidence that regular exposure to microbes originating from nature can be beneficial for children, but evidence that these approaches can associate with health later in life is still missing.

Increasing contact with nature can also be important for adults, but it is unclear if this is due to microbial exposures, or some other benefits provided by nature. Interesting evidence arises from immigrant studies showing that moving from low-income country to high-income country leads to increasing risk of non-communicable diseases. The changes in gut microbiome can be important as microbiome tends to westernize when immigrating from low-income country to high-income country (Vangay et al. 2018). Thus, changes in microbiome may mediate the adverse effect of new environment also in adults, pointing that also adult health could be safeguarded with similar actions as in children.

5.9   The Skin Microbiota from the Perspective of Biodiversity Hypothesis

Most microbiome research has focused on gut, probably due to rapidly accumulated evidence about its importance in most, if not all, organ systems and in their health. Active epithelial layers of the gut are closely contacted with gut microbes enabling crosstalk shaping human physiology. Extraction and sequencing of bacterial DNA from fecal samples is rather easy due to high density of bacteria in samples. Skin (and airway) microbiome represents less studied biome due its assumed lesser importance in human systemic immune function. Also, technical challenges relating to the DNA extraction and sequencing of these low-biomass samples influence on popularity to study these.

From the perspective of biodiversity hypothesis both skin and airway microbiomes are highly interesting. Skin and airway microbiomes are more open for colonization from the environment than gut. Stomach acids present a strong selective force, which easily destroys colonizers. Further, anoxic circumstances select only microbes evolved to survive without oxygen. Skin microbiome includes higher number of taxonomic groups than gut microbiome and larger proportion of those are transient (i.e., not part of the permanent or core community). Skin microbiome also resembles soil microbiota while gut microbiome is very distinct from that (Parfrey et al. 2014) indicating that air-borne microbes constitute a significant proportion of skin microbiome. Interestingly, soil microbes transferred to human skin can partly persist on skin a full day (Bateman 2017) indicating both that environmental microbes can modify human skin microbiome, at least short-term, and that composition of our skin microbiome is likely to be largely influenced by surrounding microbial milieu.

Biodiversity hypothesis does not make assumptions whether environmental microbes stimulate human immune system through skin, airways or gut. All these habitats provide ground for communication between microbes and immune system. Previously skin microbiome was suspected to only have a local effect on immune cells, but actually microbes on skin can produce systemic immune responses (Belkaid and Segre 2014). Interplay between skin microbes and epidermal cells regulates immune networks, controls tissue integrity and holds homeostasis of keratinocytes. Thus, skin microbes are central in controlling the barrier function of the skin, being therefore important in the development of skin diseases (Nakatsuji et al. 2017). Thus, openness of skin for colonization from environment and the role of skin microbes in human immune function suggest that skin microbiome is interesting candidate for linking biological diversity and human health.

5.10 Evidence from Other Mammals

Health of humans can have surprising similarities with health of other mammals. For example, pet dogs are more likely to be obese if their owner is obese, more likely to be stressed if owner is stressed and even more likely to be allergic if owner is suffering from allergies (Lehtimäki et al. 2018b). Pet dogs can be relevant model animals to understand the health-impacts of human living environments as their shorter life span, less complex lifestyles and similar disease burden makes them appropriate and easier to study than humans. Skin microbiome of dogs was associated with the living environment and lifestyle of their owners. Dogs living in rural areas in large families and having also other pets around were less likely to develop allergies while dogs living in urban areas living with single persons were more likely to become allergic. Interestingly, allergic dogs had human skin related microbes enriched in their skin (Lehtimäki et al. 2018b) corresponding to the composition of urban environmental microbiomes. Interestingly, dogs and their owners tend to have simultaneous risk of developing allergic diseases (Lehtimäki et al. 2020a), i.e., allergic dog-owners were more likely to have allergic pets. Dogs and their owners partly shared their skin microbiomes, but their gut microbiotas are distinct indicating that environmental or skin related microbes are more likely to explain similarities in allergy risk than gut microbes.

Regular contact between pet dogs and their owners or living in the same household can explain the similarity of their skin microbiomes. In comprehensive comparison between skin microbiotas in humans, other primates and several mammalian orders showed that humans were most distinct from others and their skin microbiota was least diverse (Ross et al. 2018). However, people included to the study only represented urban and western people, which may have influenced on their distance from other, often exotic mammals living in different geographic regions. In another study, human skin microbiome did not correspond to the skin microbiome of their cattle in rural Madagascar (Manus et al. 2017). The contact between humans and cattle is probably less close than between owners and pet dogs sharing sometimes even bed. Yet, the skin microbiota in the angles of both Malagasy people and their cattle were similar, suggesting that living environment is important determinant of skin microbial communities in both species.

Captive mammals have a higher risk in developing chronic diseases that their wild relatives. For example, cardiovascular condition is common in captive great apes. Captive animals have dissimilar gut microbiome than their wild relatives, which likely reflects dissimilar diet and living environment (McKenzie et al. 2017). Changes in the microbiome has been suggested to mediate the adverse health effect of captivity. Thus, mammalian species tend to develop similar diseases as humans in response to factors corresponding to modern human life. Captive animals have been compared to people living in modern cities with limited access to natural environments and traditional diets.

5.11 Biodiversity and Human Health

Importance of both macroscopic and microscopic biological diversity for human health is debated. Scientist have suggested that (macroscopic) biodiversity is likely to be important for human health due to accumulating evidence (discussed earlier) showing that nature in living environment supports human health. Yet, scientific evidence on potential benefits provided by biodiversity is still scarce, mainly because actual exposure to biodiversity is hard to measure. Here, the current evidence is shortly described.

Few studies have attempted different ways of measuring biodiversity instead of just overall greenness in human living environments and associated that to human health. A pioneering study from New-Zealand measured the amount of different natural land cover types, which was used as a proxy of vegetation diversity, in living environments of 50 000 children. Children were followed from birth to adults. Study found that increasing vegetation diversity associated with a reduced risk of asthma (Donovan et al. 2018) supporting the beneficial role of biodiversity. Similar research approach was adopted in Australian study in which associations between vegetation groups and hospital admissions due to respiratory diseases were studied at continental scale. Higher diversity of major vegetation groups within a region decreased regional public hospital admissions due to respiratory diseases (Liddicoat et al. 2018). In rural Finland, diversity of native, flowering plants at home yard was associated with a reduced risk of allergic sensitization in teenagers (Hanski et al. 2012). In Denmark, the number of red-listed species in children's living environments was used a proxy of biodiversity. The risk of severe asthma decreased if nearby environments were biodiverse, but for other types of asthma, no association was discovered (Winnicki et al. 2022). These studies and previously presented studies on environmental microbial exposures indoors and outdoors suggest that biodiversity exposure can be beneficial to human health and thus support biodiversity hypothesis.

As mentioned earlier, biodiversity hypothesis does not suggest that higher diversity of human microbiomes is essential for health. However, this has been common hypothesis in human microbiome research. For many diseases, it has been suggested that decreasing diversity of gut microbiome supports diseases development. This idea was fueled by notion that diversity of gut microbiome is lower in westernized populations who have higher rates of non-communicable diseases when compared to traditional populations with lower risk of these diseases (Sonnenburg and Sonnenburg 2019). However, both increasing and decreasing diversity are reported from diseased individuals, and, even more regularly, no significant diversity differences between healthy and diseased individuals are discovered. However, there is some evidence that lower diversity prior the onset of disease can increase the susceptibility of person to develop non-communicable disease (Karkman et al. 2017). Thus, mixed findings can partly be explained with cross-sectional study designs. Moreover, most studies have focused on westernized populations with lower microbial (gut) diversity as a starting point, which may have impacted on findings. Therefore, the role of diversity in human (gut) microbiome in health and disease remains open, but in outer microbial exposures indoors and outdoors, diversity can be important determinant. Moreover, diverse outer exposures, even if important, do not necessarily translate into diverse human microbiome. Competition and other selective pressures control the number of species in human microbiome regardless of constant colonization by transient members.

5.12 Microbiome Functions as a Part of Total Exposome

Prior twenty-first century, genetics was considered by many as the most important determinant of non-communicable diseases such as cardiovascular diseases and cancers. However, genetic determinism did not find support. Instead, the development of non-communicable diseases is largely influenced by non-genetic, environmental factors, which can be very personalized creating a challenging complexity for research. Non-communicable diseases develop to people with genetic susceptibility, but only if exposed to adverse environment. In medicine, 'environment' usually implies everything external or non-self, basically 'non-genetic factors' including medications, diet, lifestyles and other. This far in this chapter, 'environment' have mean the geographical place or its characters. However, introduction of exposome concept requires looking 'environment' with wider lenses.

The simultaneous exposures to multiple environmental factors are central in exposome concept. It means the total environmental exposures of a person during a lifetime, from prenatal period onwards (Wild 2005). According to the concept, human health is a result of all *lifetime* environmental exposures complementing the genetic susceptibility. Non-communicable diseases usually develop slowly in response to numerous adverse exposures and this mixture widely varies between people. The total exposome of a person builds on three overlapping components. External exposome implies factors outside of a body and can be divided into general and specific external exposome. General external exposome includes social, environmental, and physiological factors such as living environment, geographic region, climate and stress. Specific external exposome includes factors often addressed in epidemiological research such as pollution, tobacco, lifestyle and occupation. Internal exposome is the last component of exposome and compromises from, e.g., metabolism, inflammation, hormones, morphology, and also, microbiome (Wild 2012).

Microbiome is a part of the human exposome. Therefore, considering microbiome as a single disease-promoting or -protecting factor can be far too simplified. For example, urban children were protected from atopic diseases in case both diverse microbiome and diverse set of allergens were present in their homes while neither of these alone reduced the risk (Lynch et al. 2014). This is not an example about exposome study but shows that adding just one explanatory factor more draws more complete picture about disease etiology. Microbiome, as well as other factors included to the internal exposome, can be central in disease development as it may mediate the influences of external exposome. 'Microbial exposome' has been suggested as a distinct component of exposome, which can combine microbial exposures coming from mother, diet, indoor and outdoor air and whether those influence humans through skin, airways or gut (Renz et al. 2017).

5.13 Human Health and Wellbeing Depend on Health of Natural Systems

Earlier sections in this chapter have discussed how humans are mentally and physically healthier when able to visit in green, biodiverse environments, and that microbial exposures can partly mediate the health effects of green environments. Moreover, not just humans, but also other mammals benefit from similar exposures. These ideas are central for 'planetary health' concept that suggests dependence of human health from the health of natural systems. Concept was first presented *The Rockefeller foundation-Lancet commission on planetary health* during 2015 and has rapidly received a large interest from researchers and society. According to the authors of original paper, current human health and wellbeing, which are regardless of many health issues probably better than ever in human history, has been achieved by over-exploitation of natural resources. Therefore, current wellbeing is not sustainable and unless civilization learns how to disentangle health from consumption of limited resources, a dramatic decline in human health and wellbeing is expected during the coming decades (Whitmee et al. 2015). Both exposome and planetary health concepts are guiding the thinking towards the complexity and interlinkages of multiple positive and negative factors in human health research. As in exposome concept, also in planetary health concept, the role of microbiome is considered important. Scientific evidence about linkages between human health and environmental microbial exposures are often provided as examples about planetary health. Besides examples provided in this chapter, microbiome as a component of ecosystem supports functioning of natural systems, which provides essential health and wellbeing benefits for humans (Cavicchioli et al. 2019).

5.14 Key Points

- Non-communicable diseases explain most of the global burden of disease.
- Biodiversity is currently declining at unprecedented scales.
- Biodiversity hypothesis suggests that declining biological diversity and increasing burden of non-communicable diseases are linked via decreasing exposure to immune-stimulating environmental microbes that are maintained by biodiverse ecosystems.
- Hygiene hypothesis and old friends hypothesis are related to biodiversity hypothesis.

- Farming-related indoor microbiome decreases the risk of asthma and atopic diseases via immune-stimulation.
- Urban, built environments harbors homogenous environmental microbiome, which probably do not provide a sufficient immune stimulation potentially associated with increasing risk of asthma and atopic diseases in urban areas.
- As skin and airway microbiomes are open for colonization from the environmental and skin can impact on systemic immune function, they can potentially link biodiversity exposure and human health.
- Microbial exposures can be especially important for infants and small children.
- Focusing only on microbial exposures can be misleading as microbiome presents only one component of human lifetime exposures, i.e., exposome, which together impact human health.
- Popular planetary health concept states that human health is intimately linked to the health of biotic systems on Earth.

5.15　Summary and Conclusion

Biodiversity hypothesis suggests that decline of biological diversity contributes to increasing burden of non-communicable diseases. Link between these global megatrends is suggested to be limited exposure to beneficial, immune-stimulating environmental microbes which provide essential immune-stimulation. Humans, as well as all animals, have evolved surrounded by immense microbial diversity and during millions of years of co-evolution, have developed an intimate dependency to some of these microbial partners. Urban environments and westernized lifestyle may disrupt the exposure to a large proportion of microbial life. This may have caused increasing susceptibility of urban individuals to develop asthma and atopic diseases while people living in rural areas or farms are still exposed to protective microbial exposures that associate with better immunoregulation.

Skin mediates external information to individual. Skin microbes are one source of information. Composition of microbial exposure is defined by many factors, but importantly by the surrounding environment. Already newborn babies experience dissimilar microbial exposures depending on their living environment and this shapes their skin microbiome. This influences the messages travelling from the skin to immune system that tries to answer properly to the current environment in order to maximize the fitness of an individual. Therefore, skin can be the mediator of the associations suggested by biodiversity hypothesis.

Even though biodiversity hypothesis and current evidence appears plausible, scientific evidence remain limited. The complex associations biodiversity hypothesis suggests are hard to address by research, and more longitudinal, experimental, and interventional studies would be needed to strengthen the evidence. Regardless of current knowledge gaps, ongoing decline of biodiversity is alarming from the perspective of the hypothesis. Urgent actions are needed to safeguard biodiversity on Earth to ensure possibility of next generations to live in health-supporting environments.

References

Adams RI, Bhangar S, Dannemiller KC, Eisen JA, Fierer N, Gilbert JA, Green JL, Marr LC, Miller SL, Siegel JA, Stephens B, Waring MS, Bibby K. Ten questions concerning the microbiomes of buildings. Build Environ. 2016;109:224–34. https://doi.org/10.1016/j.buildenv.2016.09.001.

Amoah AS, Obeng BB, May L, Kruize YC, Larbi IA, Kabesch M, Wilson MD, Hartgers FC, Boakye DA, Yazdanbakhsh M. Urban–rural differences in the gene expression profiles of Ghanaian children. Genes Immun. 2014;15:313–9. https://doi.org/10.1038/gene.2014.21.

Antonelli M, Donelli D, Barbieri G, Valussi M, Maggini V, Firenzuoli F. Forest volatile organic compounds and their effects on human health: a state-of-the-art review. Int J Environ Res Public Health. 2020;17:6506. https://doi.org/10.3390/ijerph17186506.

Barberán A, Ladau J, Leff JW, Pollard KS, Menninger HL, Dunn RR, Fierer N. Continental-scale distributions of dust-associated bacteria and fungi. Proc Natl Acad Sci. 2015;112:5756–61. https://doi.org/10.1073/pnas.1420815112.

Baruch Z, Liddicoat C, Cando-Dumancela C, Laws M, Morelli H, Weinstein P, Young JM, Breed MF. Increased plant species richness associates with greater soil bacterial diversity in urban green spaces. Environ Res. (2020);110425. https://doi.org/10.1016/j.envres.2020.110425.

Bateman A. The dynamics of microbial transfer and persistence on human skin. 2017.

Belkaid Y, Segre JA. Dialogue between skin microbiota and immunity. Science. 2014;346:954–9. https://doi.org/10.1126/science.1260144.

Bianconi A, Longo G, Coa AA, Fiore M, Gori D. Impacts of urban green on cardiovascular and cerebrovascular diseases—a systematic review and meta-analysis. Int J Environ Res Public Health. 2023;20:5966. https://doi.org/10.3390/ijerph20115966.

Blaser MJ. The microbiome revolution. J Clin Invest. 2014;124:4162–5. https://doi.org/10.1172/JCI78366.

Cameron EK, Martins IS, Lavelle P, Mathieu J, Tedersoo L, Bahram M, Gottschall F, Guerra CA, Hines J, Patoine G, Siebert J, Winter M, Cesarz S, Ferlian O, Kreft H, Lovejoy TE, Montanarella L, Orgiazzi A, Pereira HM, Phillips HRP, Settele J, Wall DH, Eisenhauer N. Global mismatches in aboveground and belowground biodiversity. Conserv Biol. 2019;33:1187–92. https://doi.org/10.1111/cobi.13311.

Cavicchioli R, Ripple WJ, Timmis KN, Azam F, Bakken LR, Baylis M, Behrenfeld MJ, Boetius A, Boyd PW, Classen AT, Crowther TW, Danovaro R, Foreman CM, Huisman J, Hutchins DA, Jansson JK, Karl DM, Koskella B, Welch DBM, Martiny JBH, Moran MA, Orphan VJ, Reay DS, Remais JV, Rich VI, Singh BK, Stein LY, Stewart FJ, Sullivan MB, van Oppen MJH, Weaver SC, Webb EA, Webster NS. Scientists' warning to humanity: microorganisms and climate change. Nat Rev Microbiol. 2019;17:569–86. https://doi.org/10.1038/s41579-019-0222-5.

Collaborators GCD, Monasta L, Ronfani L. Global, regional, and national age-sex-specific mortality for 282 causes of death in 195 countries and territories, 1980–2017: a systematic analysis for the Global Burden of Disease Study 2017. Lancet Lond Engl. 2017;392, 1736–88. https://doi.org/10.1016/S0140-6736(18)32203-7

Donovan GH, Gatziolis D, Longley I, Douwes J. Vegetation diversity protects against childhood asthma: results from a large New Zealand birth cohort. Nat Plants. 2018;4:358–64. https://doi.org/10.1038/s41477-018-0151-8.

Donovan GH, Michael YL, Gatziolis D, Mannetje A, 't, Douwes, J.,. Association between exposure to the natural environment, rurality, and attention-deficit hyperactivity disorder in children in

New Zealand: a linkage study. Lancet Planet Health. 2019;3:e226–34. https://doi.org/10.1016/S2542-5196(19)30070-1.

Ege MJ, Mayer M, Normand A-C, Genuneit J, Cookson WOCM, Braun-Fahrländer C, Heederik D, Piarroux R, von Mutius E. Exposure to environmental microorganisms and childhood asthma. N Engl J Med. 2011;364:701–9. https://doi.org/10.1056/NEJMoa1007302.

Fujimura KE, Demoor T, Rauch M, Faruqi AA, Jang S, Johnson CC, Boushey HA, Zoratti E, Ownby D, Lukacs NW, Lynch SV. House dust exposure mediates gut microbiome *Lactobacillus* enrichment and airway immune defense against allergens and virus infection. Proc Natl Acad Sci. 2014;111:805–10. https://doi.org/10.1073/pnas.1310750111.

Gehring U, Strikwold M, Schram-Bijkerk D, Weinmayr G, Genuneit J, Nagel G, Wickens K, Siebers R, Crane J, Doekes G, Domenicantonio RD, Nilsson L, Priftanji A, Sandin A, El-Sharif N, Strachan D, Hage MV, Mutius EV, Brunekreef B. Asthma and allergic symptoms in relation to house dust endotoxin: phase two of the International Study on Asthma and Allergies in Childhood (ISAAC II). Clin Exp Allergy. 2008;38:1911–20. https://doi.org/10.1111/j.1365-2222.2008.03087.x.

Gluckman PD, Hanson MA, Cooper C, Thornburg KL. Mechanisms of Disease: Effect of In Utero and Early-Life Conditions on Adult Health and Disease. N. Engl. J. Med. 2008;359, 61–73 Boston. https://doi.org/10.1056/NEJMra0708473.

Grönroos M, Parajuli A, Laitinen OH, Roslund MI, Vari HK, Hyöty H, Puhakka R, Sinkkonen A. Short-term direct contact with soil and plant materials leads to an immediate increase in diversity of skin microbiota. MicrobiologyOpen. 2019;8: e00645. https://doi.org/10.1002/mbo3.645.

Gupta S, Hjelmsø MH, Lehtimäki J, Li X, Mortensen MS, Russel J, Trivedi U, Rasmussen MA, Stokholm J, Bisgaard H, Sørensen SJ. Environmental shaping of the bacterial and fungal community in infant bed dust and correlations with the airway microbiota. Microbiome. 2020;8:115. https://doi.org/10.1186/s40168-020-00895-w.

Hanski I, von Hertzen L, Fyhrquist N, Koskinen K, Torppa K, Laatikainen T, Karisola P, Auvinen P, Paulin L, Mäkelä MJ, Vartiainen E, Kosunen TU, Alenius H, Haahtela T. Environmental biodiversity, human microbiota, and allergy are interrelated. Proc Natl Acad Sci. 2012;109:8334–9. https://doi.org/10.1073/pnas.1205624109.

Healy DB, Ryan CA, Ross RP, Stanton C, Dempsey EM. Clinical implications of preterm infant gut microbiome development. Nat Microbiol. 2022;7:22–33. https://doi.org/10.1038/s41564-021-01025-4.

Karkman A, Lehtimäki J, Ruokolainen L. The ecology of human microbiota: dynamics and diversity in health and disease. Ann N Y Acad Sci. 2017;1399:78–92. https://doi.org/10.1111/nyas.13326.

Kirjavainen PV, Karvonen AM, Adams RI, Täubel M, Roponen M, Tuoresmäki P, Loss G, Jayaprakash B, Depner M, Ege MJ, Renz H, Pfefferle PI, Schaub B, Lauener R, Hyvärinen A, Knight R, Heederik DJJ, von Mutius E, Pekkanen J. Farm-like indoor microbiota in non-farm homes protects children from asthma development. Nat Med. 2019;25:1089–95. https://doi.org/10.1038/s41591-019-0469-4.

Konijnendijk C, Devkota D, Mansourian S, Wildburger C. Forests and trees for human health: pathways, impacts, challenges and response options. (n.d.).

Lee-Sarwar K. The farm-like effect: rural exposures in early life, the microbiome, and asthma. J Allergy Clin Immunol. 2021. https://doi.org/10.1016/j.jaci.2021.04.020.

Lehtimäki J, Karkman A, Laatikainen T, Paalanen L, von Hertzen L, Haahtela T, Hanski I, Ruokolainen L. Patterns in the skin microbiota differ in children and teenagers between rural and urban environments. Sci Rep. 2017;7:45651. https://doi.org/10.1038/srep45651.

Lehtimäki J, Laatikainen T, Karkman A, von Hertzen L, Haahtela T, Hanski I, Ruokolainen L. Nature-oriented daycare diversifies skin microbiota in children—no robust association with allergies. Pediatr Allergy Immunol. 2018a;29:318–21. https://doi.org/10.1111/pai.12872.

Lehtimäki J, Sinkko H, Hielm-Björkman A, Salmela E, Tiira K, Laatikainen T, Mäkeläinen S, Kaukonen M, Uusitalo L, Hanski I, Lohi H, Ruokolainen L. Skin microbiota and allergic symptoms associate with exposure to environmental microbes. Proc Natl Acad Sci. 2018b;115:4897–902. https://doi.org/10.1073/pnas.1719785115.

Lehtimäki J, Sinkko H, Hielm-Björkman A, Laatikainen T, Ruokolainen L, Lohi H. Simultaneous allergic traits in dogs and their owners are associated with living environment, lifestyle and microbial exposures. Sci Rep. 2020a;10:21954. https://doi.org/10.1038/s41598-020-79055-x.

Lehtimäki J, Thorsen J, Rasmussen MA, Hjelmsø M, Shah S, Mortensen MS, Trivedi U, Vestergaard G, Bønnelykke K, Chawes BL, Brix S, Sørensen SJ, Bisgaard H, Stokholm J. Urbanized microbiota in infants, immune constitution and later risk of atopic diseases. J Allergy Clin Immunol. 2020b. https://doi.org/10.1016/j.jaci.2020.12.621.

Lehtimäki J, Gupta S, Hjelmsø M, Shah S, Thorsen J, Rasmussen MA, Soverini M, Li X, Russel J, Trivedi U, Brix S, Bønnelykke K, Chawes BL, Bisgaard H, Sørensen SJ, Stokholm J. Fungi and bacteria in the beds of rural and urban infants correlate with later risk of atopic diseases. Clin Exp Allergy. 2023. https://doi.org/10.1111/cea.14414.

Liddicoat C, Waycott M, Weinstein P. Environmental change and human health: can environmental proxies inform the biodiversity hypothesis for protective microbial-human contact? Bioscience. 2016;66:1023–34. https://doi.org/10.1093/biosci/biw127.

Liddicoat C, Bi P, Waycott M, Glover J, Lowe AJ, Weinstein P. Landscape biodiversity correlates with respiratory health in Australia. J Environ Manage. 2018;206:113–22. https://doi.org/10.1016/j.jenvman.2017.10.007.

Liu X-X, Ma X-L, Huang W-Z, Luo Y-N, He C-J, Zhong X-M, Dadvand P, Browning MHEM, Li L, Zou X-G, Dong G-H, Yang B-Y. Green space and cardiovascular disease: a systematic review with meta-analysis. Environ Pollut. 2022;301: 118990. https://doi.org/10.1016/j.envpol.2022.118990.

Lynch SV, Wood RA, Boushey H, Bacharier LB, Bloomberg GR, Kattan M, O'Connor GT, Sandel MT, Calatroni A, Matsui E, Johnson CC, Lynn H, Visness CM, Jaffee KF, Gergen PJ, Gold DR, Wright RJ, Fujimura K, Rauch M, Busse WW, Gern JE. Effects of early-life exposure to allergens and bacteria on recurrent wheeze and atopy in urban children. J Allergy Clin Immunol. 2014;134:593-601.e12. https://doi.org/10.1016/j.jaci.2014.04.018.

Manus MB, Yu JJ, Park LP, Mueller O, Windsor SC, Horvath JE, Nunn CL. Environmental influences on the skin microbiome of humans and cattle in rural Madagascar. Evol Med Public Health. 2017;2017:144–53. https://doi.org/10.1093/emph/eox013.

Matricardi PM. Prevalence of atopy and asthma in eastern versus Western Europe: why the difference? Ann Allergy Asthma Immunol Off Publ Am Coll Allergy Asthma Immunol. 2001;87, 24–7. https://doi.org/10.1016/s1081-1206(10)62336-8.

McCall LI, Callewaert C, Zhu Q, Song SJ, Bouslimani A, Minich JJ, Ernst M, Ruiz-Calderon JF, Cavallin H, Pereira HS, Novoselac A, Hernandez J, Rios R, Branch OH, Blaser MJ, Paulino LC, Dorrestein PC, Knight R, Dominguez-Bello MG. Home chemical and microbial transitions across urbanization. Nat Microbiol. 2019;1–8. https://doi.org/10.1038/s41564-019-0593-4.

McKenzie VJ, Song SJ, Delsuc F, Prest TL, Oliverio AM, Korpita TM, Alexiev A, Amato KR, Metcalf JL, Kowalewski M, Avenant NL, Link A, Di Fiore A, Seguin-Orlando A, Feh C, Orlando L, Mendelson JR, Sanders J, Knight R. The effects of captivity on the mammalian gut microbiome. Integr Comp Biol. 2017;57:690–704. https://doi.org/10.1093/icb/icx090.

Mhuireach G, Johnson BR, Altrichter AE, Ladau J, Meadow JF, Pollard KS, Green JL. Urban greenness influences airborne bacterial community composition. Sci Total Environ. 2016;571:680–7. https://doi.org/10.1016/j.scitotenv.2016.07.037.

Nakatsuji T, Chen TH, Narala S, Chun KA, Two AM, Yun T, Shafiq F, Kotol PF, Bouslimani A, Melnik AV, Latif H, Kim J-N, Lockhart A, Artis K, David G, Taylor P, Streib J, Dorrestein PC, Grier A, Gill SR, Zengler K, Hata TR, Leung DYM, Gallo RL. Antimicrobials from human skin commensal bacteria protect against Staphylococcus aureus and are deficient in atopic dermatitis. Sci Transl Med. 2017;9. https://doi.org/10.1126/scitranslmed.aah4680.

Ottman N, Ruokolainen L, Suomalainen A, Sinkko H, Karisola P, Lehtimäki J, Lehto M, Hanski I, Alenius H, Fyhrquist N. Soil exposure modifies the gut microbiota and supports immune tolerance in a mouse model. J Allergy Clin Immunol. 2019;143:1198-1206.e12. https://doi.org/10.1016/j.jaci.2018.06.024.

Parajuli A, Grönroos M, Siter N, Puhakka R, Vari HK, Roslund MI, Jumpponen A, Nurminen N, Laitinen OH, Hyöty H, Rajaniemi J, Sinkkonen A. Urbanization reduces transfer of diverse environmental microbiota indoors. Front Microbiol. 2018;9. https://doi.org/10.3389/fmicb.2018.00084.

Parfrey LW, Walters WA, Lauber CL, Clemente JC, Berg-Lyons D, Teiling C, Kodira C, Mohiuddin M, Brunelle J, Driscoll M, Fierer N, Gilbert JA, Knight R. Communities of microbial eukaryotes in the mammalian gut within the context of environmental eukaryotic diversity. Front Microbiol. 2014;5. https://doi.org/10.3389/fmicb.2014.00298.

Pimm SL, Jenkins CN, Abell R, Brooks TM, Gittleman JL, Joppa LN, Raven PH, Roberts CM, Sexton JO. The biodiversity of species and their rates of extinction, distribution, and protection. Science. 2014;344:1246752. https://doi.org/10.1126/science.1246752.

Prober SM, Leff JW, Bates ST, Borer ET, Firn J, Harpole WS, Lind EM, Seabloom EW, Adler PB, Bakker JD, Cleland EE, DeCrappeo NM, DeLorenze E, Hagenah N, Hautier Y, Hofmockel KS, Kirkman KP, Knops JMH, La Pierre KJ, MacDougall AS, McCulley RL, Mitchell CE, Risch AC, Schuetz M, Stevens CJ, Williams RJ, Fierer N. Plant diversity predicts beta but not alpha diversity of soil microbes across grasslands worldwide. Ecol Lett. 2015;18:85–95. https://doi.org/10.1111/ele.12381.

Renz H, Holt PG, Inouye M, Logan AC, Prescott SL, Sly PD. An exposome perspective: early-life events and immune development in a changing world. J Allergy Clin Immunol. 2017;140:24–40. https://doi.org/10.1016/j.jaci.2017.05.015.

Robinson JM, Cando-Dumancela C, Antwis RE, Cameron R, Liddicoat C, Poudel R, Weinstein P, Breed MF. Exposure to airborne bacteria depends upon vertical stratification and vegetation complexity. Sci Rep. 2021;11:9516. https://doi.org/10.1038/s41598-021-89065-y.

Rojas-Rueda D, Nieuwenhuijsen MJ, Gascon M, Perez-Leon D, Mudu P. Green spaces and mortality: a systematic review and meta-analysis of cohort studies. Lancet Planet Health. 2019;3:e469–77. https://doi.org/10.1016/S2542-5196(19)30215-3.

Rook GA. Regulation of the immune system by biodiversity from the natural environment: an ecosystem service essential to health. Proc Natl Acad Sci. 2013;110:18360–7. https://doi.org/10.1073/pnas.1313731110.

Rook G, Bäckhed F, Levin BR, McFall-Ngai MJ, McLean AR. Evolution, human-microbe interactions, and life history plasticity. The Lancet. 2017;390:521–30. https://doi.org/10.1016/S0140-6736(17)30566-4.

Roslund MI, Parajuli A, Hui N, Puhakka R, Grönroos M, Soininen L, Nurminen N, Oikarinen S, Cinek O, Kramná L, Schroderus A-M, Laitinen OH, Kinnunen T, Hyöty H, Sinkkonen A, Cerrone D, Grönroos M, Laitinen OH, Luukkonen A, Mäkelä I, Nurminen N, Oikarinen S, Parajuli A, Puhakka R, Roslund MI, Saarenpää M, Soininen L, Rajaniemi J, Hyöty H, Sinkkonen A. A Placebo-controlled double-blinded test of the biodiversity hypothesis of immune-mediated diseases: environmental microbial diversity elicits changes in cytokines and increase in T regulatory cells in young children. Ecotoxicol Environ Saf. 2022;242: 113900. https://doi.org/10.1016/j.ecoenv.2022.113900.

Roslund MI, Puhakka R, Grönroos M, Nurminen N, Oikarinen S, Gazali AM, Cinek O, Kramná L, Siter N, Vari HK, Soininen L, Parajuli A, Rajaniemi J, Kinnunen T, Laitinen OH, Hyöty H, Sinkkonen A, Group A. Biodiversity intervention enhances immune regulation and health-associated commensal microbiota among daycare children. Sci Adv. 2020;6, eaba2578. https://doi.org/10.1126/sciadv.aba2578.

Ross AA, Müller KM, Weese JS, Neufeld JD. Comprehensive skin microbiome analysis reveals the uniqueness of human skin and evidence for phylosymbiosis within the class Mammalia. Proc Natl Acad Sci. 2018;115:E5786–95. https://doi.org/10.1073/pnas.1801302115.

Ruokolainen L, von Hertzen L, Fyhrquist N, Laatikainen T, Lehtomäki J, Auvinen P, Karvonen AM, Hyvärinen A, Tillmann V, Niemelä O, Knip M, Haahtela T, Pekkanen J, Hanski I. Green areas around homes reduce atopic sensitization in children. Allergy. 2015;70:195–202. https://doi.org/10.1111/all.12545.

Schuijs MJ, Willart MA, Vergote K, Gras D, Deswarte K, Ege MJ, Madeira FB, Beyaert R, van Loo G, Bracher F, von Mutius E, Chanez P, Lambrecht BN, Hammad H. Farm dust and endotoxin protect against allergy through A20 induction in lung epithelial cells. Science. 2015;349:1106–10. https://doi.org/10.1126/science.aac6623.

Selway CA, Mills JG, Weinstein P, Skelly C, Yadav S, Lowe A, Breed MF, Weyrich LS. Transfer of environmental microbes to the skin and respiratory tract of humans after urban green space exposure. Environ Int. 2020;145: 106084. https://doi.org/10.1016/j.envint.2020.106084.

Sonnenburg ED, Sonnenburg JL. The ancestral and industrialized gut microbiota and implications for human health. Nat Rev Microbiol. 2019;17:383–90. https://doi.org/10.1038/s41579-019-0191-8.

Stein MM, Hrusch CL, Gozdz J, Igartua C, Pivniouk V, Murray SE, Ledford JG, Marques Dos Santos M, Anderson RL, Metwali N, Neilson JW, Maier RM, Gilbert JA, Holbreich M, Thorne PS, Martinez FD, von Mutius E, Vercelli D, Ober C, Sperling AI. Innate immunity and asthma risk in Amish and Hutterite farm children. N Engl J Med. 2016;375:411–21. https://doi.org/10.1056/NEJMoa1508749.

Stokholm J, Blaser MJ, Thorsen J, Rasmussen MA, Waage J, Vinding RK, Schoos A-MM, Kunøe A, Fink NR, Chawes BL, Bønnelykke K, Brejnrod AD, Mortensen MS, Al-Soud WA, Sørensen SJ, Bisgaard H. Maturation of the gut microbiome and risk of asthma in childhood. Nat Commun. 2018;9:141. https://doi.org/10.1038/s41467-017-02573-2.

Strachan DP. Hay fever, hygiene, and household size. BMJ. 1989;299:1259–60. https://doi.org/10.1136/bmj.299.6710.1259.

Strachan DP. Family size, infection and atopy: the first decade of the "hygiene hypothesis." Thorax. 2000;55:S2–10.

Tilman D, Isbell F, Cowles JM. Biodiversity and ecosystem functioning. Annu Rev Ecol Evol Syst. 2014;45:471–93. https://doi.org/10.1146/annurev-ecolsys-120213-091917.

Vangay P, Johnson AJ, Ward TL, Al-Ghalith GA, Shields-Cutler RR, Hillmann BM, Lucas SK, Beura LK, Thompson EA, Till LM, Batres R, Paw B, Pergament SL, Saenyakul P, Xiong M, Kim AD, Kim G, Masopust D, Martens EC, Angkurawaranon C, McGready R, Kashyap PC, Culhane-Pera KA, Knights D. US immigration westernizes the human gut microbiome. Cell. 2018;175:962-972.e10. https://doi.org/10.1016/j.cell.2018.10.029.

Vartiainen E, Petäys T, Haahtela T, Jousilahti P, Pekkanen J. Allergic diseases, skin prick test responses, and IgE levels in North Karelia, Finland, and the Republic of Karelia, Russia. J Allergy Clin Immunol. 2002;109:643–8. https://doi.org/10.1067/mai.2002.123307.

von Hertzen L, Hanski I, Haahtela T. Natural immunity. EMBO Rep. 2011;12:1089–93. https://doi.org/10.1038/embor.2011.195.

von Mutius E, Martinez FD, Fritzsch C, Nicolai T, Roell G, Thiemann HH. Prevalence of asthma and atopy in two areas of West and East Germany. Am J Respir Crit Care Med. 1994;149:358–64. https://doi.org/10.1164/ajrccm.149.2.8306030.

White MP, Alcock I, Grellier J, Wheeler BW, Hartig T, Warber SL, Bone A, Depledge MH, Fleming LE. Spending at least 120 minutes a week in nature is associated with good health and wellbeing. Sci Rep. 2019;9:1–11. https://doi.org/10.1038/s41598-019-44097-3.

Whitmee S, Haines A, Beyrer C, Boltz F, Capon AG, de Souza Dias BF, Ezeh A, Frumkin H, Gong P, Head P, Horton R, Mace GM, Marten R, Myers SS, Nishtar S, Osofsky SA, Pattanayak SK, Pongsiri MJ, Romanelli C, Soucat A, Vega J, Yach D. Safeguarding human health in the Anthropocene epoch: report of The Rockefeller Foundation-Lancet Commission on planetary health. The Lancet. 2015;386:1973–2028. https://doi.org/10.1016/S0140-6736(15)60901-1.

Wild CP. Complementing the genome with an "exposome": the outstanding challenge of environmental exposure measurement in molecular epidemiology. Cancer Epidemiol Prev Biomark. 2005;14:1847–50. https://doi.org/10.1158/1055-9965.EPI-05-0456.

Wild CP. The exposome: from concept to utility. Int J Epidemiol. 2012;41:24–32. https://doi.org/10.1093/ije/dyr236.

Winnicki MH, Dunn RR, Winther-Jensen M, Jess T, Allin KH, Bruun HH. Does childhood exposure to biodiverse greenspace reduce the risk of developing asthma? Sci Total Environ. 2022;850: 157853. https://doi.org/10.1016/j.scitotenv.2022.157853.

Chapter 6
Microbiome in Patients with Atopic Dermatitis

Eva Maria Rehbinder, Alexis Rapin, and Niki Ubags

Abstract Patients with atopic dermatitis often have an altered microbiota with decreased microbial diversity and increased colonization of *Staphylococcus aureus* *(S. aureus)*, especially in lesional skin. Whether this dysbiosis is a cause or consequence of atopic dermatitis is still unclear. However, it is known that atopic skin is characterized by increased transepidermal water loss and decreased pH, both indicators of impaired skin barrier function. This defective skin barrier is also associated with lower level of antimicrobial peptides, which further facilitates the colonization and entry of pathogens. Atopic dermatitis most often develops during infancy, when the immune system is still maturing, and early skin microbial colonization and establishment can influence this immune maturation. As the microbiome can be influenced by a number of both endogenous and exogenous factors, it has been hypothesised that variations in the microbial community of the skin during infancy could impact the development of atopic disease. Therapy targeting the gut microbiome through probiotics has been widely studied, but with different approaches and varying results. Directly targeting the skin microbiota is less studied but shows promising results with decreased colonization of *S. aureus* and improvement of the severity. In this chapter we review the available literature on what is known about the skin microbiota in atopic dermatitis patients. We will cover the development of the skin microbiota and its influence on the immune system, the characteristics of atopic skin microbiota and

---

First author has coordinated the book chapter, last author is senior author, otherwise all three authors have contributed equally.

E. M. Rehbinder (✉)
Department of Dermatology and Venerology, Oslo University Hospital, Oslo, Norway
e-mail: e.m.rehbinder@medisin.uio.no

Faculty of Medicine, Institute of Clinical Medicine, University of Oslo, Oslo, Norway

A. Rapin
Laboratory of Integrative Systems Physiology, Ecole Polytechnique Fédérale de Lausanne (EPFL), CH-1015 Lausanne, Switzerland

N. Ubags
Faculty of Biology and Medicine, University of Lausanne, Service de Pneumologie, CHUV, Lausanne, Switzerland

how it is affected by treatment, as well as discuss potential therapies targeting the gut and skin microbiome in atopic dermatitis treatment and prevention.

Keywords Atopic dermatitis · Eczema · Microbiota · Microbiome · Skin barrier · Lesional skin · Immune system · Treatment · Prevention

6.1 Development of Skin Microbiota and Atopic Dermatitis

6.1.1 Skin Microbiome Development and Health

The skin microbiota undergoes drastic changes from the day an infant is born. It has been proposed that exposure to bacterial communities may start *in utero* (Steel et al. 2005; Aagaard et al. 2014; Leiby et al. 2018; Lauder et al. 2016; He et al. 2020; Stinson et al. 2020). However, growing evidence rather point towards a womb without live bacteria prior to labour, in uncomplicated pregnancies (Lim et al. 2018; Rehbinder et al. 2018; Perez-Munoz et al. 2017; Liu et al. 2020; Kennedy et al. 2023, 2021). Although the healthy fetus is most likely protected from direct influence of microbial stimuli (Kennedy et al. 2023; Archer et al. 2023) findings of a diverse set of microbially-derived metabolites in the intestines of second-trimester terminated fetuses may be linked to and indirect microbial role in fetal immune system development (Archer et al. 2023; Li et al. 2020).

During the first days after birth, rapid surface colonization of the skin coincides with significant changes in the skin barrier function (Trompette and Ubags 2023). During this short period, the newborn skin largely differ from adult skin in structure, function, and biochemical composition (Stamatas et al. 2010). Indeed, the skin microbiota is highly variable within the first few weeks or even months of life, but rather evolves over the first year and likely beyond. Timely and proper establishment of a healthy skin microbiome composed of commensal, or non-pathogenic microorganisms, is thought to be instrumental in maintaining skin barrier function and preventing colonization by opportunistic pathogens. The microbial colonization of infant skin is expected to critically affect the development of the skin barrier function, in particular the maturation of the skin immunity and development of the larger immune system (Capone et al. 2011). We elaborate on this topic in the next paragraphs.

Immediately following birth, the skin microbiome composition depends mainly on the birth mode (discussed below) and does not exhibit body-site specificity (Dominguez-Bello et al. 2010, 2016; Chu et al. 2017, Rapin et al. 2023). During the first months of life, the infant skin microbiome is mainly composed of the genera *Staphylococcus*, *Streptococcus* and *Corynebacterium* (Fig. 6.1) (Rapin et al. 2023; Schneider and Nelson 2019) and starts to demonstrate body-site specificity (Chu et al. 2017; Kennedy et al. 2017; Younge et al. 2018). Subsequently, the diversity and biomass of the skin microbiome increases throughout childhood (Fig. 6.1)

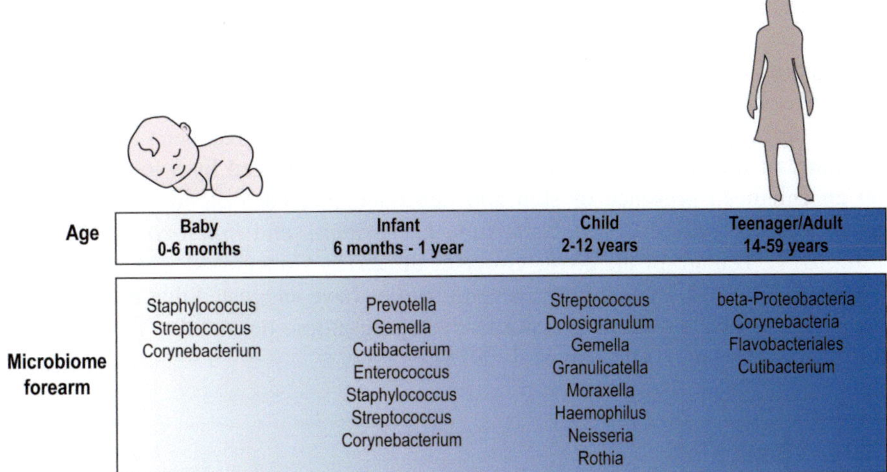

Fig. 6.1 Healthy infant, child and adult skin microbiomes of the forearm. Over time the skin microbiome changes. In early life (0–6 months), the forearm microbiome is dominated by 3 genera (*Staphylococcus, Streptococcus* and *Corynebacterium*). In the months and years that follow, these 3 genera become less abundant, and more genera are detected in a greater abundance. At puberty and towards adulthood the forearm microbiome stabilizes and becomes less diverse. Adapted from paper by Schneider AM, Nelson AM. Skin microbiota: Friend or foe in pediatric skin health and skin disease. Pediatr Dermatol. 2019 Nov;36(6):815–822. https://doi.org/10.1111/pde.13955. Epub 2019 Oct 6. PMID: 31588632

(Capone et al. 2011; Schneider and Nelson 2019), and young children have a more diverse skin microbiome compared to adults (Oh et al. 2012; Schneider and Nelson 2019). Towards adulthood the topographical and temporal differences in the skin microbiome (Gao et al. 2007; Costello et al. 2009; Grice et al. 2009) become more pronounced, and overall remains relatively stable over time in one individual (Grice et al. 2009; Costello et al. 2009).

6.1.2   Factors Influencing Skin Microbiota Composition

Skin microbiota composition can be influenced by a variety of endogenous and exogenous factors, including, but not limited to, birth mode, antibiotics usage, and environmental exposures. In this part, we will discuss the influence of these factors on the skin microbiome composition in early life and adulthood, and their effect on the development of atopic dermatitis.

6.1.2.1 Gestational Age

Preterm birth has been shown to affect the functional development of the infant skin (Stamatas et al. Ped Derm 2010; Nikolovski et al. JID 2008). Moreover, compared to term birth, premature birth (<37 weeks gestational age) has been associated to variations of the skin microbiome composition characterized by a lower diversity and an enhanced presence of skin and gut-associated bacteria such as *Staphylococcus, Streptococcus, Corynebacterium, Escherichia,* and *Enterococcus*; (Pammi et al. 2017; Younge et al. 2018; Groer et al. 2015; Underwood and Sohn 2017; Schoch et al. 2023). Interestingly, several studies have suggested that preterm birth is associated with a decreased risk of developing atopic dermatitis (Tronnes et al. 2013; Siltanen et al. 2001; Zhu et al. 2018).

6.1.2.2 Birth Mode

Over the past decade, several different studies demonstrated that the delivery mode affects the neonate's skin microbiome. Dominguez-Bello and colleagues provided the first evidence that, immediately after birth, children delivered via vaginal birth have bacterial communities which resemble the mother's vaginal microbiome (*Lactobacillus, Prevotella* or *Sneathia* spp), whereas children born via caesarean section acquire bacterial communities similar to the mother's skin microbiome (*Staphylococcus, Corynebacterium* and *Cutibacterium*) (Dominguez-Bello et al. 2010, Rapin et al. 2023). Moreover, by 6–12 weeks of age the difference in the infant skin microbiome based on delivery mode is no longer present (Chu et al. 2017, Rapin et al. 2023), suggesting that although the infant skin microbiome is affected by the delivery mode immediately after birth, this is likely a short-lived effect. However, the potential long-term effects of this initial differential seeding of bacterial communities on the skin remain to be elucidated (Rapin et al. 2023).

6.1.2.3 Antibiotics

The use of oral antibiotics alters the gut microbial composition (Patangia et al. 2022), which may in turn influence immune responses in other mucosal tissues including the skin (Zheng et al. 2020, Campbell et al. 2023). Antibiotics use has been inconsistently linked to an increased incidence of atopic diseases (Droste et al. 2000; Farooqi and Hopkin 1998; McKeever et al. 2002; Schmitt et al. 2010; Yamamoto-Hanada et al. 2017; Kusel et al. 2008; Slob et al. 2020; Ng et al. 2023), and most studies have focused on the use of antibiotics in early life. Although it is known that oral antibiotics usage affects the gut microbiome directly, which may consequently alter local and systemic immune responses, few studies investigated the potential direct effects of oral antibiotics on the skin microbiome composition in humans. Among them, one study including 14 healthy adults, demonstrated that systemic antibiotics had direct long-lasting effects on skin microbial communities including expansion of antimicrobial resistant bacteria (Jo et al. 2021).

Antibiotics are commonly used in the management of atopic dermatitis with the goal to reduce *S. aureus* infection, as this is associated with atopic dermatitis severity. A systematic review of randomized controlled trials concluded that while anti-staphylococcal agents were more efficient in reducing the abundance of *Staphylococci* on the skin in atopic dermatitis patients compared to controls. However, this reduction in *Staphylococci* did not lead to clinical improvement of atopic dermatitis (Bath-Hextall et al. 2010).

6.1.2.4 Environment

The environment also influences the microbial composition of the skin (Grice et al. 2008, Hanski et al. 2012, Callewaert et al. 2020b, Skowron et al. 2021). Extrinsic factors such as UV radiation, climate, physical activity, air and water pollution, hygiene, beauty routine and exposure to chemicals may influence the skin microbiome by affecting its microenvironment, including the availability of nutrients for microorganisms (Skowron et al. 2021). A study performed in India observed a predominance of Proteobacteria on the skin of subjects living in a rural environment, while Firmicutes was more abundant in those living in urban areas (Ramadan et al. 2019). Urban living is associated with higher incidence of atopic dermatitis (Haahtela et al. 2015; Lynch et al. 2014), and in children with AD, Firmicutes has been found to have a higher abundance than in adolescents and adults (Ramadan et al. 2019). Actinobacteria is the bacterial phylum showing the lowest relative abundance on the skin in all age groups in both healthy individuals and atopic dermatitis patients, and a significantly higher relative abundance of this phylum is observed in AD patients compared to healthy individuals, both in adolescents and adults (Ramadan et al. 2019). A change in environment can also have beneficial effects on the skin microbiome in children with atopic dermatitis. The skin microbial composition was significantly altered in children with difficult to treat atopic dermatitis following 6-weeks of alpine climate treatment. In particular, an increase in shannon diversity and a decrease in *S. aureus* abundance load was observed in both lesional and non-lesional skin (van Mierlo et al. 2019). This suggests that the environment may not only influence the development of atopic dermatitis, but also the progression of the disease.

6.2   Skin Microbiota and Immune Responses in Atopic Dermatitis

The microbial colonization of mucosal surfaces is tightly linked to the development and maturation of the immune system (Gensollen et al. 2016). Cutaneous immune responses together with the structural barrier of the skin form a double line of defence against invading pathogens. Over the past years, it has become evident that colonization of the skin in early life is imperative for adequate immune maturation and development of skin barrier function (Scharschmidt et al. 2015, 2017; Ubags et al. 2020; Trompette and Ubags 2023; Cha et al. 2024), and sets its immunological tone. Altogether, the joint maturation of the skin microbiome, the immunity and skin barrier function may set the path to either health or disease.

Cutaneous bacteria are located throughout the epidermal layers and in the hair follicles, of which the latter being the preferred colonization site for commensals (Lange-Asschenfeldt et al. 2011; Montes and Wilborn 1969). The colonization of hair follicle by commensal microbes in the neonate has been associated with T regulatory cell migration via chemokine interactions (e.g., Ccl20-Ccr6) (Scharschmidt et al. 2015). In turn, this influx of T regulatory cells mediates tolerance to skin commensal microbes (e.g. *Staphylococcus epidermidis)* in early but not adult life (Scharschmidt et al. 2017). Recent evidence shows that the skin commensal microbiome may also lead to dynamic postnatal priming of type 2 innate lymphoid cells (ILC2s) in the first weeks of life (Cha et al. 2024).

Moreover, it has been demonstrated that the murine neonatal immune system can discriminate between a colonizing commensal and a pathogen to selectively enable tolerance to commensal species (Xing and Naik 2019; Leech et al. 2019). In addition, recent evidence from murine studies indicates that age and microbiome can determine the nature and severity of allergic skin disease via variations in tissue immune cell coordination (Ubags et al. 2020). In this study, formation of the skin microbiome in early life was shown to drive cutaneous chemokine production and seeding of the skin with antigen presenting cells, which consequently allowed mature antigen presenting cells to localize inflammation to the site of allergen exposure.

It has become increasingly clear that the immune profile associated with atopic dermatitis can differ across ages (Brunner et al. 2018; Czarnowicki et al. 2020). Early-onset paediatric atopic dermatitis is characterized by a Th2/Th17/Th22 driven inflammatory response and lacks the upregulation of Th1 responses that are observed in adult atopic dermatitis (Brunner et al. 2018). Moreover, unique disease endotypes have been observed in infants, toddlers, children, adolescents, and adults (Czarnowicki et al. 2020). However, there is limited evidence from human studies that these immune profiles in different age categories are associated with a specific skin microbiome signature. Although *S. aureus* is strongly linked to the pathogenesis of atopic dermatitis, the role of *Staphylococci* in the establishment of atopic dermatitis had not been investigated until recently. Kennedy and colleagues studied the temporal transition of the skin microbiome in early life and the dysbiosis observed in atopic dermatitis patients. They demonstrated that colonization with commensal *Staphylococci* at 2 months of age could be protective of atopic dermatitis development at 1 year of age (Kennedy et al. 2017).

Using whole metagenome profiling Chng and colleagues demonstrated that skin microbial composition in atopic dermatitis can enhance the risk for atopic dermatitis exacerbations by influencing the cutaneous microenvironment and immune responses (Chng et al. 2016). Specifically, an enrichment in nitrogen, proline and arginine metabolism pathways was observed in the skin of atopic dermatitis patients. These pathways are linked to ammonia production. It is suggested that the atopic dermatitis microbiome utilizes this ammonia to create a less favorable microenvironment for skin commensals, thereby establishing ideal living conditions for *S. aureus,* and other opportunistic pathogens to initiate flares (Chng et al. 2016; Knor et al. 2011). Moreover, reduced production of antimicrobial peptides (Ong et al. 2002) and decreased filaggrin expression (van Drongelen et al. 2014) can also facilitate *S. aureus* colonization (Rippke et al. 2004).

6.3 Skin Microbiota Composition in Atopic Dermatitis Patients

The atopic skin, independent of the presence of dermatitis, is usually dry (Bohme et al. 2000; Rehbinder et al. 2019), with lower levels of natural moisturizing factor and lipids, and exhibits changes in skin barrier proteins (Elias et al. 2008; Yang et al. 2020) that all lead to an impaired skin barrier reflected by increased transepidermal water loss (Werner and Lindberg 1985; Flohr et al. 2010; Rehbinder et al. 2019). In atopic skin, transepidermal water loss is higher in lesional skin than in non-lesional skin (Eberlein-Konig et al. 2000; Werner and Lindberg 1985; Rehbinder et al. 2019), and higher levels of transepidermal water loss is associated with higher skin pH (Eberlein-Konig et al. 2000).

An enhanced skin pH is associated with higher serine protease activity, leading to extracellular corneodesmosomal protein cleavage and decreased corneocyte adhesion and desquamation (Elias et al. 2008). Overall, the defective skin barrier, together with an alkaline milieu and reduced levels of antimicrobial peptides, perturbs the skin homeostasis and facilitates the colonization and entry of pathogens as well as skin microbial dysbiosis (Bradley et al. 2016; Pothmann et al. 2019; Kim and Kim 2019) (Fig. 6.2).

6.3.1 Atopic Lesional and Non-lesional Skin

The microbial diversity is often lower in atopic skin, compared to healthy skin (Kong et al. 2012; Shi et al. 2016; Ramadan et al. 2019; Byrd et al. 2017, Hrestak et al.

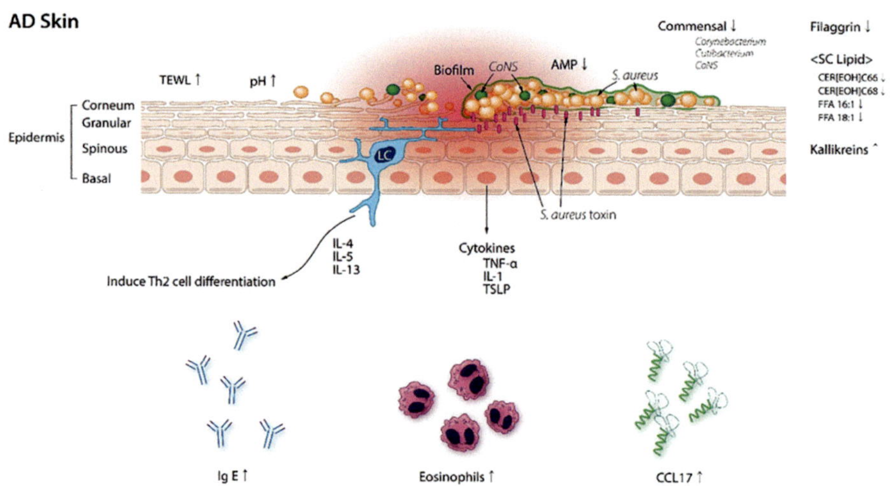

Fig. 6.2 Epidermal barrier disruption in atopic dermatitis skin. Trans-epidermal water loss (TEWL), pH, serum IgE, serum thymus and activated cytokine (TARC/CCL17), and eosinophils are significantly elevated in AD patients. Filaggrin and stratum corneum (SC) lipid composition, and serine protease (Kallikreins) are also altered in AD, allowing *S. aureus* colonization. With the decrease in coagulase-negative *Staphylococci* (CoNS) and its antimicrobial peptides (AMP), *S. aureus* proliferates and also forms biofilms. AD: Atopic dermatitis; CER: Ceramide; FFA: Free fatty acid; IL: Interleukin; *S. aureus*: *Staphylococcus aureus*; TNF: Tumor necrosis factor; TSLP: Thymic stromal lymphopoietin. Reprinted under the creative commons attribution license. Kim, J. E.; Kim, H. S. Microbiome of the Skin and Gut in Atopic Dermatitis (AD): Understanding the Pathophysiology and Finding Novel Management Strategies. *J. Clin. Med.* **2019**, *8*, 444

2022), especially in predilections sites of atopic dermatitis, such as the antecubital and popliteal fossa (Kong et al. 2012). Inter-individual variations in term of skin microbial composition tend to be larger in paediatric populations than in adolescents, with adult populations presenting the lowest inter-individual variations (Shi et al. 2016; Ramadan et al. 2019). The most dominant bacterial phyla on the skin are Firmicutes, Proteobacteria, Actinobacteria and Bacteriodetes (Grice et al. 2008). The relative abundance of the different phyla in the skin is influenced by the body site (for example moist, dry, or sebaceous areas) (Hrestak et al. 2022; Grice and Segre 2011), as well as the age (Rapin et al. 2023, Luna 2020) of the individual.

On the genus level around 15 genera have been found to predominate in the skin of both healthy individuals and atopic dermatitis patients, the most common being *Cutibacterium* (formerly known as *Propionibacterium*), *Corynebacterium*, *Staphylococcus* and *Streptococcus* (Shi et al. 2016; Ramadan et al. 2019). *Staphylococci* are significantly more abundant in both lesional and non-lesional skin of individuals with atopic dermatitis compared to the skin of healthy individuals (Shi et al. 2016; Ramadan et al. 2019). In adolescents *Cutibacterium* is dominating, mainly explained by its lipophilic nature in the sebum rich pubertal skin, while *Streptococci* become more abundant in the adult population. Although clear differences in skin bacterial community composition were found between different age groups in healthy individuals and atopic dermatitis patients (Shi et al. 2016, Ramadan et al. 2019, Luna 2020, Barnes et al. 2022), at present the limited number of studies focusing on the skin microbiome in atopic dermatitis patients permit little conclusive observations due to differences in study design and methods as well as inconsistent results. Figure 6.3 depicts the current notion on how skin microbiota differs between healthy skin and skin with atopic dermatitis (Hrestak et al. 2022). However, the effect of atopic dermatitis on the bacterial community variation is relatively small compared to the much larger general inter-individual variations in bacterial communities that are typically observed (Barnes et al. 2022, Rapin et al. 2023).

A lower skin microbial diversity has been associated with AD, including at non-lesional sites. Not surprisingly, the lowest diversity and largest shifts in microbiome composition were found in inflamed eczematous skin lesions (Kong et al. 2012; Shi et al. 2016; Paller et al. 2019; Ramadan et al. 2019). Culture-based studies have shown that atopic dermatitis lesions were typically colonized with *Staphylococcus aureus*, which was also more commonly found in non-lesional skin compared with the skin of healthy subjects (Leyden et al. 1974). These findings were confirmed by culture-independent metagenomic studies based on high-throughput sequencing of the bacterial 16S rRNA gene, which highlighted higher relative abundances of *Staphylococci* species during atopic dermatitis flares, in particular *S. aureus* and *S.*

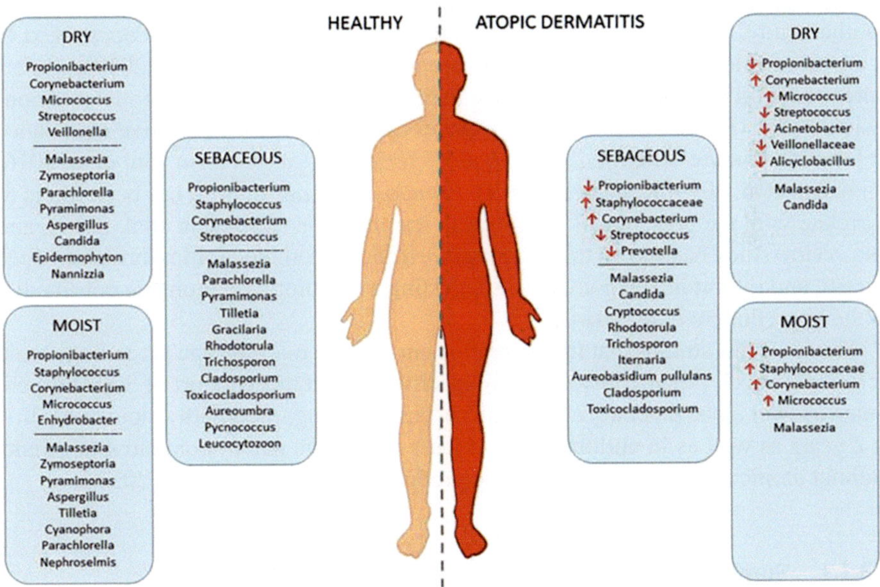

Fig. 6.3 Skin microbiota composition in healthy skin versus skin affected by atopic dermatitis. Reprinted under the creative commons attribution license. Hrestak, D.; Matijašić, M.; Čipčić Paljetak, H.; Ledić Drvar, D.; Ljubojević Hadžavdić, S.; Perić, M. Skin Microbiota in Atopic Dermatitis. Int. J. Mol. Sci. 2022, 23, 3503. https://doi.org/10.3390/ijms23073503

epidermidis (Kong et al. 2012; Shi et al. 2016; Fyhrquist et al. 2019; Moosbrugger-Martinz et al. 2020).

In atopic dermatitis patients, filaggrin, a skin barrier protein, is often reduced, either due to mutations in the gene encoding for filaggrin, or as a result of inflammation. This alteration in the skin barrier integrity together with reduction in certain ceramide subspecies are also correlated with *S. aureus* colonization (Emmert et al. 2020).

While *S. aureus* is largely considered as an opportunistic pathogen, *S. epidermidis* is regarded as a commensal and represents the dominant *Staphylococci* species on the skin of healthy controls (Lai et al. 2010; Kong et al. 2012; Shi et al. 2016; Ramadan et al. 2019), although it can also cause nosocomial infections resistant to antibiotics (Landemaine et al. 2023). The presence of *S. epidermidis* has been proposed to have a protective function against the development of atopic dermatitis in infants (Kennedy et al. 2017). Additionally, the increase of *S. epidermidis* in lesional skin may represent a compensatory attempt to control the destructive behavior of *S. aureus* (Kong et al. 2012). While *S. epidermidis* isolates from atopic or healthy skin may have opposite effect on skin cells, the exact interplay between different strains of S. epidermidis and the host cell in health and disease is still unclear (Landemaine et al. 2023). Moreover, interestingly, shotgun metagenomics have demonstrated that during flares, atopic dermatitis patients are usually colonized with a single *S. aureus* strain, suggesting the outgrowth of a single, dominant, strain (Byrd et al. 2017). In another study, *S. caprae* was found to be the most abundant *Staphylococcus* next to *S. aureus*, while *S. epidermidis* was underrepresented (Ramadan et al. 2019), while a third study did not show any difference in *S. epidermidis* between lesional and non-lesional skin (Kwon et al. 2019). Species found to decrease in relative abundance in lesional skin are *Streptococci*, *Corynebacteria* and *Cutibacteria* (Shi et al. 2016; Ramadan et al. 2019; Kong et al. 2012). *Pseudomonas aeruginosa* has been found to correlate with the presence of *S. aureus* in lesional skin (Ramadan et al. 2019), and one *in vitro* study has shown that *P. aeruginosa* could promote biofilm formation by *S. aureus*, and inhibit its phagocytosis, suggesting a symbiotic relationship detrimental to the host (Fugere et al. 2014).

There are few studies that find alterations in the skin microbiome preceding atopic dermatitis development, however a prospective Danish birth cohort of 300 children, found a lower alpha diversity at 2 months in children diagnosed with atopic dermatitis at 2 years as well as in children with at least one atopic parent compared to infants without atopic dermatitis and no atopic predisposition (Halling et al. 2023).

6.3.1.1 Staphylococcus Aureus

For several decades, it has been established that atopic dermatitis patients are commonly colonized with *S. aureus*, however the number of atopic dermatitis patients colonized have varied considerably from 30% to nearly 100% between different studies (Leyden et al. 1974; Totte et al. 2016). A large meta-analysis from 2016 demonstrated that the pooled prevalence of *S. aureus* colonization was 70% for lesional skin, 39% for non-lesional skin and 62% for the nose in atopic dermatitis patients versus 23% of healthy controls being *S. aureus* carriers in the nose (Totte et al. 2016).

Staphylococcus aureus, a member of the Firmicutes phylum, is a Gram-positive, round shaped bacterium where some of its strains produce staphyloxanthin, the characteristic yellow pigment. It is a facultative anaerobe, acting bosth as a commensal and as an opportunistic pathogen, largely depending on the strain. *Staphylococcus aureus* abundance on atopic skin increases during flares and decreases with recovery, returning to the same state of diversity as before the flare (Kong et al. 2012). *Staphylococcus aureus* secretes different factors that can aggravate inflammation in atopic dermatitis patients and compromise barrier function, as detailed in Table 6.1. The majority of *S. aureus* isolates from atopic dermatitis patients secrete superantigens, such as Staphylococcal enterotoxin (SE) and Toxic Shock Syndrome Toxin-1 (TSST-1), which are involved in hyper-activation of T-cells and cytokine release leading to significant inflammation (Gonzalez et al. 2017; Paller et al. 2019; Wan and Chen 2020), and specific IgE against these molecules are often observed (Travers 2014). Furthermore, in atopic dermatitis, resistance to treatment with topical steroids, such as dexamethasone, has been associated with higher levels of superantigens (Gonzalez et al. 2017). The *Staphylococcal* alpha toxin also forms direct pores on keratinocytes, destroying the barrier which is further potentiated through the presence of Th2 cytokines (Gonzalez et al. 2017; Kim and Kim 2019). *Staphylococcus aureus* also degrades filaggrin through increased serine protein activity, and induces decreased expression of filaggrin in both lesional and non-lesional skin (Gonzalez et al. 2017; Dahal et al. 2024).

Table 6.1 Mechanisms of *S. aureus* mediated severity in atopic dermatitis adapted from Kim J. E., Kim H. S.

Virulence factors	Mechanisms for increased atopic dermatitis severity
α-toxin	Directly forms pores in ketatinocytes, eroding the integrity of the epidermal barrier
Protease	Facilitate dissolution of the stratum corneum
Staphylococcal superantigens (SEA, SEB, SEC, TSST-1)	Trigger B cell expansion and cytokine release from keratinocytes Non-specific APC-mediated T cell activation
Protein A	Triggers inflammatory response from keratinocytes through the tumor necrosis factor receptor 1 (TNFR1)
PSM α	Stimulates keratinocyte production of IL-36, and Th17 inflammation
PSM γ (δ-toxin)	Stimulates dermal mast cells and induces skin inflammation

Microbiome of the Skin and Gut in Atopic Dermatitis (AD): Understanding the Pathophysiology and Finding Novel Management Strategies. J Clin Med. 2019 Apr 2;8(4):444. https://doi.org/10.3390/jcm8040444. PMID: 30987008; PMCID: PMC6518061

SEA, SEB, SEC Staphylococcal enterotoxin A, B, C; TSST-1 toxic shock syndrome toxin-1; *PSM* Phenol soluble modulin; *APC* antigen presenting cells

Other important virulence factors are proteases secreted by *S. aureus*, including V8 protease and exfoliative toxins A and B which are also involved in degrading the skin barrier (Gonzalez et al. 2017; Kim and Kim 2019). Pro-inflammatory staphylococcal lipoproteins provoke keratinocyte apoptosis with the subsequent expression of Thymic stromal lymphopietin (TSLP) resulting in a strong itch response as well as recruitment of Th2 cytokines, thereby further down-regulating the local antimicrobial peptides production (Gonzalez et al. 2017; Kim and Kim 2019).

The propensity of *S. aureus* to form biofilms also contributes to atopic dermatitis severity (Gonzalez et al. 2021) by shielding *S. aureus* from the innate immune response, especially against macrophage phagocytosis and neutrophils (Fig. 6.4). It has also been shown that *S. aureus* biofilms inhibit terminal differentiation and stimulate apoptosis of keratinocytes (Gonzalez et al. 2017; Wan and Chen 2020).

The directionality of the causality between *S. aureus* outgrowth and flare remains to be elucidated. While it has been shown that *S. aureus* present in already established

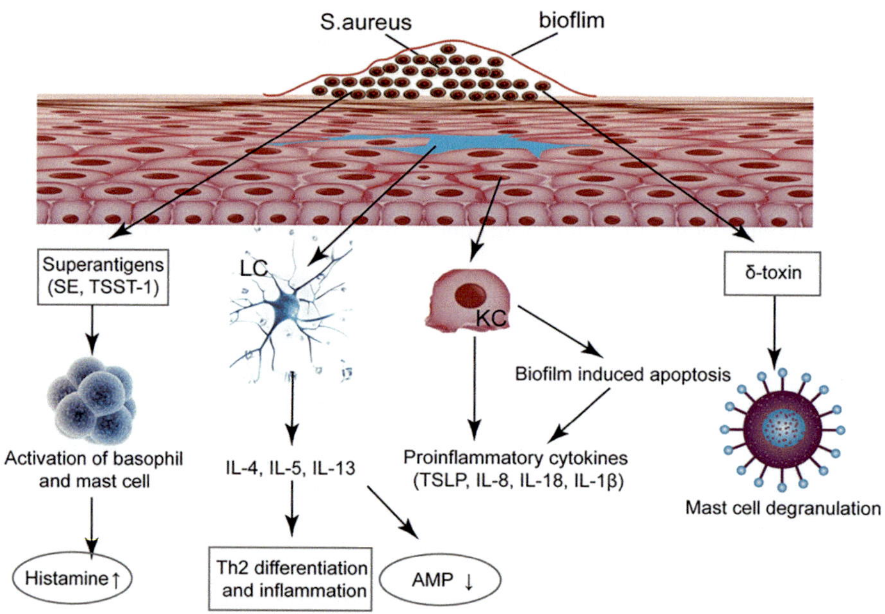

Fig. 6.4 Pathogenic role of *Staphylococcus aureus* involved in atopic dermatitis. *S. aureus* expresses superantigens, such as SE and TSST-1, which activate basophils and mast cell and cause histamine release; *S. aureus* activates LC releasing IL-4, IL-5, and IL-13, which induces AMP reduction and Th2 differentiation and inflammation; *S. aureus* stimulates KC releasing proinflammatory cytokines including TSLP, IL-8, IL-18, and IL-1β and biofilm can induce KC apoptosis releasing inflammatory cytokines; *S. aureus* can release δ-toxin inducing mast cell degranulation. SE staphylococcal enterotoxin, TSST-1 toxic shock syndrome toxin-1, LC Langerhans cell, TSLP thymic stromal lymphopoietin, IL interleukin, KC keratinocyte. Reprinted with permission from Springer Nature. Wan, P., Chen, J. A Calm, Dispassionate Look at Skin Microbiota in Atopic Dermatitis: An Integrative Literature Review. *Dermatol Ther (Heidelb)* **10,** 53–61 (2020). https://doi.org/10.1007/s13555-020–00352-4

atopic dermatitis can further drive the inflammation (Kobayashi et al. 2015; Kim and Kim 2019; Paller et al. 2019; Wan and Chen 2020), few studies have demonstrated an *S. aureus* outgrowth prior to the debut of atopic dermatitis. In a study of 149 infants, *S. aureus* was more prevalent on the skin in those that later developed atopic dermatitis (Meylan et al. 2017), which was in contrast to no increase of *S. aureus* prior to atopic dermatitis debut in 50 infants (Kennedy et al. 2017). However, some studies have found that downregulation of filaggrin expression increases *S. aureus* colonization (Clausen et al. 2017; Miyake et al. 2022), including the findings in a longitudinal study with 326 young children with atopic dermatitis where lower expression of filaggrin in non-lesional skin positively mediated future *S. aureus* colonization (Dahal et al. 2024).

6.3.1.2 Fungi and Viruses

Studies characterizing the fungal communities, or mycobiome, in atopic dermatitis patients with culture-independent sequencing techniques are only emerging, probably due to the technical challenges fungi pose compared to bacteria, which have been widely investigated with such methods (Han et al. 2018). Fungal diversity appears to be less influenced by atopic dermatitis, especially in non-lesional skin where it is comparable to the skin of healthy controls (Moosbrugger-Martinz et al. 2020).

The most dominant fungal phyla in both healthy individuals and atopic dermatitis patients has been found to be Basidiomycota (Sugita et al. 2003; Zhang et al. 2011; Chng et al. 2016; Moosbrugger-Martinz et al. 2020), with some exceptions on specific body locations, such as in the popliteal fossa where Ascomycota are more abundant (Moosbrugger-Martinz et al. 2020; Han et al. 2018). The *Malassezia* species, belonging to the Basidiomycota phylum, is the most dominant microorganism of the skin mycobiome (Tuor and LeibundGut-Landmann 2023). Recent studies showed that this phylum is less abundant in atopic dermatitis patients compared to healthy controls (Bjerre et al. 2017; Moosbrugger-Martinz et al. 2020; Nowicka and Nawrot 2019). However, there is evidence that certain *Malassezia* species are enriched in atopic dermatitis patients, such as *M. dermatis, M. globosa and M. restricta* (Zhang et al. 2011; Chng et al. 2016; Han et al. 2018). The exact role of *Malassezia* in atopic dermatitis pathogenesis is not completely clear, however in atopic dermatitis patients dominated by a dermatitis in the sebaceous areas of the head and neck, a sensitization towards *Malassezia* is frequent (Darabi et al. 2009; Nowicka and Nawrot 2019) (see Fig. 6.5 for details).

Although antifungal treatment may improve the symptoms in patients with head and neck dermatitis, it appears that topical steroids have the same effect (Broberg and Faergemann 1995). In contrast to a decreased diversity in *Malassezia* species in atopic dermatitis patients, there is an increased diversity in non-*Malassezia* species, with increased abundance of *Aspergillus, Candida Albicans* and *Cryptococcus diffluens* (Sugita et al. 2003; Zhang et al. 2011; Bjerre et al. 2017; Han et al. 2018) compared to healthy controls. Fungal microbiota is also affected by the epidermal barrier integrity

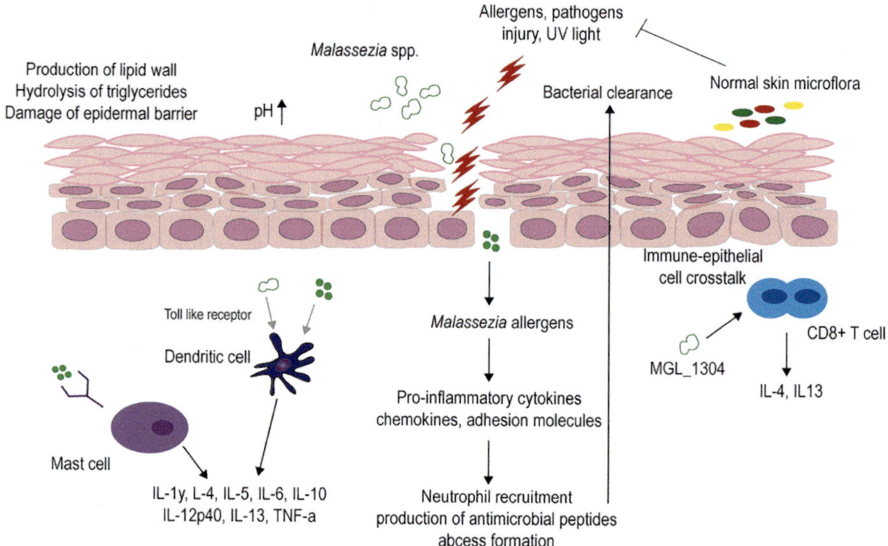

Fig. 6.5 Mechanisms of *Malassezia* spp invasion in atopic dermatitis. Adapted from paper by Nowicka D., Nawrot U. Contribution of *Malassezia* spp. to the development of atopic dermatitis. Mycoses. 2019 Jul;62(7):588–596. https://doi.org/10.1111/myc.12913. Epub 2019 May 15. PMID: 30908750

and alterations in skin pH, TEWL, and lipid composition play a part in the changes seen in fungal composition seen in atopic dermatitis (Kim and Kim 2019).

In addition to bacterial and fungal dysbiosis, patients with atopic dermatitis are more susceptible to common viral skin infections, often with a more severe or persistent course than in individuals with healthy skin (Weidinger et al. 2018), such as pox virus, herpes simplex virus, human papilloma virus or vaccinia virus (Kobayashi and Nagao 2019). There are very few studies on skin virome in relation to atopic dermatitis patients. A small study with 10 atopic dermatitis patients and 5 controls found site-specific dysbiosis involving bacteria, fungi and virus, where Staphylococcus phages were more abundant in lesional samples (Bjerre et al. 2021). Increased human papillomavirus and bacteriophages in lesional and non-lesional atopic dermatitis skin was reported in an abstract (Zaramela et al. 2019), and phage-terapy has been described in mice models (Natarelli et al. 2023).

6.3.2 Skin Microbiota and Atopic Dermatitis Severity

Bacterial diversity on the skin is inversely correlated with the severity score SCORAD (SCOring Atopic Dermatitis), suggesting that severe atopic dermatitis is associated with decreased microbial diversity in the skin (Byrd et al. 2017; Kong et al. 2012; Rauer et al. 2023). In lesional skin, microbial alpha diversity Evenness rather than

Richness has been found to be negatively correlated with atopic dermatitis severity (Rauer et al. 2023; Demessant-Flavigny et al. 2023). The dysbiosis observed in atopic skin has mainly been driven by an increase in relative *S. aureus* abundance, which was positively correlated with SCORAD (Byrd et al. 2017; Kong et al. 2012; Tauber et al. 2016; Rauer et al. 2023). The severity of atopic dermatitis has been found to be positively correlated with the colonization rate and density of *S. aureus* in lesional skin (Totte et al. 2016; Kwon et al. 2019; Alsterholm et al. 2017; Zheng et al. 2019), as well as its ability to form biofilms (Kim and Kim 2019; Gonzalez et al. 2021), while *S. hominis* is negatively correlated with atopic dermatitis severity (Demessant-Flavigny et al. 2023). In 18 patients with varying age the microbial diversity showed only a weak correlation with atopic dermatitis severity in the antecubital fossa (Kwon et al. 2019).

The perioral microbial diversity was correlated to atopic dermatitis severity in infants where a significant decreased abundance of Bacteroidetes and Fusobacterium was linked to increasing disease severity. *Corynebacterium simulans* and *Prevotella melaninogenica* were positively and negatively correlated with atopic dermatitis severity (Zheng et al. 2019). The ratio of two *Malassezia* species seems to vary according to atopic dermatitis severity. *Malassezia restricta* predominates over *Malassezia globosa* in mild to moderate severity, while in severe atopic dermatitis patients the ratio approximates to 1 (Zhang et al. 2011).

6.3.3 Effect of Atopic Dermatitis Treatment on the Skin Microbiota

Daily emollients are recommended in the treatment of atopic dermatitis patients, and have been shown to improve skin barrier, prevent skin infection and reduce flares, which in turn has a corticosteroid-sparing effect (Darmstadt et al. 2014; van Zuuren et al. 2017). A few studies have found that the use of emollients decreases the skin pH and increases the bacterial richness as well as the diversity (Seite et al. 2014; Glatz et al. 2018; Xu et al. 2020; Capone et al. 2023). Emollients containing colloidal oatmeal have been found to decrease *S. aureus* and increase microbial diversity, both in vitro (Liu-Walsh et al. 2021) and in vivo (Capone et al. 2020). A small study observed that *Streptococcus salivarius* was especially increased in the emollient group versus the controls (Glatz et al. 2018). *S. Salivarius* has been shown to decrease pro-inflammatory cytokines and dampen Th-2 mediated response (Eyerich and Novak 2013). The use of emollients may also have a positive impact on the mycobiome, as it has been reported to increase its diversity in non-lesional skin of atopic dermatitis patients (Chandra et al. 2018).

Topical steroids are the standard of care treatment for flares in atopic dermatitis patients (Wollenberg et al. 2022) and quickly cause local vasocontriction, inhibit proliferation and inflammation, and lead to immunosuppression (Bolognia et al. 2008). Studies have shown that treatment with topical steroids alone reduce *S.*

aureus colonization (Kong et al. 2012; Gonzalez et al. 2016; Kwon et al. 2019) in addition to increasing the bacterial diversity (Kong et al. 2012; Gonzalez et al. 2016) alone, without an additive effect of neither bleach baths (Gonzalez et al. 2016) or narrow-band UVB treatment (Kwon et al. 2019). The topical application of the calcineurin inhibitor tacrolimus on atopic dermatitis lesions, another commonly used anti-inflammatory agent, was associated with increased diversity, and increased abundances of certain genera including *Dermacoccus, Pseudomonas, Corynebacterium, Proteus, Micrococcus Luteus* and *Lactococcus* (Wongpiyabovorn et al. 2019).

UVB radiation has known antimicrobial properties and studies have found an effect in increasing microbial diversity and reducing *S. aureus* colonization in atopic dermatitis patients where UVB-treatment has been applied without the concomitant treatment of topical steroids (Dotterud et al. 2008; Silva et al. 2006). However, another study only found a transient shift towards higher microbial diversity in lesional skin after UVB-treatment, but no changes in *S. aureus* colonization was observed (Lossius et al. 2022). Glycerol, a humectant often used in emollients in concentrations of 20–30%, has been shown to have antimicrobial properties in *in vitro* studies, and in study comparing the application of 85% glycerol and NB-UVB showed similar results in *S. aureus* eradication (Youssef et al. 2020). Coal tar, one of the oldest topical therapies with antimicrobial properties has been found to reduce *Staphylococcus* species, however not specifically *S. aureus*, and additionally increase *Cutibacterium* when applied as atopic dermatitis treatment (Smits et al. 2020). Although a small study has found that antibacterial treatment with bleach bath and the application of the antiseptic cream mupirocin intranasally improves atopic dermatitis severity (Huang et al. 2009), a systematic review did not find any evidence that commonly used antistaphylococcal interventions are beneficial in the treatment of atopic dermatitis without clinical superinfection. Moreover, there was no significant difference between topical steroids alone and combination of topical steroids with topical antibiotics (Bath-Hextall et al. 2010). Targeting inflammation seems promising as a therapeutic strategy to improve atopic dermatitis severity while reducing the *S. aureus* colonization and increasing skin microbial diversity. Dupilumab, an IL-4 and IL-13 inhibitor for treatment of moderate to severe atopic dermatitis has been found to improve the dysbiosis in both lesional and non-lesional skin with decrease in *S. aureus* and increased microbial diversity (Bieber 2020, Callewaert et al. 2020a, Hartmann et al. 2023), with similar findings reported for the IL-13 inhibitor, Tralokinumab (Beck et al. 2023). Other, more experimental atopic dermatitis therapies that have been shown to influence the skin microbiome by mainly targeting *S. aureus* include climatotherapy (Brandwein et al. 2019), textiles with antimicrobial properties (Lopes et al. 2015), gentian violet (Krzysiek et al. 2023), niclosamide (Weiss et al. 2022), indolicidin derivative (antimicrobial peptide) (Niemeyer-van der Kolk et al. 2020), bleach baths (Gonzalez et al. 2016) and coal tar (Smits et al. 2020).

6.4 Microbiome in Other Organs in Patients with Atopic Dermatitis

Given that the human body is a complex organism in which inter-organ interaction and crosstalk is imperative for the maintenance of its health, it is important to consider the involvement of other mucosal surfaces in the disease setting. Patients with atopic dermatitis often suffer from a wide range of allergic diseases including food allergies, allergic rhinitis and allergic asthma, suggestive of a crosstalk between the different organ systems affected, including the intestine and upper and lower respiratory tract (Nibbering and Ubags 2020). In this section, we will provide an overview of how these organ systems are affected in atopic dermatitis and how they are involved in disease development and progression, with a focus on the microbiome.

6.4.1 Atopic Dermatitis and the Gut Microbiome

In recent years, it has become increasingly clear that alterations of the gut microbiome in early life are linked to the development of allergic disease (Gensollen and Blumberg 2017; Bisgaard et al. 2011; Simonyte Sjodin et al. 2019). Moreover, it has been demonstrated that the intestinal microbiome is altered in subjects with atopic dermatitis (Lee et al. 2018, Saoin et al. 2018, Wopereis et al. 2018, Abrahamsson et al. 2012, Kirjavainen et al. 2002, Watanabe et al. 2003, Mah et al. 2006, Penders et al. 2006, Penders et al. 2007, van Nimwegen et al. 2011). Specifically, gut microbiome diversity was observed to be decreased in infants who developed atopic dermatitis at 6 months (Forno et al. 2008) and 2 years of age (Abrahamsson et al. 2012). In line with this, analysis of the gut microbiome composition in the CHILD birth cohort study indicated that increased bacterial diversity in 3 months old infants was associated with a protective effect on the development of allergic diseases at 1 year of age, including atopic dermatitis (Boutin et al. 2020). Alterations in bacterial diversity of the gut microbiome were linked to a decrease in Bacteroidetes phyla and more specifically *Bacteroides* genus in 1 month old infants (Abrahamsson et al. 2012). Moreover, colonization with *Clostridium difficile* was associated with a higher risk for the development of atopic dermatitis and other allergic diseases in analysis of the KOALA birth cohort study (Penders et al. 2007). Together this suggests an important influence of the gut microbial composition in the development of atopic dermatitis in early life.

The first indications for the mechanisms underlying the link between the gut microbiome composition and atopic dermatitis development and progression are associated with altered bacterial metabolite production, and in particular short-chain fatty acids (SCFA). Analysis of SCFA levels in fecal content of children enrolled in the PASTURE birth cohort study revealed a trend towards a lower atopic dermatitis incidence in children with high butyrate levels (Roduit et al. 2019). Moreover, the abundance of *Faecalibacterium prausnitzii*, a poor butyrate producer, was found increased in the gut of subjects with atopic dermatitis and concomitantly faecal butyrate levels were found to be reduced (Song et al. 2016). Interestingly, Cait and colleagues observed that the gut microbiome of infants who developed allergic disease in childhood have a reduced genetic potential for butyrate fermentation (Cait et al. 2019). It has been shown that SCFA can affect haematopoiesis, which leads to a dampening in Th2 immune responses in other allergic diseases such as allergic asthma (Trompette et al. 2014). High fiber diet feeding and increased SCFA can improve epidermal barrier integrity by altering the mitochondrial metabolism of epidermal keratinocytes and the production of key structural components of the skin (Trompette et al. 2022). Ultimately, this led to limited allergen sensitization via the skin and reduced development of atopic dermatitis like skin inflammation.

Further evidence of a gut-skin axis mediated by systemic modulation of immunity was found in the reported negative association between *H. pylori*, known for promoting gastric ulcers or cancer, and atopic dermatitis. Studies in mice further showed that *H. pylori* exhibits a systemic anti-inflammatory effect by promoting T regulatory cells proliferation. More generally, the reduced prevalence of *H. pylori* across populations has been proposed to underlie the allergic disease epidemic observed in developed areas, in the context of the "hygiene hypothesis" (Arnold et al. 2011; Blaser and Falkow 2009). In contrast, inflammatory bowel diseases, which are characterized by a chronic inflammation of the intestine and a dysbiosis, are often accompanied with skin manifestation in which Th1, Th2 and Th17 immunity are involved (Huang et al. 2012). Altogether, this suggests that the gut microbiome could lead to opposite effects on the skin depending on whether it promotes or suppresses inflammation systemically.

6.5 Skin Microbiota as Target in Atopic Dermatitis Therapy

6.5.1 Topical Treatments

A few studies show promising results concerning topical application of either bacterial strains or lysates to improve the microbial dysbiosis and atopic dermatitis severity (Habeebuddin et al. 2022). Most of the studies use different vehicles containing different probiotic strains, including Lactobacilli, Bifidobacteria, Streptococci, Roseomonas, Vitreoscilla and Nitrosomonas, and have found decrease in atopic dermatitis severity, and in *S. aureus* colonization (Seité et al. 2017; Blanchet-Rethore et al. 2017; Myles et al. 2020; Silverberg et al. 2023). Coagulase-negative *Staphylococcus* (CoNS) collected from healthy skin was found to have antimicrobial properties and reduced *S. aureus* colonization both in murine and human skin. This was not however true for the strains collected from lesional atopic dermatitis skin (Nakatsuji et al. 2021a, 2021b). Moisturizers containing lysates of *Vitreoscilla filiformis* have been shown to significantly reduce episodes of flare-ups and normalize skin microbiota in atopic dermatitis patients (Gueniche et al. 2008). A recent study with almost 400 participants investigating a cream containing a mixture of prebiotics and postbiotics found decrease in atopic dermatitis severity scores, however they did not include a control group (Gelmetti et al. 2023).

6.5.2 Oral Probiotics and Prebiotics

Beside topical interventions on the skin microbiome, oral probiotic products with systemic effects have been proposed to prevent and improve skin conditions (Al-Ghazzewi and Tester 2014).

6.5.2.1 Oral Probiotics and the Treatment of Atopic Dermatitis

A number of small double-blind randomized placebo controlled clinical trials were conducted to assess the potential of various bacterial strains for the treatment of atopic dermatitis in children and adults. These studies focused on species of *Lactobacillus*, *Bifidobacterium* and *Cutibacterium* with pre-existing probiotic claims using a variety of formulations including single strains, combination of multiple strains, either as live or heat-killed bacteria, and in the form of drinks, fermented yogurts or enriched diets administered over 4–12 week periods (Isolauri et al. 2008; Rosenfeldt et al. 2003; Viljanen et al. 2005; Matsumoto et al. 2014, 2007; Roessler et al. 2008; Drago et al. 2011; Inoue et al. 2014; Moroi et al. 2011). The results ranged from no to moderate positive effects on atopic dermatitis symptoms. The mechanisms underlying possible effects on the skin are not fully deciphered, but are proposed to involve a systemic regulation of type 2 immunity through an increased production of intestinal SCFAs that promote the differentiation of T regulatory cells (O'Neill et al. 2016; Lee et al. 2018). Interestingly, one study using a strain of *Bifidobacterium animalis* suggested that higher intestinal levels of kynurenic acid, a product of tryptophan metabolism, which were associated with the probiotic supplementation in a small group of subjects, may mediate an antipruritic effect through neuro-modulation (Matsumoto et al. 2014). In line with this possibility, variations in the gut microbiome composition were associated with variations of circulating levels of neuroendocrines associated with atopic dermatitis symptoms. Altogether, this suggests that a gut-brain-skin axis could be exploited for therapeutic interventions (Jin et al. 2014; Cryan and Dinan 2012; O'Neill et al. 2016; Sinha et al. 2021). Overall, the power of these clinical trials was largely limited by small cohort sizes and the fact that the observed effect of oral probiotics may be confounded in the effect of standard atopic dermatitis treatments, which were not discontinued during the trials. Systematic meta-analyses of Randomized Controlled Trials highlighted that only weak evidence support a positive effect of probiotics on SCORAD in children with atopic dermatitis, and that such effect may depend not only on the probiotic strain, or combination of strains, but also on the children´s age and living location (Panduru et al. 2015; Chang et al. 2016; Huang et al. 2017; Xue et al. 2023).

6.5.2.2   Oral Probiotics and the Prevention of Atopic Dermatitis

Studies in mice have shown that beyond its immunomodulatory aspects, the microbiome plays an important role in the development and maturation of the host immune system, and that perturbation of the gut microbiome in early life can affect the immune system in a way that persists into adulthood (Al-Asmakh and Zadjali 2015; Gensollen and Blumberg 2017; Gensollen et al. 2016; Olszak et al. 2012). As atopic dermatitis typically establishes during childhood, it has been proposed that perturbations in the establishment of the microbiome in early life may lead to the onset of the disease (Gensollen and Blumberg 2017). In this context, interventions aiming at preventing the development of allergic disorders in children using live bacteria supplementation in babies or in mothers during the gestation period, were investigated in a number of double-blind, placebo controlled randomized clinical trials, and led to mixed results (Kalliomaki et al. 2001, 2003; Rautava et al. 2002; Kukkonen et al. 2007; Taylor et al. 2007; Wickens et al. 2008). Interestingly, despite the lack of conclusive results, a meta-analysis from 2008 suggested that the potential benefit of probiotic supplementation may be higher for preventive interventions than for the therapeutic treatment of established atopic dermatitis in children. However, it was mentioned that this observation may be due to the fact that the study size was generally larger for trials for preventive interventions compared to trials for treatments (Lee et al. 2008; Dotterud et al. 2010; Wickens et al. 2012, 2018; Enomoto et al. 2014; Bertelsen et al. 2014; Allen et al. 2014; Simpson et al. 2015; Cabana et al. 2017; Schmidt et al. 2019). Although based on relatively weak evidences and while the underlying mechanisms remain to be understood, systematic reviews and meta-analyses showed that probiotics, including strains of *Lactobacillus, Bifidobacterium and Cutibacterium* may reduce the risk of atopic dermatitis when administered prenatally or within the first months of life, and not when administered later in life (Fiocchi et al. 2015; Cuello-Garcia et al. 2015; Li et al. 2019; Amalia et al. 2020; Tan-Lim et al. 2021; Panduru et al. 2015; Doege et al. 2012; Pelucchi et al. 2012; Mansfield et al. 2014; Cao et al. 2015; Zuccotti et al. 2015; Anania et al. 2022).

6.6   Concluding Remarks

Patients with atopic dermatitis more often present with a dysbiotic skin microbiome compared to healthy individuals. The lowest microbial diversity is found in the lesional atopic skin, however non-lesion skin is also affected. *Staphylococcus aureus* is thriving in atopic dermatitis lesions and its pathogenic properties exacerbate the disease, further driving the inflammatory response. Treating the inflammation in itself is efficient in reducing the *S. aureus* load and restoring a more diverse microbiome.

Moreover, promising studies trying to enhance commensal skin bacteria in atopic dermatitis lesions may lead to novel topical steroid sparing therapies. However, atopic dermatitis is a complex disease with different phenotypes and endotypes, and identifying the patients who may benefit from microbiome targeted therapy will likely be difficult. The skin microbiome in atopic dermatitis patients remains a relatively new field of study and is dominated by small clinical studies focusing on specific age groups, sampling sites and analysis methods. Some results, such as regarding the *S. aureus* role in lesional skin, have been quite consistent, whereas others, such as the effects of microbiome targeted interventions, have not. Therefore, it is imperative for the field to conduct larger studies to determine whether promoting a more balanced skin microbiome could potentially prevent or treat already established atopic dermatitis.

References

Aagaard K, Ma J, Antony KM, Ganu R, Petrosino J, Versalovic J. The placenta harbors a unique microbiome. Sci Transl Med. 2014;6:237ra65.

Abrahamsson TR, Jakobsson HE, Andersson AF, Bjorksten B, Engstrand L, Jenmalm MC. Low diversity of the gut microbiota in infants with atopic eczema. J Allergy Clin Immunol. 2012;129:434–40, 440 e1–2.

Al-Asmakh M, Zadjali F. Use of germ-free animal models in microbiota-related research. J Microbiol Biotechnol. 2015;25:1583–8.

Al-Ghazzewi FH, Tester RF. Impact of prebiotics and probiotics on skin health. Benef Microbes. 2014;5:99–107.

Allen SJ, Jordan S, Storey M, Thornton CA, Gravenor MB, Garaiova I, Plummer SF, Wang D, Morgan G. Probiotics in the prevention of eczema: a randomised controlled trial. Arch Dis Child. 2014;99:1014–9.

Alsterholm M, Strombeck L, Ljung A, Karami N, Widjestam J, Gillstedt M, Ahren C, Faergemann J. Variation in *Staphylococcus aureus* colonization in relation to disease severity in adults with atopic dermatitis during a five-month follow-up. Acta Derm Venereol. 2017;97:802–7.

Amalia N, Orchard D, Francis KL, King E. Systematic review and meta-analysis on the use of probiotic supplementation in pregnant mother, breastfeeding mother and infant for the prevention of atopic dermatitis in children. Australas J Dermatol. 2020;61:e158–73.

Anania C, Brindisi G, Martinelli I, Bonucci E, D'orsi M, Ialongo S, Nyffenegger A, Raso T, Spatuzzo M, de Castro G, Zicari AM, Carraro C, Piccioni MG, Olivero F.. Probiotics function in preventing atopic dermatitis in children. Int J Mol Sci. 2022;23.

Archer D, Perez-Munoz ME, Tollenaar S, Veniamin S, Cheng CC, Richard C, Barreda DR, Field CJ, Walter J. The importance of the timing of microbial signals for perinatal immune system development. Microbiome Res Rep. 2023;2:11.

Arnold IC, Dehzad N, Reuter S, Martin H, Becher B, Taube C, Muller A. Helicobacter pylori infection prevents allergic asthma in mouse models through the induction of regulatory T cells. J Clin Invest. 2011;121:3088–93.

Barnes CJ, Clausen ML, Asplund M, Rasmussen L, Olesen CM, Yüsel YT, Andersen PS, Litman T, Hansen AJ, Agner T. Temporal and spatial variation of the skin-associated bacteria from healthy participants and atopic dermatitis patients. mSphere. 2022;7:e0091721.

Bath-Hextall FJ, Birnie AJ, Ravenscroft JC, Williams HC. Interventions to reduce Staphylococcus aureus in the management of atopic eczema: an updated Cochrane review. Br J Dermatol. 2010;163:12–26.

Beck LA, Bieber T, Weidinger S, Tauber M, Saeki H, Irvine AD, Eichenfield LF, Werfel T, Arlert P, Jiang L, Røpke M, Paller AS. Tralokinumab treatment improves the skin microbiota by increasing the microbial diversity in adults with moderate-to-severe atopic dermatitis: Analysis of microbial diversity in ECZTRA 1, a randomized controlled trial. J Am Acad Dermatol. 2023;88:816–23.

Bertelsen RJ, Brantsaeter AL, Magnus MC, Haugen M, Myhre R, Jacobsson B, Longnecker MP, Meltzer HM, London SJ. Probiotic milk consumption in pregnancy and infancy and subsequent childhood allergic diseases. J Allergy Clin Immunol. 2014;133(165–71):e1-8.

Bieber T. Targeting T2 inflammation by dupilumab impacts on the microbiomic "menage a trois" of atopic dermatitis. J Invest Dermatol. 2020;140:15–7.

Bisgaard H, Li N, Bonnelykke K, Chawes BL, Skov T, Paludan-Muller G, Stokholm J, Smith B, Krogfelt KA. Reduced diversity of the intestinal microbiota during infancy is associated with increased risk of allergic disease at school age. J Allergy Clin Immunol. 2011;128:646–52 e1–5.

Bjerre RD, Bandier J, Skov L, Engstrand L, Johansen JD. The role of the skin microbiome in atopic dermatitis: a systematic review. Br J Dermatol. 2017;177:1272–8.

Bjerre RD, Holm JB, Palleja A, Sølberg J, Skov L, Johansen JD. Skin dysbiosis in the microbiome in atopic dermatitis is site-specific and involves bacteria, fungus and virus. BMC Microbiol. 2021;21:256.

Blanchet-Rethore S, Bourdes V, Mercenier A, Haddar CH, Verhoeven PO, Andres P. Effect of a lotion containing the heat-treated probiotic strain *Lactobacillus johnsonii* NCC 533 on *Staphylococcus aureus* colonization in atopic dermatitis. Clin Cosmet Investig Dermatol. 2017;10:249–57.

Blaser MJ, Falkow S. What are the consequences of the disappearing human microbiota? Nat Rev Microbiol. 2009;7:887–94.

Bohme M, Svensson A, Kull I, Wahlgren CF. Hanifin's and Rajka's minor criteria for atopic dermatitis: which do 2-year-olds exhibit? J Am Acad Dermatol. 2000;43:785–92.

Bolognia J, Jorizzo JL, Rapini RP. Dermatology, Mosby/Elsevier; 2008.

Boutin RCT, Sbihi H, Dsouza M, Malhotra R, Petersen C, Dai D, Sears MR, Moraes TJ, Becker AB, Azad MB, Mandhane PJ, Subbarao P, Finlay BB, Turvey SE. Mining the infant gut microbiota for therapeutic targets against atopic disease. Allergy. 2020;75:2065–8.

Bradley CW, Morris DO, Rankin SC, Cain CL, Misic AM, Houser T, Mauldin EA, Grice EA. Longitudinal evaluation of the skin microbiome and association with microenvironment and treatment in canine atopic dermatitis. J Invest Dermatol. 2016;136:1182–90.

Brandwein M, Fuks G, Israel A, Sabbah F, Hodak E, Szitenberg A, Harari M, Steinberg D, Bentwich Z, Shental N, Meshner S. Skin microbiome compositional changes in atopic dermatitis accompany dead sea climatotherapy. Photochem Photobiol. 2019;95:1446–53.

Broberg A, Faergemann J. Topical antimycotic treatment of atopic dermatitis in the head/neck area. A double-blind randomised study. Acta Derm Venereol. 1995;75:46–9.

Brunner PM, Israel A, Zhang N, Leonard A, Wen HC, Huynh T, Tran G, Lyon S, Rodriguez G, Immaneni S, Wagner A, Zheng X, Estrada YD, Xu H, Krueger JG, Paller AS, Guttman-Yassky E. Early-onset pediatric atopic dermatitis is characterized by TH2/TH17/TH22-centered inflammation and lipid alterations. J Allergy Clin Immunol. 2018;141:2094–106.

Byrd AL, Deming C, Cassidy SKB, Harrison OJ, Ng WI, Conlan S, Program NCS, Belkaid Y, Segre JA, Kong HH. *Staphylococcus aureus* and Staphylococcus epidermidis strain diversity underlying pediatric atopic dermatitis. Sci Transl Med. 2017;9.

Cabana MD, Mckean M, Caughey AB, Fong L, Lynch S, Wong A, Leong R, Boushey HA, Hilton JF. Early probiotic supplementation for eczema and asthma prevention: a randomized controlled trial. Pediatrics. 2017;140.

Cait A, Cardenas E, Dimitriu PA, Amenyogbe N, Dai D, Cait J, Sbihi H, Stiemsma L, Subbarao P, Mandhane PJ, Becker AB, Moraes TJ, Sears MR, Lefebvre DL, Azad MB, Kollmann T, Turvey SE, Mohn WW. Reduced genetic potential for butyrate fermentation in the gut microbiome of infants who develop allergic sensitization. J Allergy Clin Immunol. 2019;144(1638–1647): e3.

Callewaert C, Nakatsuji T, Knight R, Kosciolek T, Vrbanac A, Kotol P, Ardeleanu M, Hultsch T, Guttman-Yassky E, Bissonnette R, Silverberg JI, Krueger J, Menter A, Graham NMH, Pirozzi G, Hamilton JD, Gallo RL. IL-4Ralpha blockade by dupilumab decreases *Staphylococcus aureus* colonization and increases microbial diversity in atopic dermatitis. J Invest Dermatol. 2020a;140(191–202): e7.

Callewaert C, Ravard Helffer K, Lebaron P.. Skin Microbiome and its Interplay with the environment. Am J Clin Dermatol. 2020b;21:4–11.

Campbell C, Kandalgaonkar MR, Golonka RM, Yeoh BS, Vijay-Kumar M, Saha P. Crosstalk between gut microbiota and host immunity: impact on inflammation and immunotherapy. Biomedicines. 2023;11.

Cao L, Wang L, Yang L, Tao S, Xia R, Fan W. Long-term effect of early-life supplementation with probiotics on preventing atopic dermatitis: a meta-analysis. J Dermatolog Treat. 2015;26:537–40.

Capone KA, Dowd SE, Stamatas GN, Nikolovski J. Diversity of the human skin microbiome early in life. J Invest Dermatol. 2011;131:2026–32.

Capone K, Kirchner F, Klein SL, Tierney NK. Effects of colloidal oatmeal topical atopic dermatitis cream on skin microbiome and skin barrier properties. J Drugs Dermatol. 2020;19:524–31.

Capone KA, Friscia DL, Nikolovski J, Telofski LS, Stamatas GN. A randomized clinical study on the effects of emollient use on the developing infant skin microbiome and metabolome. Exp Dermatol. 2023;32:75–7.

Cha J, Kim TG, Bhae E, Gwak HJ, Ju Y, Choe YH, Jang IH, Jung Y, Moon S, Kim T, Lee W, Park JS, Chung YW, Yang S, Kang YK, Hyun YM, Hwang GS, Lee WJ, Rho M, Ryu JH. Skin microbe-dependent TSLP-ILC2 priming axis in early life is co-opted in allergic inflammation. Cell Host Microbe. 2024.

Chandra J, Retuerto M, Seite S, Martin R, Kus M, Ghannoum MA, Baron E, Mukherjee PK. Effect of an emollient on the mycobiome of atopic dermatitis patients. J Drugs Dermatol. 2018;17:1039–48.

Chang YS, Trivedi MK, Jha A, Lin YF, Dimaano L, Garcia-Romero MT. Synbiotics for prevention and treatment of atopic dermatitis: a meta-analysis of randomized clinical trials. JAMA Pediatr. 2016;170:236–42.

Chng KR, Tay AS, Li C, Ng AH, Wang J, Suri BK, Matta SA, McGovern N, Janela B, Wong XF, Sio YY, Au BV, Wilm A, de Sessions PF, Lim TC, Tang MB, Ginhoux F, Connolly JE, Lane EB, Chew FT, Common JE, Nagarajan N. Whole metagenome profiling reveals skin microbiome-dependent susceptibility to atopic dermatitis flare. Nat Microbiol. 2016;1:16106.

Chu DM, Ma J, Prince AL, Antony KM, Seferovic MD, Aagaard KM. Maturation of the infant microbiome community structure and function across multiple body sites and in relation to mode of delivery. Nat Med. 2017;23:314–26.

Clausen ML, Edslev SM, Andersen PS, Clemmensen K, Krogfelt KA, Agner T. *Staphylococcus aureus* colonization in atopic eczema and its association with filaggrin gene mutations. Br J Dermatol. 2017;177:1394–400.

Costello EK, Lauber CL, Hamady M, Fierer N, Gordon JI, Knight R. Bacterial community variation in human body habitats across space and time. Science. 2009;326:1694–7.

Cryan JF, Dinan TG. Mind-altering microorganisms: the impact of the gut microbiota on brain and behaviour. Nat Rev Neurosci. 2012;13:701–12.

Cuello-Garcia CA, Brozek JL, Fiocchi A, Pawankar R, Yepes-Nunez JJ, Terracciano L, Gandhi S, Agarwal A, Zhang Y, Schunemann HJ. Probiotics for the prevention of allergy: a systematic review and meta-analysis of randomized controlled trials. J Allergy Clin Immunol. 2015;136:952–61.

Czarnowicki T, He H, Canter T, Han J, Lefferdink R, Erickson T, Rangel S, Kameyama N, Kim HJ, Pavel AB, Estrada Y, Krueger JG, Paller AS, Guttman-Yassky E. Evolution of pathologic T-cell subsets in patients with atopic dermatitis from infancy to adulthood. J Allergy Clin Immunol. 2020;145:215–28.

Dahal A, Chang WC, Almasri C, Johansson E, Hurd M, Velasquez V, Grashel B, Spagna D, Jenkins S, Morgan D, Satish L, Martin LJ, Biagini JM, Khurana Hershey GK. Temporal relationships between Staphylococcus aureus colonization, filaggrin expression, and pediatric atopic dermatitis. Allergy. 2024;79:104–15.

Darabi K, Hostetler SG, Bechtel MA, Zirwas M. The role of Malassezia in atopic dermatitis affecting the head and neck of adults. J Am Acad Dermatol. 2009;60:125–36.

Darmstadt GL, Ahmed S, Ahmed AS, Saha SK. Mechanism for prevention of infection in preterm neonates by topical emollients: a randomized, controlled clinical trial. Pediatr Infect Dis J. 2014;33:1124–7.

Demessant-Flavigny AL, Connétable S, Kerob D, Moreau M, Aguilar L, Wollenberg A. Skin microbiome dysbiosis and the role of Staphylococcus aureus in atopic dermatitis in adults and children: a narrative review. J Eur Acad Dermatol Venereol. 2023;37(Suppl 5):3–17.

Doege K, Grajecki D, Zyriax BC, Detinkina E, Zueulenburg C, Buhling KJ. Impact of maternal supplementation with probiotics during pregnancy on atopic eczema in childhood—a meta-analysis. Br J Nutr. 2012;107:1–6.

Dominguez-Bello MG, Costello EK, Contreras M, Magris M, Hidalgo G, Fierer N, Knight R. Delivery mode shapes the acquisition and structure of the initial microbiota across multiple body habitats in newborns. Proc Natl Acad Sci U S A. 2010;107:11971–5.

Dominguez-Bello MG, De Jesus-Laboy KM, Shen N, Cox LM, Amir A, Gonzalez A, Bokulich NA, Song SJ, Hoashi M, Rivera-Vinas JI, Mendez K, Knight R, Clemente JC. Partial restoration of the microbiota of cesarean-born infants via vaginal microbial transfer. Nat Med. 2016;22:250–3.

Dotterud LK, Wilsgaard T, Vorland LH, Falk ES. The effect of UVB radiation on skin microbiota in patients with atopic dermatitis and healthy controls. Int J Circumpolar Health. 2008;67:254–60.

Dotterud CK, Storro O, Johnsen R, Oien T. Probiotics in pregnant women to prevent allergic disease: a randomized, double-blind trial. Br J Dermatol. 2010;163:616–23.

Drago L, Iemoli E, Rodighiero V, Nicola L, de Vecchi E, Piconi S. Effects of *Lactobacillus salivarius* LS01 (DSM 22775) treatment on adult atopic dermatitis: a randomized placebo-controlled study. Int J Immunopathol Pharmacol. 2011;24:1037–48.

Droste JH, Wieringa MH, Weyler JJ, Nelen VJ, Vermeire PA, van Bever HP. Does the use of antibiotics in early childhood increase the risk of asthma and allergic disease? Clin Exp Allergy. 2000;30:1547–53.

Eberlein-Konig B, Schafer T, Huss-Marp J, Darsow U, Mohrenschlager M, Herbert O, Abeck D, Kramer U, Behrendt H, Ring J. Skin surface pH, stratum corneum hydration, trans-epidermal water loss and skin roughness related to atopic eczema and skin dryness in a population of primary school children. Acta Derm Venereol. 2000;80:188–91.

Elias PM, Hatano Y, Williams ML. Basis for the barrier abnormality in atopic dermatitis: outside-inside-outside pathogenic mechanisms. J Allergy Clin Immunol. 2008;121:1337–43.

Emmert H, Baurecht H, Thielking F, Stolzl D, Rodriguez E, Harder, I, Proksch E, Weidinger S. Stratum corneum lipidomics analysis reveals altered ceramide profile in atopic dermatitis patients across body sites with correlated changes in skin microbiome. Exp Dermatol. 2020.

Enomoto T, Sowa M, Nishimori K, Shimazu S, Yoshida A, Yamada K, Furukawa F, Nakagawa T, Yanagisawa N, Iwabuchi N, Odamaki T, Abe F, Nakayama J, Xiao JZ. Effects of bifidobacterial supplementation to pregnant women and infants in the prevention of allergy development in infants and on fecal microbiota. Allergol Int. 2014;63:575–85.

Eyerich K, Novak N. Immunology of atopic eczema: overcoming the Th1/Th2 paradigm. Allergy. 2013;68:974–82.

Farooqi IS, Hopkin JM. Early childhood infection and atopic disorder. Thorax. 1998;53:927–32.

Fiocchi A, Pawankar R, Cuello-Garcia C, Ahn K, Al-Hammadi S, Agarwal A, Beyer K, Burks W, Canonica GW, Ebisawa M, Gandhi S, Kamenwa R, Lee BW, Li H, Prescott S, Riva JJ, Rosenwasser L, Sampson H, Spigler M, Terracciano L, Vereda-Ortiz A, Waserman S, Yepes-Nunez JJ, Brozek JL, Schunemann HJ. World allergy organization-McMaster university guidelines for allergic disease prevention (GLAD-P): probiotics. World Allergy Organ J. 2015;8:4.

Flohr C, England K, Radulovic S, McLean WH, Campbel LE, Barker J, Perkin M, Lack G. Filaggrin loss-of-function mutations are associated with early-onset eczema, eczema severity and transepidermal water loss at 3 months of age. Br J Dermatol. 2010;163:1333–6.

Forno E, Onderdonk AB, McCracken J, Litonjua AA, Laskey D, Delaney ML, Dubois AM, Gold DR, Ryan LM, Weiss ST, Celedon JC. Diversity of the gut microbiota and eczema in early life. Clin Mol Allergy. 2008;6:11.

Fugere A, Lalonde Seguin D, Mitchell G, Deziel E, Dekimpe V, Cantin AM, Frost E, Malouin F. Interspecific small molecule interactions between clinical isolates of Pseudomonas aeruginosa and Staphylococcus aureus from adult cystic fibrosis patients. PLoS One. 2014;9:e86705.

Fyhrquist N, Muirhead G, Prast-Nielsen S, Jeanmougin M, Olah P, Skoog T, Jules-Clement G, Feld M, Barrientos-Somarribas M, Sinkko H, van den Bogaard EH, Zeeuwen P, Rikken G, Schalkwijk J, Niehues H, Daubener W, Eller SK, Alexander H, Pennino D, Suomela S, Tessas I, Lybeck E, Baran AM, Darban H, Gangwar RS, Gerstel U, Jahn K, Karisola P, Yan L, Hansmann B, Katayama S, Meller S, Bylesjo M, Hupe P, Levi-Schaffer F, Greco D, Ranki A, Schroder JM, Barker J, Kere J, Tsoka S, Lauerma A, Soumelis V, Nestle FO, Homey B, Andersson B, Alenius H. Microbe-host interplay in atopic dermatitis and psoriasis. Nat Commun. 2019;10:4703.

Gao Z, Tseng CH, Pei Z, Blaser MJ. Molecular analysis of human forearm superficial skin bacterial biota. Proc Natl Acad Sci U S A. 2007;104:2927–32.

Gelmetti C, Rigoni C, Cantù AM, Agolzer A, Agrusa A, Brena M, Dall'oglio F, Demichelis P, Farina S, Frasin LA, Lorenzi S, Mazzola G, Praticò M, Robotti S, Tedeschi A, Villa L, Ananiadis P, Arkoumani E, Astashonok I, Baselga Torres E, Borici S, Cano E, Cela R, Cengo A, Corella F, Cubiro Raventos X, De Jesus Silva MA, Demiraj E, Dhima E, Doci X, Domarad A, Didyk M, Dyli A, Efthimiou O, Filippi G, Flores Climente VA, Garcia Muret MP, Navarro JG, Gega M, Giakoub AN, Giakoubis V, Gica A, Gjomema M, Guri B, Janushaj E, Kanelleas A, Kanelopoulou G, Kapaj E, Kapoukranidou D, Karadima K, Katsavou A, Kotrulja L, Kyriakou A, Larios G, Lopez A, Lopez C, Manoli SM, Matvienko T, Mervic L, Mileounis K, Muja D, Nadezhda M, Panagioti D, Papakonstantis M, Papanikou M, Papathemeli D, Papigkioti K, Pivak V, Preza D, Roé E, Rogl Butina M, Serra Baldrich E, Sgouros D, Shilova A, Shllaku E, Sideris N, Sina E, Sinani A, Sourli-Chasioti F, Stankaj M, Tasioula D, Tsalmadoupis A, Tsatsou F, Tsenebi E, Tsitlakidou A, Vassis P, Vilarrassa E, Vorobey O, Voutsakis N, Yakovleva S, Yakubovskaya S, Yerygina E, Zarras A, Zenelaj V, Zenko O. Topical prebiotics/postbiotics and PRURISCORE validation in atopic dermatitis. International study of 396 patients. J Dermatolog Treat. 2023;34:2131703.

Gensollen T, Blumberg RS. Correlation between early-life regulation of the immune system by microbiota and allergy development. J Allergy Clin Immunol. 2017;139:1084–91.

Gensollen T, Iyer SS, Kasper DL, Blumberg RS. How colonization by microbiota in early life shapes the immune system. Science. 2016;352:539–44.

Glatz M, Jo JH, Kennedy EA, Polley EC, Segre JA, Simpson EL, Kong HH. Emollient use alters skin barrier and microbes in infants at risk for developing atopic dermatitis. PLoS ONE. 2018;13: e0192443.

Gonzalez ME, Schaffer JV, Orlow SJ, Gao Z, Li H, Alekseyenko AV, Blaser MJ. Cutaneous microbiome effects of fluticasone propionate cream and adjunctive bleach baths in childhood atopic dermatitis. J Am Acad Dermatol. 2016;75(481–493): e8.

Gonzalez T, Biagini Myers JM, Herr AB, Khurana Hershey GK. Staphylococcal biofilms in atopic dermatitis. Curr Allergy Asthma Rep. 2017;17:81.

Gonzalez T, Stevens ML, Baatyrbek Kyzy A, Alarcon R, He H, Kroner JW, Spagna D, Grashel B, Sidler E, Martin LJ, Biagini Myers JM, Khurana Hershey GK, Herr AB. Biofilm propensity of Staphylococcus aureus skin isolates is associated with increased atopic dermatitis severity and barrier dysfunction in the MPAACH pediatric cohort. Allergy. 2021;76:302–13.

Grice EA, Segre JA. The skin microbiome. Nat Rev Microbiol. 2011;9:244–53.

Grice EA, Kong HH, Renaud G, Young AC, Program NCS, Bouffard GG, Blakesley RW, Wolfsberg TG, Turner ML, Segre JA. A diversity profile of the human skin microbiota. Genome Res. 2008;18:1043–50.

Grice EA, Kong HH, Conlan S, Deming CB, Davis J, Young AC, Program NCS, Bouffard GG, Blakesley RW, Murray PR, Green ED, Turner ML, Segre JA. Topographical and temporal diversity of the human skin microbiome. Science. 2009;324:1190–2.

Groer MW, Gregory KE, Louis-Jacques A, Thibeau S, Walker WA. The very low birth weight infant microbiome and childhood health. Birth Defects Res C Embryo Today. 2015;105:252–64.

Gueniche A, Knaudt B, Schuck E, Volz T, Bastien P, Martin R, Röcken M, Breton L, Biedermann T. Effects of nonpathogenic gram-negative bacterium Vitreoscilla filiformis lysate on atopic dermatitis: a prospective, randomized, double-blind, placebo-controlled clinical study. Br J Dermatol 2008;159(6):1357–63. https://doi.org/10.1111/j.1365-2133.2008.08836.x. Epub 2008 Sep 15. PMID: 18795916

Haahtela T, Laatikainen T, Alenius H, Auvinen P, Fyhrquist N, Hanski I, von Hertzen L, Jousilahti P, Kosunen TU, Markelova O, Makela MJ, Pantelejev V, Uhanov M, Zilber E, Vartiainen E. Hunt for the origin of allergy—comparing the Finnish and Russian Karelia. Clin Exp Allergy. 2015;45:891–901.

Habeebuddin M, Karnati RK, Shiroorkar PN, Nagaraja S, Asdaq SMB, Khalid Anwer M, Fattepur S. Topical probiotics: more than a skin deep. Pharmaceutics. 2022;14.

Halling AS, Fritz BG, Gerner T, Rinnov MR, Bay L, Knudgaard MH, Ravn NH, Trautner S, Ruge IF, Olesen C, Díiaz-Pinées Cort I, Skov L, Sørensen N, Møller Rønnstad AT, Thomsen SF, Egeberg A, Jakasa I, Kezic S, Bjarnsholt T, Thyssen JP. Reduced Skin microbiome diversity in infancy is associated with increased risk of atopic dermatitis in high-risk children. J Invest Dermatol. 2023;143:2030–8.e6.

Han SH, Cheon HI, Hur MS, Kim MJ, Jung WH, Lee YW, Choe YB, Ahn KJ. Analysis of the skin mycobiome in adult patients with atopic dermatitis. Exp Dermatol. 2018;27:366–73.

Hanski I, von Hertzen L, Fyhrquist N, Koskinen K, Torppa K, Laatikainen T, Karisola P, Auvinen P, Paulin L, Makela MJ, Vartiainen E, Kosunen TU, Alenius H, Haahtela T. Environmental biodiversity, human microbiota, and allergy are interrelated. Proc Natl Acad Sci U S A. 2012;109:8334–9.

Hartmann J, Moitinho-Silva L, Sander N, Harder I, Häsler R, Rodriguez E, Haufe E, Kleinheinz A, Abraham S, Heratizadeh A, Weisshaar E, Schäkel K, Handrick C, Augustin M, Wollenberg A, Staubach-Renz P, Ertner K, Sticherling M, Schwarz B, Quist S, Wiemers F, Schenck F, Wildberger J, Tittmann L, Lieb W, Schmitt J, Werfel T, Weidinger S. Dupilumab but not cyclosporine treatment shifts the microbiome toward a healthy skin flora in patients with moderate-to-severe atopic dermatitis. Allergy. 2023;78:2290–300.

He Q, Kwok LY, Xi X, Zhong Z, Ma T, Xu H, Meng H, Zhao F, Zhang H. The meconium microbiota shares more features with the amniotic fluid microbiota than the maternal fecal and vaginal microbiota. Gut Microbes. 2020;12:1794266.

Hrestak D, Matijašić M, Čipčić paljetak H, Ledić Drvar D, Ljubojević Hadžavdić S, Perić M. Skin microbiota in atopic dermatitis. Int J Mol Sci. 2022;23.

Huang JT, Abrams M, Tlougan B, Rademaker A, Paller AS. Treatment of Staphylococcus aureus colonization in atopic dermatitis decreases disease severity. Pediatrics. 2009;123:e808–14.

Huang BL, Chandra S, Shih DQ. Skin manifestations of inflammatory bowel disease. Front Physiol. 2012;3:13.

Huang R, Ning H, Shen M, Li J, Zhang J, Chen X. Probiotics for the treatment of atopic dermatitis in children: a systematic review and meta-analysis of randomized controlled trials. Front Cell Infect Microbiol. 2017;7:392.

Inoue Y, Kambara T, Murata N, Komori-Yamaguchi J, Matsukura S, Takahashi Y, Ikezawa Z, Aihara M. Effects of oral administration of *Lactobacillus acidophilus* L-92 on the symptoms and serum cytokines of atopic dermatitis in Japanese adults: a double-blind, randomized, clinical trial. Int Arch Allergy Immunol. 2014;165:247–54.

Isolauri E, Salminen S, Nutrition AMI. Probiotics: use in allergic disorders: a Nutrition, Allergy, Mucosal Immunology, and Intestinal Microbiota (NAMI) Research Group Report. J Clin Gastroenterol. 2008;42(Suppl 2):S91–6.

Jin UH, Lee SO, Sridharan G, Lee K, Davidson LA, Jayaraman A, Chapkin RS, Alaniz R, Safe S. Microbiome-derived tryptophan metabolites and their aryl hydrocarbon receptor-dependent agonist and antagonist activities. Mol Pharmacol. 2014;85:777–88.

Jo JH, Harkins CP, Schwardt NH, Portillo JA, Zimmerman MD, Carter CL, Hossen MA, Peer CJ, Polley EC, Dartois V, Figg WD, Moutsopoulos NM, Segre JA, Kong HH. Alterations of human skin microbiome and expansion of antimicrobial resistance after systemic antibiotics. Sci Transl Med. 2021;13:eabd8077.

Kalliomaki M, Salminen S, Arvilommi H, Kero P, Koskinen P, Isolauri E. Probiotics in primary prevention of atopic disease: a randomised placebo-controlled trial. Lancet. 2001;357:1076–9.

Kalliomaki M, Salminen S, Poussa T, Arvilommi H, Isolauri E. Probiotics and prevention of atopic disease: 4-year follow-up of a randomised placebo-controlled trial. Lancet. 2003;361:1869–71.

Kennedy EA, Connolly J, Hourihane JO, Fallon PG, McLean WHI, Murray D, Jo JH, Segre JA, Kong HH, Irvine AD. Skin microbiome before development of atopic dermatitis: early colonization with commensal staphylococci at 2 months is associated with a lower risk of atopic dermatitis at 1 year. J Allergy Clin Immunol. 2017;139:166–72.

Kennedy KM, Gerlach MJ, Adam T, Heimesaat MM, Rossi L, Surette MG, Sloboda DM, Braun T. Fetal meconium does not have a detectable microbiota before birth. Nat Microbiol. 2021;6:865–73.

Kennedy KM, de Goffau MC, Perez-Munoz ME, Arrieta MC, Backhed F, Bork P, Braun T, Bushman FD, Dore J, de Vos WM, Earl AM, Eisen JA, Elovitz MA, Ganal-Vonarburg SC, Ganzle MG, Garrett WS, Hall LJ, Hornef MW, Huttenhower C, Konnikova L, Lebeer S, Macpherson AJ, Massey RC, McHardy AC, Koren O, Lawley TD, Ley RE, O'Mahony L, O'Toole PW, Pamer EG, Parkhill J, Raes J, Rattei T, Salonen A, Segal E, Segata N, Shanahan F, Sloboda DM, Smith GCS, Sokol H, Spector TD, Surette MG, Tannock GW, Walker AW, Yassour M, Walter J. Questioning the fetal microbiome illustrates pitfalls of low-biomass microbial studies. Nature. 2023;613:639–49.

Kim JE, Kim HS. Microbiome of the skin and gut in atopic dermatitis (AD): understanding the pathophysiology and finding novel management strategies. J Clin Med. 2019;8.

Kirjavainen PV, Arvola T, Salminen SJ, Isolauri E. Aberrant composition of gut microbiota of allergic infants: a target of bifidobacterial therapy at weaning? Gut. 2002;51:51–5.

Knor T, Meholjic-Fetahovic A, Mehmedagic A. Stratum corneum hydration and skin surface pH in patients with atopic dermatitis. Acta Dermatovenerol Croat. 2011;19:242–7.

Kobayashi T, Nagao K. Host-microbial dialogues in atopic dermatitis. Int Immunol. 2019;31:449–56.

Kobayashi T, Glatz M, Horiuchi K, Kawasaki H, Akiyama H, Kaplan DH, Kong HH, Amagai M, Nagao K. Dysbiosis and *staphylococcus aureus* colonization drives inflammation in atopic dermatitis. Immunity. 2015;42:756–66.

Kong HH, Oh J, Deming C, Conlan S, Grice EA, Beatson MA, Nomicos E, Polley EC, Komarow HD, Program NCS, Murray PR, Turner ML, Segre JA. Temporal shifts in the skin microbiome associated with disease flares and treatment in children with atopic dermatitis. Genome Res. 2012;22:850–9.

Krzysiek J, Żurawska-Olszewska J, Szczerba I, Lesiak A, Pastuszak-Lewandoska D, Grzegorczyk J, Ciążyńska M, Narbutt J. Shift in skin microbiota of children with atopic dermatitis after topical gentian violet application. Postepy Dermatol Alergol. 2023;40:308–14.

Kukkonen K, Savilahti E, Haahtela T, Juntunen-Backman K, Korpela R, Poussa T, Tuure T, Kuitunen M. Probiotics and prebiotic galacto-oligosaccharides in the prevention of allergic diseases: a randomized, double-blind, placebo-controlled trial. J Allergy Clin Immunol. 2007;119:192–8.

Kusel MM, de Klerk N, Holt PG, Sly PD. Antibiotic use in the first year of life and risk of atopic disease in early childhood. Clin Exp Allergy. 2008;38:1921–8.

Kwon S, Choi JY, Shin JW, Huh CH, Park KC, Du MH, Yoon S, Na JI. Changes in lesional and non-lesional skin microbiome during treatment of atopic dermatitis. Acta Derm Venereol. 2019;99:284–90.

Lai Y, Cogen AL, Radek KA, Park HJ, Macleod DT, Leichtle A, Ryan AF, di Nardo A, Gallo RL. Activation of TLR2 by a small molecule produced by Staphylococcus epidermidis increases antimicrobial defense against bacterial skin infections. J Invest Dermatol. 2010;130:2211–21.

Landemaine L, da Costa G, Fissier E, Francis C, Morand S, Verbeke J, Michel ML, Briandet R, Sokol H, Gueniche A, Bernard D, Chatel JM, Aguilar L, Langella P, Clavaud C, Richard ML. Staphylococcus epidermidis isolates from atopic or healthy skin have opposite effect on skin cells: potential implication of the AHR pathway modulation. Front Immunol. 2023;14:1098160.

Lange-Asschenfeldt B, Marenbach D, Lang C, Patzelt A, Ulrich M, Maltusch A, Terhorst D, Stockfleth E, Sterry W, Lademann J. Distribution of bacteria in the epidermal layers and hair follicles of the human skin. Skin Pharmacol Physiol. 2011;24:305–11.

Lauder AP, Roche AM, Sherrill-Mix S, Bailey A, Laughlin AL, Bittinger K, Leite R, Elovitz MA, Parry S, Bushman FD. Comparison of placenta samples with contamination controls does not provide evidence for a distinct placenta microbiota. Microbiome. 2016;4:29.

Lee J, Seto D, Bielory L. Meta-analysis of clinical trials of probiotics for prevention and treatment of pediatric atopic dermatitis. J Allergy Clin Immunol. 2008;121(116–121): e11.

Lee SY, Lee E, Park YM, Hong SJ. Microbiome in the gut-skin axis in atopic dermatitis. Allergy Asthma Immunol Res. 2018;10:354–62.

Leech JM, Dhariwala MO, Lowe MM, Chu K, Merana GR, Cornuot C, Weckel A, Ma JM, Leitner EG, Gonzalez JR, Vasquez KS, Diep BA, Scharschmidt TC. Toxin-triggered interleukin-1 receptor signaling enables early-life discrimination of pathogenic versus commensal skin bacteria. Cell Host Microbe. 2019;26(795–809): e5.

Leiby JS, McCormick K, Sherrill-Mix S, Clarke EL, Kessler LR, Taylor LJ, Hofstaedter CE, Roche AM, Mattei LM, Bittinger K, Elovitz MA, Leite R, Parry S, Bushman FD. Lack of detection of a human placenta microbiome in samples from preterm and term deliveries. Microbiome. 2018;6:196.

Leyden JJ, Marples RR, Kligman AM. Staphylococcus aureus in the lesions of atopic dermatitis. Br J Dermatol. 1974;90:525–30.

Li L, Han Z, Niu X, Zhang G, Jia Y, Zhang S, He C. Probiotic supplementation for prevention of atopic dermatitis in infants and children: a systematic review and meta-analysis. Am J Clin Dermatol. 2019;20:367–77.

Li Y, Toothaker JM, Ben-Simon S, Ozeri L, Schweitzer R, Mccourt BT, Mccourt CC, Werner L, Snapper SB, Shouval DS, Khatib S, Koren O, Agnihorti S, Tseng G, Konnikova L. In utero human intestine harbors unique metabolome, including bacterial metabolites. JCI Insight. 2020;5.

Lim ES, Rodriguez C, Holtz LR. Amniotic fluid from healthy term pregnancies does not harbor a detectable microbial community. Microbiome. 2018;6:87.

Liu Y, Li X, Zhu B, Zhao H, Ai Q, Tong Y, Qin S, Feng Y, Wang Y, Wang S, Ma J, Yang H. Midtrimester amniotic fluid from healthy pregnancies has no microorganisms using multiple methods of microbiologic inquiry. Am J Obstet Gynecol. 2020;223:248 e1–248 e21.

Liu-Walsh F, Tierney NK, Hauschild J, Rush AK, Masucci J, Leo GC, Capone KA. Prebiotic colloidal oat supports the growth of cutaneous commensal bacteria including *S. Epidermidis* and enhances the production of lactic acid. Clin Cosmet Investig Dermatol. 2021;14:73–82.

Lopes C, Soares J, Tavaria F, Duarte A, Correia O, Sokhatska O, Severo M, Silva D, Pintado M, Delgado L, Moreira A. Chitosan coated textiles may improve atopic dermatitis severity by modulating skin staphylococcal profile: a randomized controlled trial. PLoS ONE. 2015;10: e0142844.

Lossius AH, Sundnes O, Ingham AC, Edslev SM, Bjørnholt JV, Lilje B, Bradley M, Asad S, Haraldsen G, Skytt-Andersen P, Holm J, Berents TL. Shifts in the skin microbiota after UVB treatment in adult atopic dermatitis. Dermatology. 2022;238:109–20.

Luna PC. Skin microbiome as years go by. Am J Clin Dermatol. 2020.

Lynch SV, Wood RA, Boushey H, Bacharier LB, Bloomberg GR, Kattan M, O'Connor GT, Sandel MT, Calatroni A, Matsui E, Johnson CC, Lynn H, Visness CM, Jaffee KF, Gergen PJ, Gold DR, Wright RJ, Fujimura K, Rauch M, Busse WW, Gern JE. Effects of early-life exposure to allergens and bacteria on recurrent wheeze and atopy in urban children. J Allergy Clin Immunol. 2014;134(593–601): e12.

Mah KW, Bjorksten B, Lee BW, van Bever HP, Shek LP, Tan TN, Lee YK, Chua KY. Distinct pattern of commensal gut microbiota in toddlers with eczema. Int Arch Allergy Immunol. 2006;140:157–63.

Mansfield JA, Bergin SW, Cooper JR, Olsen CH. Comparative probiotic strain efficacy in the prevention of eczema in infants and children: a systematic review and meta-analysis. Mil Med. 2014;179:580–92.

Matsumoto M, Aranami A, Ishige A, Watanabe K, Benno Y. LKM512 yogurt consumption improves the intestinal environment and induces the T-helper type 1 cytokine in adult patients with intractable atopic dermatitis. Clin Exp Allergy. 2007;37:358–70.

Matsumoto M, Ebata T, Hirooka J, Hosoya R, Inoue N, Itami S, Tsuji K, Yaginuma T, Muramatsu K, Nakamura A, Fujita A, Nagakura T. Antipruritic effects of the probiotic strain LKM512 in adults with atopic dermatitis. Ann Allergy Asthma Immunol. 2014;113(209–216): e7.

McKeever TM, Lewis SA, Smith C, Collins J, Heatlie H, Frischer M, Hubbard R. Early exposure to infections and antibiotics and the incidence of allergic disease: a birth cohort study with the West Midlands General Practice Research Database. J Allergy Clin Immunol. 2002;109:43–50.

Meylan P, Lang C, Mermoud S, Johannsen A, Norrenberg S, Hohl D, Vial Y, Prod'hom G, Greub G, Kypriotou M, Christen-Zaech S. Skin colonization by staphylococcus aureus precedes the clinical diagnosis of atopic dermatitis in infancy. J Invest Dermatol. 2017.

Miyake R, Iwamoto K, Sakai N, Matsunae K, Aziz F, Sugai M, Takahagi S, Tanaka A, Hide M. Uptake of *Staphylococcus aureus* by keratinocytes is reduced by interferon-fibronectin pathway and filaggrin expression. J Dermatol. 2022;49:1148–57.

Montes LF, Wilborn WH. Location of bacterial skin flora. Br J Dermatol. 1969;81(Suppl 1):23+.

Moosbrugger-Martinz V, Hackl H, Gruber R, Pilecky M, Knabl L, Orth-Holler D, Dubrac S. First evidences of distinguishable bacterial and fungal dysbiosis in the skin of patients with Atopic Dermatitis or Netherton Syndrome. J Invest Dermatol. 2020.

Moroi M, Uchi S, Nakamura K, Sato S, Shimizu N, Fujii M, Kumagai T, Saito M, Uchiyama K, Watanabe T, Yamaguchi H, Yamamoto T, Takeuchi S, Furue M. Beneficial effect of a diet containing heat-killed Lactobacillus paracasei K71 on adult type atopic dermatitis. J Dermatol. 2011;38:131–9.

Myles IA, Castillo CR, Barbian KD, Kanakabandi K, Virtaneva K, Fitzmeyer E, Paneru M, Otaizo-Carrasquero F, Myers TG, Markowitz TE, Moore IN, Liu X, Ferrer M, Sakamachi Y, Garantziotis S, Swamydas M, Lionakis MS, Anderson ED, Earland NJ, Ganesan S, Sun AA, Bergerson JRE, Silverman RA, Petersen M, Martens CA, Datta SK. Therapeutic responses to Roseomonas mucosa in atopic dermatitis may involve lipid-mediated TNF-related epithelial repair. Sci Transl Med. 2020;12.

Nakatsuji T, Gallo RL, Shafiq F, Tong Y, Chun K, Butcher AM, Cheng JY, Hata TR. Use of autologous bacteriotherapy to treat *Staphylococcus aureus* in patients with atopic dermatitis: a randomized double-blind clinical trial. JAMA Dermatol. 2021a;157:978–82.

Nakatsuji T, Hata TR, Tong Y, Cheng JY, Shafiq F, Butcher AM, Salem SS, Brinton SL, Rudman Spergel AK, Johnson K, Jepson B, Calatroni A, David G, Ramirez-Gama M, Taylor P, Leung DYM, Gallo RL. Development of a human skin commensal microbe for bacteriotherapy of atopic dermatitis and use in a phase 1 randomized clinical trial. Nat Med. 2021b;27:700–9.

Natarelli N, Gahoonia N, Sivamani RK. Bacteriophages and the microbiome in dermatology: the role of the phageome and a potential therapeutic strategy. Int J Mol Sci. 2023;24.

Ng WZJ, van Hasselt J, Aggarwal B, Manoharan A. Association between adult antibiotic use, microbial dysbiosis and atopic conditions—a systematic review. J Asthma Allergy. 2023;16:1115–32.

Nibbering B, Ubags NDJ. Microbial interactions in the atopic march. Clin Exp Immunol. 2020;199:12–23.

Niemeyer-van der Kolk T, van der Wall H, Hogendoorn GK, Rijneveld R, Luijten S, van Alewijk D, van den Munckhof EHA, de Kam ML, Feiss GL, Prens EP, Burggraaf J, Rissmann R, van Doorn

MBA. Pharmacodynamic effects of topical omiganan in patients with mild to moderate atopic dermatitis in a randomized, placebo-controlled, phase II trial. Clin Transl Sci. 2020;13:994–1003.

Nowicka D, Nawrot U. Contribution of Malassezia spp. to the development of atopic dermatitis. Mycoses. 2019;62:588–96.

Oh J, Conlan S, Polley EC, Segre JA, Kong HH. Shifts in human skin and nares microbiota of healthy children and adults. Genome Med. 2012;4:77.

Olszak T, An D, Zeissig S, Vera MP, Richter J, Franke A, Glickman JN, Siebert R, Baron RM, Kasper DL, Blumberg RS. Microbial exposure during early life has persistent effects on natural killer T cell function. Science. 2012;336:489–93.

O'Neill CA, Monteleone G, McLaughlin JT, Paus R. The gut-skin axis in health and disease: a paradigm with therapeutic implications. BioEssays. 2016;38:1167–76.

Ong PY, Ohtake T, Brandt C, Strickland I, Boguniewicz M, Ganz T, Gallo RL, Leung DY. Endogenous antimicrobial peptides and skin infections in atopic dermatitis. N Engl J Med. 2002;347:1151–60.

Paller AS, Kong HH, Seed P, Naik S, Scharschmidt TC, Gallo RL, Luger T, Irvine AD. The microbiome in patients with atopic dermatitis. J Allergy Clin Immunol. 2019;143:26–35.

Pammi M, O'Brien JL, Ajami NJ, Wong MC, Versalovic J, Petrosino JF. Development of the cutaneous microbiome in the preterm infant: a prospective longitudinal study. PLoS ONE. 2017;12: e0176669.

Panduru M, Panduru NM, Salavastru CM, Tiplica GS. Probiotics and primary prevention of atopic dermatitis: a meta-analysis of randomized controlled studies. J Eur Acad Dermatol Venereol. 2015;29:232–42.

Patangia DV, Anthony Ryan C, Dempsey E, Paul Ross R, Stanton C. Impact of antibiotics on the human microbiome and consequences for host health. Microbiologyopen. 2022;11:e1260.

Pelucchi C, Chatenoud L, Turati F, Galeone C, Moja L, Bach JF, la Vecchia C. Probiotics supplementation during pregnancy or infancy for the prevention of atopic dermatitis: a meta-analysis. Epidemiology. 2012;23:402–14.

Penders J, Stobberingh EE, Thijs C, Adams H, Vink C, van Ree R, van den Brandt PA. Molecular fingerprinting of the intestinal microbiota of infants in whom atopic eczema was or was not developing. Clin Exp Allergy. 2006;36:1602–8.

Penders J, Thijs C, van den Brandt PA, Kummeling I, Snijders B, Stelma F, Adams H, van Ree R, Stobberingh EE. Gut microbiota composition and development of atopic manifestations in infancy: the KOALA Birth Cohort Study. Gut. 2007;56:661–7.

Perez-Munoz ME, Arrieta MC, Ramer-Tait AE, Walter J. A critical assessment of the "sterile womb" and "in utero colonization" hypotheses: implications for research on the pioneer infant microbiome. Microbiome. 2017;5:48.

Pothmann A, Illing T, Wiegand C, Hartmann AA, Elsner P. The microbiome and atopic dermatitis: a review. Am J Clin Dermatol. 2019;20:749–61.

Ramadan M, Solyman S, Yones M, Abdallah Y, Halaby H, Hanora A. Skin microbiome differences in atopic dermatitis and healthy controls in Egyptian children and adults, and association with serum immunoglobulin E. OMICS. 2019;23:247–60.

Rapin A, Rehbinder EM, Macowan M, Pattaroni C, Lodrup Carlsen KC, Harris NL, Jonassen CM, Landro L, Lossius AH, Nordlund B, Rudi K, Skjerven HO, Cathrine Staff A, Soderhall C, Ubags N, Vettukattil R, Marsland BJ. The skin microbiome in the first year of life and its association with atopic dermatitis. Allergy. 2023;78:1949–63.

Rauer L, Reiger M, Bhattacharyya M, Brunner PM, Krueger JG, Guttman-Yassky E, Traidl-Hoffmann C, Neumann AU. Skin microbiome and its association with host cofactors in determining atopic dermatitis severity. J Eur Acad Dermatol Venereol. 2023;37:772–82.

Rautava S, Kalliomaki M, Isolauri E. Probiotics during pregnancy and breast-feeding might confer immunomodulatory protection against atopic disease in the infant. J Allergy Clin Immunol. 2002;109:119–21.

Rehbinder EM, Lodrup Carlsen KC, Staff AC, Angell IL, Landro L, Hilde K, Gaustad P, Rudi K. Is amniotic fluid of women with uncomplicated term pregnancies free of bacteria? Am J Obstet Gynecol. 2018;219:289 e1–289 e12.

Rehbinder EM, Winger AJ, Landro L, Asarnoj A, Berents TL, Carlsen KH, Hedlin G, Jonassen CM, Nordlund B, Sandvik L, Skjerven HO, Soderhall C, Vettukattil R, Carlsen KCL, Study G. Dry skin and skin barrier in early infancy. Br J Dermatol. 2019.

Rippke F, Schreiner V, Doering T, Maibach HI. Stratum corneum pH in atopic dermatitis: impact on skin barrier function and colonization with *Staphylococcus aureus*. Am J Clin Dermatol. 2004;5:217–23.

Roduit C, Frei R, Ferstl R, Loeliger S, Westermann P, Rhyner C, Schiavi E, Barcik W, Rodriguez-Perez N, Wawrzyniak M, Chassard C, Lacroix C, Schmausser-Hechfellner E, Depner M, von Mutius E, Braun-Fahrlander C, Karvonen AM, Kirjavainen PV, Pekkanen J, Dalphin JC, Riedler J, Akdis C, Lauener R, O'mahony L, Group PES. High levels of butyrate and propionate in early life are associated with protection against atopy. Allergy. 2019;74:799–809.

Roessler A, Friedrich U, Vogelsang H, Bauer A, Kaatz M, Hipler UC, Schmidt I, Jahreis G. The immune system in healthy adults and patients with atopic dermatitis seems to be affected differently by a probiotic intervention. Clin Exp Allergy. 2008;38:93–102.

Rosenfeldt V, Benfeldt E, Nielsen SD, Michaelsen KF, Jeppesen DL, Valerius NH, Paerregaard A. Effect of probiotic Lactobacillus strains in children with atopic dermatitis. J Allergy Clin Immunol. 2003;111:389–95.

Saoin S, Wisitponchai T, Intachai K, Chupradit K, Moonmuang S, Nangola S, Kitidee K, Fanhchaksai K, Lee VS, Hong SS, Boulanger P, Chuankhayan P, Chen CJ, Tayapiwatana C. Deciphering critical amino acid residues to modify and enhance the binding affinity of ankyrin scaffold specific to capsid protein of human immunodeficiency virus type 1. Asian Pac J Allergy Immunol. 2018;36:126–35.

Scharschmidt TC, Vasquez KS, Truong HA, Gearty SV, Pauli ML, Nosbaum A, Gratz IK, Otto M, Moon JJ, Liese J, Abbas AK, Fischbach MA, Rosenblum MD. A wave of regulatory T Cells into neonatal skin mediates tolerance to commensal microbes. Immunity. 2015;43:1011–21.

Scharschmidt TC, Vasquez KS, Pauli ML, Leitner EG, Chu K, Truong HA, Lowe MM, Rodriguez RS, Ali N, Laszik ZG, Sonnenburg JL, Millar SE, Rosenblum MD. Commensal microbes and hair follicle morphogenesis coordinately drive treg migration into neonatal skin. Cell Host Microbe. 2017;21:467–77 e5.

Schmidt RM, Pilmann Laursen R, Bruun S, Larnkjær A, Molgaard C, Michaelsen KF, Host A. Probiotics in late infancy reduce the incidence of eczema: a randomized controlled trial. Pediatr Allergy Immunol. 2019;30:335–40.

Schmitt J, Schmitt NM, Kirch W, Meurer M. Early exposure to antibiotics and infections and the incidence of atopic eczema: a population-based cohort study. Pediatr Allergy Immunol. 2010;21:292–300.

Schneider AM, Nelson AM. Skin microbiota: friend or foe in pediatric skin health and skin disease. Pediatr Dermatol. 2019;36:815–22.

Schoch JJ, Gauthier J, Gharaibeh RZ, Jobin C, Bohannon M, Neu J, Parker L. Skin microbiome sampling in the preterm neonate. Pediatr Dermatol. 2023;40:129–31.

Seite S, Flores GE, Henley JB, Martin R, Zelenkova H, Aguilar L, Fierer N. Microbiome of affected and unaffected skin of patients with atopic dermatitis before and after emollient treatment. J Drugs Dermatol. 2014;13:1365–72.

Seité S, Zelenkova H, Martin R. Clinical efficacy of emollients in atopic dermatitis patients—relationship with the skin microbiota modification. Clin Cosmet Investig Dermatol. 2017;10:25–33.

Shi B, Bangayan NJ, Curd E, Taylor PA, Gallo RL, Leung DY, Li H. The skin microbiome is different in pediatric versus adult atopic dermatitis. J Allergy Clin Immunol. 2016;138:1233–6.

Siltanen M, Kajosaari M, Pohjavuori M, Savilahti E. Prematurity at birth reduces the long-term risk of atopy. J Allergy Clin Immunol. 2001;107:229–34.

Silva SH, Guedes AC, Gontijo B, Ramos AM, Carmo LS, Farias LM, Nicoli JR. Influence of narrow-band UVB phototherapy on cutaneous microbiota of children with atopic dermatitis. J Eur Acad Dermatol Venereol. 2006;20:1114–20.

Silverberg JI, Lio PA, Simpson EL, Li C, Brownell DR, Gryllos I, Ng-Cashin J, Krueger T, Swaidan VR, Bliss RL, Kim HD. Efficacy and safety of topically applied therapeutic ammonia oxidising bacteria in adults with mild-to-moderate atopic dermatitis and moderate-to-severe pruritus: a randomised, double-blind, placebo-controlled, dose-ranging, phase 2b trial. EClinicalMedicine. 2023;60: 102002.

Simonyte Sjodin K, Hammarstrom ML, Ryden P, Sjodin A, Hernell O, Engstrand L, West CE. Temporal and long-term gut microbiota variation in allergic disease: a prospective study from infancy to school age. Allergy. 2019;74:176–85.

Simpson MR, Dotterud CK, Storro O, Johnsen R, Oien T. Perinatal probiotic supplementation in the prevention of allergy related disease: 6 year follow up of a randomised controlled trial. BMC Dermatol. 2015;15:13.

Sinha S, Lin G, Ferenczi K. The skin microbiome and the gut-skin axis. Clin Dermatol. 2021;39:829–39.

Skowron K, Bauza-Kaszewska J, Kraszewska Z, Wiktorczyk-Kapischke N, Grudlewska-Buda K, Kwiecińska-Piróg J, Wałecka-Zacharska E, Radtke L, Gospodarek-Komkowska E. Human skin microbiome: impact of intrinsic and extrinsic factors on skin microbiota. Microorganisms. 2021;9.

Slob EM, Brew BK, Vijverberg SJ, Kats CJ, Longo C, Pijnenburg MW, van Beijsterveldt TC, Dolan CV, Bartels M, Magnusson P, Lichtenstein P, Gong T, Koppelman GH, Almqvist C, Boomsma DI, Maitland-van der Zee AH. Early-life antibiotic use and risk of asthma and eczema: results of a discordant twin study. Eur Respir J. 2020;55.

Smits JPH, Ederveen THA, Rikken G, van den Brink NJM, Van Vlijmen-Willems I, Boekhorst J, Kamsteeg M, Schalkwijk J, van Hijum S, Zeeuwen P, van den Bogaard EH. Targeting the cutaneous microbiota in atopic dermatitis by coal tar via AHR-dependent induction of antimicrobial peptides. J Invest Dermatol. 2020;140(415–424): e10.

Song H, Yoo Y, Hwang J, Na YC, Kim HS. *Faecalibacterium prausnitzii* subspecies-level dysbiosis in the human gut microbiome underlying atopic dermatitis. J Allergy Clin Immunol. 2016;137:852–60.

Stamatas GN, Nikolovski J, Luedtke MA, Kollias N, Wiegand BC. Infant skin microstructure assessed in vivo differs from adult skin in organization and at the cellular level. Pediatr Dermatol. 2010;27:125–31.

Steel JH, Malatos S, Kennea N, Edwards AD, Miles L, Duggan P, Reynolds PR, Feldman RG, Sullivan MH. Bacteria and inflammatory cells in fetal membranes do not always cause preterm labor. Pediatr Res. 2005;57:404–11.

Stinson L, Hallingstrom M, Barman M, Viklund F, Keelan J, Kacerovsky M, Payne M, Jacobsson B. Comparison of bacterial DNA profiles in mid-trimester amniotic fluid samples from preterm and term deliveries. Front Microbiol. 2020;11:415.

Sugita T, Saito M, Ito T, Kato Y, Tsuboi R, Takeuchi S, Nishikawa A. The basidiomycetous yeasts *Cryptococcus diffluens* and *C. liquefaciens* colonize the skin of patients with atopic dermatitis. Microbiol Immunol. 2003;47:945–50.

Tan-Lim CSC, Esteban-Ipac NAR, Recto MST, Castor MAR, Casis-Hao RJ, Nano ALM. Comparative effectiveness of probiotic strains on the prevention of pediatric atopic dermatitis: a systematic review and network meta-analysis. Pediatr Allergy Immunol. 2021;32:1255–70.

Tauber M, Balica S, Hsu CY, Jean-Decoster C, Lauze C, Redoules D, Viode C, Schmitt AM, Serre G, Simon M, Paul CF. Staphylococcus aureus density on lesional and nonlesional skin is strongly associated with disease severity in atopic dermatitis. J Allergy Clin Immunol. 2016;137(1272–1274): e3.

Taylor AL, Dunstan JA, Prescott SL. Probiotic supplementation for the first 6 months of life fails to reduce the risk of atopic dermatitis and increases the risk of allergen sensitization in high-risk children: a randomized controlled trial. J Allergy Clin Immunol. 2007;119:184–91.

Totte JE, van der Feltz WT, Hennekam M, van Belkum A, van Zuuren EJ, Pasmans SG. Prevalence and odds of Staphylococcus aureus carriage in atopic dermatitis: a systematic review and meta-analysis. Br J Dermatol. 2016;175:687–95.

Travers JB. Toxic interaction between Th2 cytokines and *Staphylococcus aureus* in atopic dermatitis. J Invest Dermatol. 2014;134:2069–71.

Trompette A, Ubags ND. Skin barrier immunology from early life to adulthood. Mucosal Immunol. 2023;16:194–207.

Trompette A, Gollwitzer ES, Yadava K, Sichelstiel AK, Sprenger N, Ngom-Bru C, Blanchard C, Junt T, Nicod LP, Harris NL, Marsland BJ. Gut microbiota metabolism of dietary fiber influences allergic airway disease and hematopoiesis. Nat Med. 2014;20:159–66.

Trompette A, Pernot J, Perdijk O, Alqahtani RAA, Domingo JS, Camacho-Munoz D, Wong NC, Kendall AC, Wiederkehr A, Nicod LP, Nicolaou A, von Garnier C, Ubags NDJ, Marsland BJ. Gut-derived short-chain fatty acids modulate skin barrier integrity by promoting keratinocyte metabolism and differentiation. Mucosal Immunol. 2022;15:908–26.

Tronnes H, Wilcox AJ, Lie RT, Markestad T, Moster D. The association of preterm birth with severe asthma and atopic dermatitis: a national cohort study. Pediatr Allergy Immunol. 2013;24:782–7.

Tuor M, Leibundgut-Landmann S. The skin mycobiome and intermicrobial interactions in the cutaneous niche. Curr Opin Microbiol. 2023;76: 102381.

Ubags ND, Trompette A, Pernot J, Nibbering B, Wong NC, Pattaroni C, Rapin A, Nicod LP, Harris NL, Marsland BJ. Microbiome-induced antigen-presenting cell recruitment coordinates skin and lung allergic inflammation. J Allergy Clin Immunol. 2020.

Underwood MA, Sohn K. The microbiota of the extremely preterm infant. Clin Perinatol. 2017;44:407–27.

van Drongelen V, Haisma EM, Out-Luiting JJ, Nibbering PH, el Ghalbzouri A. Reduced filaggrin expression is accompanied by increased *Staphylococcus aureus* colonization of epidermal skin models. Clin Exp Allergy. 2014;44:1515–24.

van Mierlo MMF, Totte JEE, Fieten KB, van den Broek TJ, Schuren FHJ, Pardo LM, Pasmans S. The influence of treatment in alpine and moderate maritime climate on the composition of the skin microbiome in patients with difficult to treat atopic dermatitis. Clin Exp Allergy. 2019;49:1437–45.

van Nimwegen FA, Penders J, Stobberingh EE, Postma DS, Koppelman GH, Kerkhof M, Reijmerink NE, Dompeling E, van den Brandt PA, Ferreira I, Mommers M, Thijs C. Mode and place of delivery, gastrointestinal microbiota, and their influence on asthma and atopy. J Allergy Clin Immunol. 2011;128(948–55):e1-3.

van Zuuren EJ, Fedorowicz Z, Arents BWM. Emollients and moisturizers for eczema: abridged Cochrane systematic review including GRADE assessments. Br J Dermatol. 2017;177:1256–71.

Viljanen M, Savilahti E, Haahtela T, Juntunen-Backman K, Korpela R, Poussa T, Tuure T, Kuitunen M. Probiotics in the treatment of atopic eczema/dermatitis syndrome in infants: a double-blind placebo-controlled trial. Allergy. 2005;60:494–500.

Wan P, Chen J. A calm, dispassionate look at skin microbiota in atopic dermatitis: an integrative literature review. Dermatol Ther (Heidelb). 2020;10:53–61.

Watanabe S, Narisawa Y, Arase S, Okamatsu H, Ikenaga T, Tajiri Y, Kumemura M. Differences in fecal microflora between patients with atopic dermatitis and healthy control subjects. J Allergy Clin Immunol. 2003;111:587–91.

Weidinger S, Beck LA, Bieber T, Kabashima K, Irvine AD. Atopic dermatitis. Nat Rev Dis Primers. 2018;4:1.

Weiss A, Delavenne E, Matias C, Lagler H, Simon D, Li P, Hansen JU, Dos Santos TP, Jana B, Priemel P, Bangert C, Bauer M, Eberl S, Nussbaumer-Pröll A, Anne Österreicher Z, Matzneller P, Quint T, Weber M, Nielsen HM, Rades T, Johansen HK, Westh H, Kim W, Mylonakis E, Friis C, Guardabassi L, Pace J, Lundberg CV, M'zali F, Butty P, Sørensen N, Nielsen HB, Toft-Kehler R, Guttman-Yassky E, Stingl G, Zeitlinger M, Sommer M. Topical niclosamide (ATx201) reduces Staphylococcus aureus colonization and increases Shannon diversity of the skin microbiome in atopic dermatitis patients in a randomized, double-blind, placebo-controlled Phase 2 trial. Clin Transl Med. 2022;12:e790.

Werner Y, Lindberg M. Transepidermal water loss in dry and clinically normal skin in patients with atopic dermatitis. Acta Derm Venereol. 1985;65:102–5.

Wickens K, Black PN, Stanley TV, Mitchell E, Fitzharris P, Tannock GW, Purdie G, Crane J, PROBI-OTIC STUDY, G. A differential effect of 2 probiotics in the prevention of eczema and atopy: a double-blind, randomized, placebo-controlled trial. J Allergy Clin Immunol. 2008;122:788–94.

Wickens K, Black P, Stanley TV, Mitchell E, Barthow C, Fitzharris P, Purdie G, Crane J. A protective effect of *Lactobacillus rhamnosus* HN001 against eczema in the first 2 years of life persists to age 4 years. Clin Exp Allergy. 2012;42:1071–9.

Wickens K, Barthow C, Mitchell EA, Kang J, van Zyl N, Purdie G, Stanley T, Fitzharris P, Murphy R, Crane J. Effects of *Lactobacillus rhamnosus* HN001 in early life on the cumulative prevalence of allergic disease to 11 years. Pediatr Allergy Immunol. 2018;29:808–14.

Wollenberg A, Kinberger M, Arents B, Aszodi N, Avila Valle G, Barbarot S, Bieber T, Brough HA, Calzavara Pinton P, Christen-Zäch S, Deleuran M, Dittmann M, Dressler C, Fink-Wagner AH, Fosse N, Gáspár K, Gerbens L, Gieler U, Girolomoni G, Gregoriou S, Mortz CG, Nast A, Nygaard U, Redding M, Rehbinder EM, Ring J, Rossi M, Serra-Baldrich E, Simon D, Szalai ZZ, Szepietowski JC, Torrelo A, Werfel T, Flohr C. European guideline (EuroGuiDerm) on atopic eczema - part II: non-systemic treatments and treatment recommendations for special AE patient populations. J Eur Acad Dermatol Venereol. 2022;36(11):1904–26. https://doi.org/10.1111/jdv.18429. Epub 2022 Sep 3. PMID: 36056736

Wongpiyabovorn J, Soonthornchai W, Wilantho A, Palasuk M, Payungporn S, Sodsai P, Poomipak W, Weschawalit S, Ruchusatsawat K, Baillie GS, Hirankarn N, Somboonna N. Effect of tacrolimus on skin microbiome in atopic dermatitis. Allergy. 2019;74:1400–6.

Wopereis H, Sim K, Shaw A, Warner JO, Knol J, Kroll JS. Intestinal microbiota in infants at high risk for allergy: effects of prebiotics and role in eczema development. J Allergy Clin Immunol. 2018;141(1334–1342): e5.

Xing Y, Naik S. Baby's first bacteria: discriminating colonizing commensals from pathogens. Cell Host Microbe. 2019;26:705–7.

Xu Z, Liu X, Niu Y, Shen C, Heminger K, Moulton L, Yu A, Allen T, Zhang L, Yue F, Liu J, Xu Y, Zhao H, Li L, Cambron T, Xu J, Smith E, Wei K. Skin benefits of moisturising body wash formulas for children with atopic dermatitis: a randomised controlled clinical study in China. Australas J Dermatol. 2020;61:e54–9.

Xue X, Yang X, Shi X, Deng Z. Efficacy of probiotics in pediatric atopic dermatitis: a systematic review and meta-analysis. Clin Transl Allergy. 2023;13: e12283.

Yamamoto-Hanada K, Yang L, Narita M, Saito H, Ohya Y. Influence of antibiotic use in early childhood on asthma and allergic diseases at age 5. Ann Allergy Asthma Immunol. 2017;119:54–8.

Yang G, Seok JK, Kang HC, Cho YY, Lee HS, Lee JY. Skin barrier abnormalities and immune dysfunction in atopic dermatitis. Int J Mol Sci. 2020;21.

Younge NE, Araujo-Perez F, Brandon D, Seed PC. Early-life skin microbiota in hospitalized preterm and full-term infants. Microbiome. 2018;6:98.

Youssef R, Hafez V, Elkholy Y, Mourad A. Glycerol 85% efficacy on atopic skin and its microbiome: a randomized controlled trial with clinical and bacteriological evaluation. J Dermatolog Treat. 2020:1–7.

Zaramela LBB, Ramirez-Gama M, Johnson K, Leung DYM, Zengler K. Deciphering the microbiome and virome composition of patients with Atopic Dermatitis and Eczema Herpeticum (ADEH+). J Aller Clin Immunol. 2019.

Zhang E, Tanaka T, Tajima M, Tsuboi R, Nishikawa A, Sugita T. Characterization of the skin fungal microbiota in patients with atopic dermatitis and in healthy subjects. Microbiol Immunol. 2011;55:625–32.

Zheng Y, Wang Q, Ma L, Chen Y, Gao Y, Zhang G, Cui S, Liang H, He C, Song L. Alterations in the skin microbiome are associated with disease severity and treatment in the perioral zone of the skin of infants with atopic dermatitis. Eur J Clin Microbiol Infect Dis. 2019;38:1677–85.

Zheng D, Liwinski T, Elinav E. Interaction between microbiota and immunity in health and disease. Cell Res. 2020;30:492–506.

Zhu T, Zhao J, Qu Y, Zhang L, Mu D. Association of very preterm birth with decreased risk of eczema: a systematic review and meta-analysis. J Am Acad Dermatol. 2018;78(1142–1148): e8.

Zuccotti G, Meneghin F, Aceti A, Barone G, Callegari ML, Di Mauro A, Fantini MP, Gori D, Indrio F, Maggio L, Morelli L, Corvaglia L, Italian Society of, N. Probiotics for prevention of atopic diseases in infants: systematic review and meta-analysis. Allergy. 2015;70:1356–71.

Chapter 7
Skin Microbiome in Psoriasis

Nanna Fyhrquist and Antti Lauerma

Abstract Psoriasis is an immune-mediated disease, which has been studied for decades, but its pathogenesis is still not completely understood. Psoriasis is the result of interplay between genetic factors and external triggers, wherein the cutaneous microbiota may play a critical role by responding to external triggers and interacting with the host immune system. Many studies have highlighted a crucial role for microorganisms in the pathophysiology of chronic inflammatory skin disease, however, in the case of psoriasis, a direct link between the skin microbiome and psoriasis pathogenesis remains to be established.

Keywords Psoriasis · Inflammation · Microbiome · Microbiota · IL-17 · Streptococcus · Staphylococcus · Lactobacillus · Finegoldia

7.1 Introduction

Psoriasis is a chronic inflammatory skin disease with possible autoimmune background. It has been estimated that about 125 million people in the world suffer from it, with a prevalence rate of 2–4% in the developed countries (Griffiths et al. 2021). It has significant impairment on life quality and psychosocial issues. Additionally, a minority of psoriasis patients suffer from nail psoriasis that is often related to psoriasis arthritis. Psoriasis has several clinical manifestations in skin. Most common is chronic plaque psoriasis. Other forms are psoriasis guttata (often associated with streptococcal infection as trigger), psoriasis inversa (localized in flexural areas), erythrodermic psoriasis (affects whole skin) and the most dangerous form pustular psoriasis that can be associated with fever and mortality (Zhou et al. 2022). Diseases with clinical similarity include pityriasis rubra pilaris (Abdel-Azim et al. 2017),

N. Fyhrquist (✉)
Institute of Environmental Medicine, Karolinska Institutet, Nobels Väg 13, 17177 Stockholm, Sweden
e-mail: Nanna.Fyhrquist@ki.se

A. Lauerma
Department of Dermatology, University of Helsinki, Helsinki, Finland

pustulosis palmoplantaris (Remitz et al. 1996) and parapsoriasis (Salava et al. 2017), which are separate entities.

7.2 Genetics

Psoriasis is characterized by epidermal hyperproliferation and dermal inflammation. In a clinical context, drugs affecting both hyperproliferation (e.g., retinoids which have also immunomodulatory properties and target immune cells via nuclear receptors) and inflammation (e.g., immunosuppressants and biologics) are effective in reducing the disease process. Psoriasis is under intense research, as it offers several disease processes of interest and because it is associated with comorbidities such as metabolic syndrome. Early onset psoriasis is associated with a strong genetic basis and has high heritability. Genes associated with psoriasis include NF-kB signaling genes CARD14, TNFAIP3, IL36RN and TNIP1, proangiogenic factor VEGFA, IL-17 signal transducer TRAF3IP2, epidermal growth factor stabilized protein IF27 and autophagy gene AP153 (Griffiths 2012; Zhou et al. 2022). Bioinformatic analysis reveals additional genes with yet not known participation in the pathogenesis, such as ARNTL2, GM2A, KCNJ15, UBE2F, OASL, HPSE, SH3PXD2A-AS1, MAP-17 and MPZL2 (Marwah et al. 2018).

7.3 Cytokines

Psoriasis is associated with a plethora of cytokines and receptors, which in some cases also provide means to treat the disease. The IL-23/IL-17 axis is the main driver of psoriatic skin inflammation. The IL-17 family includes six members, IL-17A, IL-17B, IL-17C, IL-17D, IL-17E and IL-17F. The most well characterized member is IL-17A, which is often referred to as "IL-17". T cells (CD4+ T helper 17 (Th17), CD8+ T cells, gammadelta T cells, invariant natural killer T cells (iNKT)) and natural killer cells (NK cells) are the main sources of IL-17A, which binds to receptors on keratinocytes and stimulates abnormal keratinocyte proliferation and barrier disruption via downregulation of adhesion molecules, as well as the production of antimicrobial peptides, and chemokines which recruit more Th17 cells, neutrophils, dendritic cells and macrophages to the site. IL-17A may also indirectly induce hyperproliferation of keratinocytes via IL-19 and IL-36. IL-17 receptors include five members, from IL-17RA to IL-17RE, out of which IL-17RA is most potent (Zhou et al. 2022). IL-17 inhibitors are now a major class of biologics in psoriasis treatment. Other cytokines of pathophysiological and pharmacological interest are IL-22 and tumor necrosis-factor alpha (TNF-alpha)) (Griffiths 2012).

7.4 Energy Metabolism

Psoriatic skin proliferates at a high rate and involves activated T cells, which require extensive energy. A major source for energy is glucose/carbohydrates. Recently the importance of glucose/carbohydrate metabolism has gained interest, as it is also associated with metabolic syndromes, e.g. diabetes mellitus, which are common comorbidities of psoriasis. In addition to abnormal glucose metabolism, amino acid metabolism, including the glutamine/glutamate pathway, is also abnormal in psoriasis. Another emerging field is lipid metabolism in psoriasis with altered levels of metabolites in psoriatic skin lesion, serum and plasma (Zhou et al. 2022).

7.5 Cell Signaling and Other Factors

Psoriasis is associated with abnormal STAT and NF-kB signaling and alterations in the MAP kinase signaling pathways. New groups of oral and parenteral kinase inhibitors have been introduced as effective treatments in psoriasis (Słuczanowska-Głąbowska et al. 2021). Of novel/recent interest are non-coding RNAs, both micro RNAs and long-chain non-coding RNAs (Zhou et al. 2022).

7.6 Antimicrobial Peptides

Antimicrobial peptides (AMPs) are found in large amounts in psoriatic skin. Psoriasis is rarely infected, which may partly be explained by AMPs amounts. Major AMPs include LL37, beta-defensins and S100 proteins, which are well characterized since the 2000's. Of interest is the fact that the same AMPs are highly expressed during cutaenous wound healing (Morizane and Gallo 2012).

7.7 The Skin Microbiome

Psoriasis is associated with the community compositions of both skin and gut microbiomes. In the gut, short-chain fatty acids (SCFAs) play a major role in regulating immunity and inflammation, as well as metabolism. Skin serves as a major barrier to the outside world and protects against invasion by pathogens. Skin and the gastrointestinal tract are colonized with microbiota immediately after birth, and the first years of life is a critical period of development and fine tuning of the immune system, and of establishment of immune tolerance against commensals. Of particular interest is the interaction between commensals, pathogens, and host derived AMPs, innate immunity and adaptive immunity. Once established, the human associated microbiome is stable and usually not undergoing major changes in the long term. Despite the longterm development of immune balance between the host and its microorganisms, various external and host factors may cause disturbance, eventually leading to dysbiosis and departure from skin homeostasis to a disease state (Celoria et al. 2023).

7.8 Skin Microbiome in Psoriasis

An early study investigated whether skin microorganisms may trigger psoriatic skin. Two microbes, *Malassezia ovalis* and *Staphylococcus epidermidis* were selected, heat-killed, and sonicated extracts were applied to skin of psoriasis patients. Patch tests resulted in skin reactions, that were psoriasis-like both clinically and histologically (Lober et al. 1982).

Another early study compared *Staphylococcus aureus* and staphylococcal toxins in patients with psoriasis, atopic dermatitis and erythroderma and healthy volunteer skin. *Staphylococcus aureus* was identified in both psoriasis and atopic dermatitis skin, and the severity of skin inflammation correlated with the enterotoxin production potential of *staphylococcus aureus* in individual patients (Tomi et al. 2005).

The first study utilizing the 16S rRNA gene sequencing/amplicon sequencing technique in psoriasis revealed that the most abundant bacterial phylum in psoriasis lesions was *Firmicutes* (46.2%), occurring at significantly higher abundance than in nonlesional or healthy skin. *Actinobacteria* was most common in healthy skin. *Propionibacterium* species (now annotated as *Cutibacterium*) were underrepresented in psoriasis lesional skin compared to healthy volunteers, while in nonlesional psoriatic skin the abundance of propionibacteria was at an intermediate level (Gao et al. PLoS One 2008).

A second amplicon sequencing study showed that the psoriasis microbiome is highly diverse. This diversity was the result of the co-occurrence of four dominant bacterial genera in psoriasis, *Corynebacterium, Propionibacterium (Cutibacterium), Staphylococcus* and *Streptococcus*. Instead, organisms such as *Cupriavidus, Flavisolibacter, Methylobacterium* and *Schelegella* were underrepresented. The study described two types of skin microbiota. The first type was characterized by abundant *Proteobacteria*, whereas the second type was characterized by abundant *Firmicutes* and *Actinobacteria*. Psoriasis lesions were frequent in individuals harboring the second type of skin microbiota (Alekseyenko et al. 2013).

Staphylococcus aureus was found to be overrepresented in both lesional and nonlesional psoriatic skin, and *Staphylococcus epidermidis* and *Cutibacterium acnes* underrepresented. In a mouse this phenomenon, i.e., abundant *S. aureus* and loss of *S. epidermidis* and *C. acnes*, is associated with Th17 immune responses (Chang et al. 2018). In another study, a high bacterial load, increased *Corynebacterium* and decreased *Cutibacterium (Propionibacterium)* was found in psoriatic lesions. Nonlesional and lesional psoriatic skin had similar skin microbiota in psoriasis and psoriatic arthritis patients, when compared to normal skin in healthy individuals (Boix-Amoros et al. 2023).

Erythrodermic psoriasis is a severe subtype of psoriasis. Patients with erythrodermic psoriasis showed high bacterial diversity, increased *S. aureus* colonization and reduced AMP production (Liu et al. 2023). Another staphylococcal strain, *S. warneri* exacerbated skin inflammation in an imiquimod-induced psoriasis-like dermatitis model in mice (Si et al. 2023).

A recent large-scale, comprehensive study of the microbiome in psoriatic skin, including skin samples from 134 patients diagnosed with plaque psoriasis, and 126 healthy volunteers, found distinct patterns of host-microbe interactions in lesional psoriatic skin compared with healthy skin. Taxa such as *Corynebacterium simulans, C. kroppenstedtii, Finegoldia* and *Neisseriaceae* were significantly more abundant in psoriatic lesions compared with healthy skin, while Lactobacilli, *Burkholderia spp* and *Cutibacterium acnes* were lower in abundance. Using feature selection and classification analysis, *C. simulans, Neisseriaceae, Lepotrichia, Corynebacterium,* and *Lactobacilli* were among the most discriminating features between healthy and psoriatic skin. To understand the interplay between disease relevant taxa, networks were inferred to illustrate co-occurrence relationships between taxa. While lesional skin is typically dominated by a single species (*Staphylococcus aureus*) in atopic dermatitis (PMID: 31619666), psoriasis lesions were characterized by the co-occurrence of multiple taxa, including *Corynebacterium* and *Finegoldia* species (Fyhrquist et al. 2019).

The same study investigated gene expression profiles in underlying skin, and by combining the microbiome and transcriptome datasets, the interplay between host and microbes could be assessed. A co-expression network constructed based on the psoriasis transcriptome, and partitioned into 12 modules, allowed identification of associations between disease relevant microbial taxa and module eigengenes. The results suggested an association between the abundance of *Corynebacterium spp* and three modules of genes which were enriched for biological functions such as cell cycling, interferon signaling, and Th1 and Th2 activation, respectively. To investigate effects of the skin microbiota and gene expression on clinical severity, feature selection was coupled with multivariate regression, ranking genes and microorganisms according to their correlation with severity scores. However, no associations were found between clinical severity and the abundance of disease relevant taxa in psoriatic lesions (Fyhrquist et al. 2019).

7.9   Conclusions

Psoriasis is a major inflammatory skin disease. Major progress has been made in management of inflammation and hyperproliferation especially with biologics. Of interest is the effect by skin and gut microbiota. Future studies will show what is the true clinical significance of skin microbiome in psoriasis.

References

Abdel-Azim NE, Ismail SA, Fathy E. Differentiation of pityriasis rubra pilaris from plaque psoriasis by dermoscopy. Arch Dermatol Res. 2017 May;309(4):311–314.

Alekseyenko AV, Perez-Perez GI, De Souza A, Strober B, Gao Z, Bihan M, Li K, Methé BA, Blaser MJ. Community differentiation of the cutaneous microbiota in psoriasis. Microbiome. 2013;1(1):31.

Boix-Amorós A, Badri MH, Manasson J, Blank RB, Haberman RH, Neimann AL, Girija PV, Jimenez Hernandez A, Heguy A, Koralov SB, Bonneau R, Clemente JC, Scher JU. Alterations in the cutaneous microbiome of patients with psoriasis and psoriatic arthritis reveal similarities between non-lesional and lesional skin. Ann Rheum Dis. 2023;82(4):507–14.

Celoria V, Rosset F, Pala V, Dapavo P, Ribero S, Quaglino P, Mastorino L. The skin microbiome and its role in psoriasis: a review. Psoriasis (Auckl). 2023;26(13):71–8.

Chang HW, Yan D, Singh R, Liu J, Lu X, Ucmak D, Lee K, Afifi L, Fadrosh D, Leech J, Vasquez KS, Lowe MM, Rosenblum MD, Scharschmidt TC, Lynch SV, Liao W. Alteration of the cutaneous microbiome in psoriasis and potential role in Th17 polarization. Microbiome. 2018;6(1):154.

Fahlén A, Engstrand L, Baker BS, Powles A, Fry L. Comparison of bacterial microbiota in skin biopsies from normal and psoriatic skin. Arch Dermatol Res. 2012;304(1):15–22.

Fry L, Baker BS, Powles AV, Fahlen A, Engstrand L. Is chronic plaque psoriasis triggered by microbiota in the skin? Br J Dermatol. 2013;169(1):47–52.

Fyhrquist N, Muirhead G, Prast-Nielsen S, Jeanmougin M, Olah P, Skoog T, Jules-Clement G, Feld M, Barrientos-Somarribas M, Sinkko H, van den Bogaard EH, Zeeuwen PLJM, Rikken G, Schalkwijk J, Niehues H, Däubener W, Eller SK, Alexander H, Pennino D, Suomela S, Tessas I, Lybeck E, Baran AM, Darban H, Gangwar RS, Gerstel U, Jahn K, Karisola P, Yan L, Hansmann B, Katayama S, Meller S, Bylesjö M, Hupé P, Levi-Schaffer F, Greco D, Ranki A, Schröder JM, Barker J, Kere J, Tsoka S, Lauerma A, Soumelis V, Nestle FO, Homey B, Andersson B, Alenius H. Microbe-host interplay in atopic dermatitis and psoriasis. Nat Commun. 2019;10(1):4703.

Gao Z, Tseng CH, Strober BE, Pei Z, Blaser MJ. Substantial alterations of the cutaneous bacterial biota in psoriatic lesions. PLoS ONE. 2008;3(7): e2719.

Griffiths CEM. Biologics for psoriasis: current evidence and future use. Br J Dermatol. 2012;167(Suppl 3):1–2

Griffiths CEM, Armstrong AW, Gudjonsson JE, Barker JNWN. Psoriasis. Lancet. 2021;397(10281):1301–15.

Liu Y, Wu X, Song P, Liu L, Zhong X, He Q, Zhang Z. Increased S. aureus colonization and reduced antimicrobial peptide expression in erythrodermic psoriasis. Int Immunopharmacol. 2023 Dec 13;127:111343.

Lober CW, Belew PW, Rosenberg EW, Bale G. Patch tests with killed sonicated microflora in patients with psoriasis. Arch Dermatol. 1982;118(5):322–5.

Marwah VS, Kinaret PAS, Serra A, Scala G, Lauerma A, Fortino V, Greco D. INfORM: Inference of NetwOrk Response Modules. Bioinformatics. 2018;34(12):2136–213.

Morin S, Tremblay A, Dumais E, Julien P, Flamand N, Pouliot R. Eicosapentaenoic acid influences the lipid profile of an in vitro psoriatic skin model produced with T cells. Biomolecules. 2023;13(9):1413.

Morizane S, Gallo RL. Antimicrobial peptides in the pathogenesis of psoriasis. J Dermatol. 2012;39(3):225–30.

Quan C, Chen XY, Li X, Xue F, Chen LH, Liu N, Wang B, Wang LQ, Wang XP, Yang H, Zheng J. Psoriatic lesions are characterized by higher bacterial load and imbalance between Cutibacterium and Corynebacterium. J Am Acad Dermatol. 2020;82(4):955–61.

Remitz A, Lauerma AI, Erkko P, Reitamo S. Delayed-type hypersensitivity in palmoplantar pustulosis: effect of cyclosporin A treatment on skin testing with recall antigens. Acta Derm Venereol. 1996;76(4):310–3.

Salava A, Pereira P, Aho V, Väkevä L, Paulin L, Auvinen P, Ranki A, Lauerma A. Skin microbiome in small- and large-plaque parapsoriasis. Acta Derm Venereol. 2017;97(6):685–91.

Si W, Li M, Wang K, Li J, Xu M, Zhou X, Bai J, Qu Z, Song G, Wu X, Guo Y, Hu H, Fu D, Yang Z, Wu M, Yan D, Song X, Tian Z. Staphylococcus warneri strain XSB102 exacerbates psoriasis and promotes keratinocyte proliferation in imiquimod-induced psoriasis-like dermatitis mice. Arch Microbiol. 2023;206(1):3.

Simard M, Tremblay A, Morin S, Rioux G, Flamand N, Pouliot R. N-eicosapentaenoyl-ethanolamine decreases the proliferation of psoriatic keratinocytes in a reconstructed psoriatic skin model. Sci Rep. 2023;13(1):1211.

Słuczanowska-Głąbowska S, Ziegler-Krawczyk A, Szumilas K, Pawlik A. Role of Janus Kinase inhibitors in therapy of psoriasis. J Clin Med. 2021;10(19):4307.

Tomi NS, Kränke B, Aberer E. Staphylococcal toxins in patients with psoriasis, atopic dermatitis, and erythroderma, and in healthy control subjects. J Am Acad Dermatol. 2005;53(1):67–72.

Zhou X, Chen Y, Cui L, Shi Y, Guo C. Advances in the pathogenesis of psoriasis: from keratinocyte perspective. Cell Death Dis. 2022;13(1):81.

Chapter 8
Studying the Skin Virome Using Metagenomics

Guilherme Augusto Maia and Björn Andersson

Abstract Virus infections are common in human skin and several skin diseases are associated with viruses. It is also possible that viruses are linked to common autoimmune diseases. Virus infections in human skin can be readily detected in metagenomic sequencing data using standard database searches, including both bacteriophages and human viruses. Virus infections differ from microbiome communities in that they are often transient and more variable. This affects both methodology and down-stream analyses. This chapter describes the characteristics of the human skin virus microbiome and outlines key considerations for studying it effectively.

Keywords Skin viruses · Virome · Metagenomics · Bioinformatics · Skin diseases · Skin cancer

8.1 Introduction

Studying the skin microbiome involves exploring the diverse community of microorganisms that inhabit the surface of the skin. This ecosystem includes bacteria, fungi, viruses, and other microbes. The skin microbiome plays a crucial role in maintaining skin health, modulating immune responses, and protecting against pathogens (Naik et al. 2012, Belkaid and Segre 2014). The studies of the skin microbiome have thus far mainly focused on bacterial communities, and to a lesser extent on fungi (Byrd et al. 2018).

There are multiple human viruses that infect skin cells, and several that are known to cause skin diseases (see below), and the bacterial communities in the skin are rich in bacteriophages. Although these viruses can be detected in shotgun metagenomics analyses from skin samples, analyzing viruses presents several difficulties. Skin samples often contain small amounts of DNA, which can result in low detection levels. This, combined with environmental exposure, makes the samples sensitive to contaminants, both from the environment and from laboratory reagents (Salter

G. A. Maia · B. Andersson (✉)
Department of Cell and Molecular Biology, Karolinska Institutet, Stockholm, Sweden
e-mail: bjorn.andersson@ki.se

© The Author(s), under exclusive license to Springer Nature Switzerland AG 2025
A. Lauerma et al. (eds.), *The Skin Microbiome Manual*,
https://doi.org/10.1007/978-3-031-82689-4_8

et al. 2014). These contaminants include viruses from other organisms, often from plants or insects, and also phages from various sources (Salter et al. 2014, Liang and Bushman 2021). In addition, skin samples often contain large amounts of human DNA sequences, which may yield false database matches to viruses due to repeats or integrated retroviral sequences.

Viral infections can manifest as chronic, transient, or dormant, with virus production occurring only under specific conditions (Virgin et al. 2009). While bacteriophages can be analyzed as a part of the stable microbiome and be associated with certain bacterial hosts, human viruses are more difficult to study, as they only occur at certain skin sites at specific times (Zárate et al. 2017).

A complete metagenomic search for viral sequences often generates a long list of viral matches, where the entries need to be carefully considered to identify true skin viruses. This process involves removing viruses known to infect other hosts, removing known laboratory contaminants, identifying human sequences, and validation through for example Polymerase Chain Reaction (PCR), as necessary.

Additional considerations regarding which viruses to include in the final analysis will depend on the biological question. For example, studies may focus on the effect of bacteriophages on skin bacterial communities, the influence of human virus infections on particular skin phenotypes, or the discovery of previously unknown skin viruses. Most analysis pipelines will provide a broad overview, followed by automated and manual selection steps to exclude contaminants and select viruses of interest (Smith et al. 2022).

8.2 Methods and Strategies for Sequencing the Skin Virome

8.2.1 Sample Collection

Sampling of skin microbiome is mostly performed using skin swabs or by cups filled with fluid. Because the microbial biomass on the skin is low, these methods provide a balanced ratio of human to microbial material, compared to skin biopsies.

The selection of skin sites for analysis will depend on the research questions. Different anatomical regions have distinct microbial communities, which may be differentially affected by viral infections and skin diseases. For an extensive search for viruses on the skin microbiome, samples can be collected from areas like the face, arms, back, and feet. In cases where a specific skin disease is studied, it is beneficial to collect samples from and around skin lesions, to capture virus infections at different stages. Due to the transient nature of many virus infections, longitudinal sampling may be necessary to capture the dynamics of virus infections and to ensure that all relevant infections are detected.

8.2.2 DNA Extraction

For virome analysis, total nucleic acid is extracted from collected skin swabs or other samples to analyze the genetic material of skin microorganisms. As with all microbiome studies, it is necessary to include blank controls to account for potential contamination from microbial and viral DNA present in laboratory reagents (Kong et al. 2017). Half of the extracted sample can undergo a reverse transcriptase treatment to specifically detect RNA viruses, while the remaining untreated portion of the sample is used to detect DNA viruses. It has previously been common to use methods to enrich for virus particles when studying viruses, using manly nuclease treatments, followed by amplification using an unspecific polymerase Chain Reaction (PCR) to increase DNA concentrations. As sequencing methods have improved, both regarding the starting amounts needed and total reads produced, this is in most cases no longer needed, which reduces bias in the microbiome data.

8.2.3 Sequencing

Shotgun metagenomics must be employed for virus microbiome studies. This indispensable method enables sequencing all the genetic material in a sample, providing a comprehensive view of the entire microbiome, including bacteria, fungi, and viruses. While PCR assays exist for common viruses, these are time-consuming and may not detect rare variants and rare or novel viruses.

8.2.4 Bioinformatics Analysis

Standard microbiome pipelines commonly use KRAKEN or similar tools for taxonomic classification of microbial taxa on the skin using sequencing data. However, these pipelines often fall short of providing a complete picture of viral content due to incomplete databases, especially because virus families are diverse and there are many newly discovered virus strains and species. This is particularly true for bacteriophages, where the diversity and complexity are great, and much is unknown. Also, databases may include sequences that hinder accurate analysis, such as Human Endogenous Retroviruses (HERVs), which in most cases originate from human DNA contamination.

To address these shortcomings, it is preferable to conduct searches using databases like GenBank, or a local virus datbase, using tools such as BLAST or DIAMOND. This is more time-consuming, but careful removal of human and bacterial reads can speed up the process. The resulting lists of hits need to be carefully examined to eliminate spurious matches, often caused by repeats or sequences that have been erroneously labelled as viruses in public databases. While it is possible to automate much of this process, a manual inspection remains essential to rectify errors. Additionally, environmental and reagent contaminants can be identified and removed by comparing them with blank controls and analyzing individual virus hits and their origins. For example, a sequence match that is 100% identical to a plant virus is unlikely to signify a human skin infection. An example of initial virome data is shown in Fig. 8.1.

8.2.5 Functional Analysis

Depending on read depth, complete or partial virus genomes can be assembled and assessed for genetic diversity. Subsequently, strain and evolutionary analysis can be performed, as well as functional analyses of viral genes. As virus families differ greatly from each other, the research questions associated with each virus will be different, but a novel genome sequence represents a good starting point for future studies.

8.2.6 Integration with Clinical Data

The relationship between virus content and skin health can be explored either by applying statistical methods to data from specific sample collections or following up the discovery of a specific virus or set of viruses by carrying out targeted assays in additional individuals. These approaches aim to identify associations between particular virus infections and skin conditions such as acne, atopic dermatitis, or psoriasis (Fyhrquist et al. 2019). However, it is important to take the dynamics of virus infection into account when carrying out such associations. Virus infections are often transient and infections may be at different stages in the specific sites sampled in each patient, adding complexity to data interpretation.

It's important to note that the term "microbiome" traditionally refers to the community of microorganisms, including bacteria, fungi, viruses, and other microbes, that inhabit a particular environment (Cho and Blaser 2012). However, the concept of the "virus microbiome" is often used interchangeably with the virome— the collection of viruses present in a particular ecosystem or, in this case, within the human body. The human virome is a complex and dynamic system that includes both pathogenic and non-pathogenic viruses (Santiago-Rodriguez and Hollister 2019).

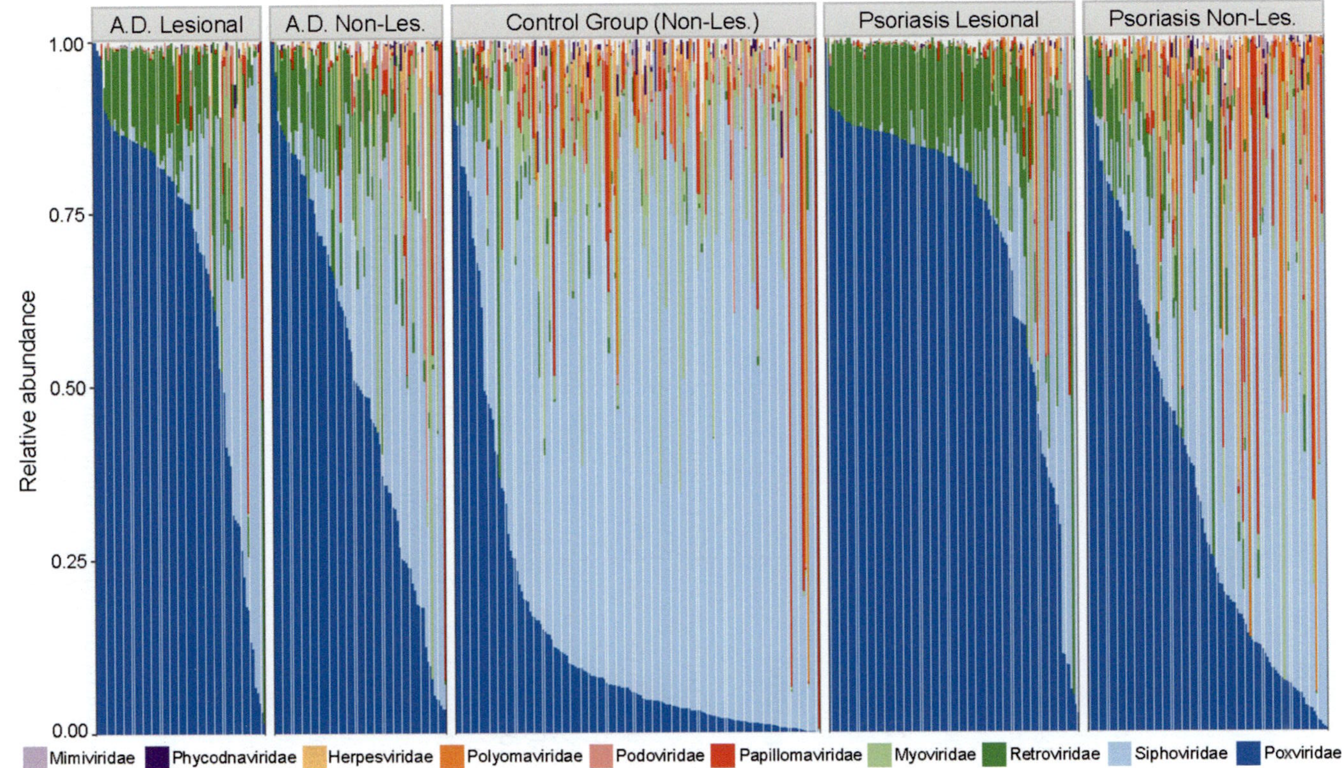

Fig. 8.1 Initial analysis data of the virus content of a set of skin samples after shotgun sequencing

8.3 Overview of the Human Virome

The study of the human virome is a rapidly evolving field, and ongoing research aims to uncover the intricacies of viral communities within the human body and their impact on health and disease.

8.3.1 Virus Types

Bacteriophages are viruses that infect bacteria. These play a role in modulating bacterial populations and influencing the bacterial composition in various body sites, such as the gut.

Eukaryotic Viruses are viruses that infect eukaryotic cells, including animals and humans. This category includes both pathogenic viruses (e.g., influenza virus, herpesviruses) and non-pathogenic viruses.

8.3.2 Locations

Viruses have the capacity to infect a multitude of different cell types throughout the human body, and they can be detected in many different sample types. This includes viruses that inhabit the skin, influencing skin health and potentially contributing to skin disorders.

The gut is a rich environment for viruses, where bacteriophages interact with the bacterial community, influencing the gut microbiota's composition and function of the gut microbiome.

The respiratory tract, alongside the gastrointestinal tract, is a common entry point for viruses. Respiratory viruses, such as influenza viruses and respiratory syncytial virus (RSV), have a great impact on human health.

Plasma or serum samples are used to detect viruses in the bloodstream. While the presence of viruses in the bloodstream is typically limited, certain conditions can lead to viremia. There are families of chronic human viruses, like anelloviruses, that circulate in the blood.

8.3.3 Impact

The composition of the human virome can change over time due to factors such as infections, exposure to new environments, and alterations in the host immune response. Also, the virome interacts with other components of the microbiome, such as bacteria and fungi, which may have implications for host health and disease.

Exposure to non-pathogenic viruses in the virome helps educate the immune system and may contribute to immune tolerance.

Imbalances or dysbiosis in the virome have been associated with various diseases, including inflammatory bowel diseases (IBD), respiratory infections, and certain skin conditions (Fyhrquist et al. 2019, Santiago-Rodriguez and Hollister 2019).

8.4 The Skin Virome

The skin is the largest organ in the human body, serving as a vital protective barrier against various external threats, including viruses. Viruses can impact the human skin in various ways, inducing a range of infections, symptoms, and conditions. Some viruses specifically target the skin or mucous membranes, while others may affect the skin as part of a broader systemic infection. Here are descriptions of viruses commonly associated with skin infection and disease.

8.4.1 Bacteriophages

Microbiome sequencing from skin samples will result in a multitude of sequences that can be identified as bacteriophages. These viruses typically originate from several different families, including Myoviridae, Podoviridae and Siphoviridae. Due to the vast diversity of bacteriophages, sequencing results will include a few perfect matches to well-studied species, numerous more distant hits, as well as entirely new species. Characterizing the complete bacteriophage microbiome is a monumental task and any analysis will only provide a partial picture of the actual phage content.

8.4.2 Human Viruses

Herpesviruses: Human skin harbors several herpesviruses, including Human herpesvirus-1 to − 5. Among these, Herpes Simplex Virus (HSV) stands out, with HSV-1 and HSV-2 causing oral and genital herpes, respectively. These viruses can cause painful blisters or sores on the skin, often in clusters. Additionally, Varicella-Zoster Virus (VZV) causes chickenpox during initial infection and may later reactivate to cause shingles, resulting in a painful rash and blisters localized to one side of the body. Other herpesviruses linked to skin issues are Human Herpesvirus 6 and 7 (HHV-6, HHV-7), associated with roseola—a viral infection primarily affecting infants and young children, causing a high fever and a rash once the fever subsides—and Epstein-Barr Virus (EBV, HHV-4), which can occasionally lead to a skin rash as a part of the infection.

Human Papillomavirus (HPV): HPV can cause various skin conditions like warts, including common warts, plantar warts (on the feet), and genital warts. Some strains of HPV are also linked to certain cancers, including cervical cancer (Dunne and Park 2013). HPV compromises numerous subtypes, many of which can be detected in skin samples. It is important to note that HPV can be present as a contaminant in reagents and laboratories. Therefore, it is advisable to include blank control samples in HPV detection assays.

Molluscum Contagiosum Virus: Infection with this virus is common and can result in small, raised, round bumps on the skin, that may appear flesh-colored, white, or pink. These lesions can be itchy and are highly contagious. This virus is commonly found in human skin samples, even from asymptomatic individuals. It is a poxvirus, and as such, has a relatively large genome that contains some repetitive sequences. The repeats found in poxviruses can be similar to repeats from other, larger genomes, which may cause spurious matches. Consequently, it is necessary to examine all poxvirus hits carefully.

Enteroviruses: Certain enteroviruses like Coxsackievirus can cause hand, foot, and mouth disease, which manifests as sores in the mouth and a rash on the hands and feet. Belonging to the Picornaviridae family, enteroviruses are RNA viruses. Therefore, these will not be detected in standard microbiome sequencing without an additional reverse transcriptase step.

Polyomaviruses: Before 2005, only two human polyomaviruses were known, both causing neurological symptoms in immunosuppressed individuals (Dalianis and Hirsch 2013). Since then, by using metagenomics methods, at least 12 additional human polyomaviruses have been discovered. Among these discoveries, Human polyomavirus 5, known as Merkel cell polyomavirus, has emerged as particularly significant. It has been linked to Merkel cell carcinoma, a rare but aggressive form of skin cancer (Dalianis and Hirsch 2013). Intriguingly, this virus is also commonly found in skin microbiome samples from healthy individuals, suggesting a complex relationship between its presence and disease development. Three others recently discovered polyomaviruses also infect human skin: Human polyomavirus 6, 7 and 10. These viruses are often found to be shed in large amounts from the skin, but their role in disease pathology remains unclear.

Dermatotropic Viruses: Some viruses have a specific affinity for skin cells, and can cause various skin conditions, like viral exanthems (rashes). Other examples include measles, rubella, and the fifth disease (erythema infectiosum), which are attributed to parvovirus B19.

8.5 Conclusions

Most viral skin infections are diagnosed based on symptom observation, clinical examination, and occasionally, specific laboratory tests or viral cultures. Emerging diagnostic techniques like metagenomics hold promise as an option, especially as sequencing costs decrease. Understanding the various viruses that can affect human skin is crucial for effective prevention, diagnosis, and treatment, as well as for research into new disease associations. Ongoing research and advancements in virology will contribute to improved strategies for managing skin infections, emphasizing the importance of multidisciplinary collaborations in dermatology and infectious disease management.

Through continued skin metagenomics studies, coupled with improved characterization using bioinformatics and validation of findings, it is likely that additional viruses that infect human skin will be discovered. Novel bacteriophages are found continuously, and other candidates for validation are often seen as either weak sequence similarities to known viruses or as sequences of unknown origin. Despite a predominant focus on known viruses by most studies, virus discovery remains important.

The key takeaway of this chapter is that the nature of the virus microbiome is fundamentally different from that of the bacterial and fungal microbiome. While the latter can be described as a community or ecosystem that is relatively stable over time, the virome is much more dynamic and variable. Virus infections are often transient and only occur in a specific location for a short time. In addition, longer-term or chronic infections go through fluctuations in activity, with periods of undetectability interspersed with high titers. This dynamic nature needs to be considered when planning virome studies, which requires adaptations to be made to both sampling and downstream analysis. For example, samples need to be carefully selected and larger sample numbers may be needed. In addition, the fluctuating titers of viruses over short periods render the relative abundance of sequenced reads less reliable for analysis. It is also important to take into account that the genome of viruses is small and is often present in small amounts in samples, making it especially important to carefully exclude contaminants from reagents and the environment. By recognizing these nuances and adapting methodologies accordingly, researchers can navigate the intricacies of the virome, leading to more comprehensive insights into viral skin infections and improved diagnostic and therapeutic approaches.

References

Belkaid Y, Segre JA. Dialogue between skin microbiota and immunity. Science. 2014;346(6212):954–9. https://doi.org/10.1126/science.1260144.

Byrd AL, Belkaid Y, Segre JA. The human skin microbiome. Nat Rev Microbiol. 2018;16(3):143–55. https://doi.org/10.1038/nrmicro.2017.157.

Cho I, Blaser MJ. The human microbiome: at the interface of health and disease. Nat Rev Genet. 2012;13(4):260–70. https://doi.org/10.1038/nrg3182.

Dalianis T, Hirsch HH. Human polyomaviruses in disease and cancer. Virology. 2013;437(2):63–72. https://doi.org/10.1016/j.virol.2012.12.015.

Dunne EF, Park IU. HPV and HPV-associated diseases. Infect Dis Clin North Am. 2013;27(4):765–78. https://doi.org/10.1016/j.idc.2013.09.001.

Fyhrquist N, Muirhead G, Prast-Nielsen S, Jeanmougin M, Olah P, Skoog T, Jules-Clement G, Feld M, Barrientos-Somarribas M, Sinkko H, van den Bogaard EH, Zeeuwen PLJM, Rikken G,

Schalkwijk J, Niehues H, Däubener W, Eller SK, Alexander H, Pennino D, Suomela S. Microbe-host interplay in atopic dermatitis and psoriasis. Nat Commun. 2019;10(1):4703. https://doi.org/10.1038/s41467-019-12253-y.

Kong HH, Andersson B, Clavel T, Common JE, Jackson SA, Olson ND, Segre JA, Traidl-Hoffmann C. Performing skin microbiome research: a method to the madness. J Invest Dermatol. 2017;137(3):561–8. https://doi.org/10.1016/j.jid.2016.10.033.

Liang G, Bushman FD. The human virome: assembly, composition and host interactions. Nat. Rev. Microbiol. (2021);19(8). https://doi.org/10.1038/s41579-021-00536-5.

Naik S, Bouladoux N, Wilhelm C, Molloy MJ, Salcedo R, Kastenmuller W, Deming C, Quinones M, Koo L, Conlan S, Spencer S, Hall JA, Dzutsev A, Kong H, Campbell DJ, Trinchieri G, Segre JA, Belkaid Y. Compartmentalized control of skin immunity by resident commensals. Science. 2012;337(6098):1115–9. https://doi.org/10.1126/science.1225152.

Salter SJ, Cox MJ, Turek EM, Calus ST, Cookson WO, Moffatt MF, Turner P, Parkhill J, Loman NJ, Walker AW. Reagent and laboratory contamination can critically impact sequence-based microbiome analyses. BMC Biology. (2014);12(1). https://doi.org/10.1186/s12915-014-0087-z.

Santiago-Rodriguez TM, Hollister EB. Human virome and disease: high-throughput sequencing for virus discovery, identification of phage-bacteria dysbiosis and development of therapeutic approaches with emphasis on the human gut. Viruses. 2019;11(7):656. https://doi.org/10.3390/v11070656.

Smith SE, Huang W, Tiamani K, Unterer M, Mirzaei MK, Deng L. Emerging technologies in the study of the virome. Curr Opin Virol. 2022;54:101231–101231. https://doi.org/10.1016/j.coviro.2022.101231.

Virgin HW, Wherry EJ, Ahmed R. Redefining chronic viral infection. Cell. 2009;138(1):30–50. https://doi.org/10.1016/j.cell.2009.06.036.

Zárate S, Taboada B, Yocupicio-Monroy M, Arias CF. Human virome. Arch Med Res. 2017;48(8):701–16. https://doi.org/10.1016/j.arcmed.2018.01.005.

Chapter 9
The Skin Microbiome: Potential for Novel Diagnostic and Therapeutic Strategies

Alexander Salava and Nanna Fyhrquist

Abstract Microbiome based-diagnostics and microbiome-targeted therapies are novel interesting strategies in the management of skin diseases. Substantial microbiome changes have been observed in skin conditions and there seems to be significant potential to use this information in clinical diagnostics. Microbiome-targeted therapies have been studied in different settings and three main concepts have evolved. First, the cutaneous microbiome can be influenced by using methods that affect the cutaneous microbiome directly, e.g., topical pro- and prebiotics. Second, healthy or modified microbiomes or single microbial strains can be relocated onto the patients' skin (transplantation or engraftments). And third, mechanisms that affect the cutaneous microbiome indirectly can be used, e.g., targeting the gut-skin axis (gastrointestinal probiotics). The skin microbiome remains an interesting area of research in developing new diagnostics or therapeutics in clinical medicine, especially dermatology. In addition, microbiome studies have had a great effect on our understanding of the pathophysiology of skin diseases.

Keywords Microbiome-based diagnostics · Microbiome-targeted therapies · Clinical medicine · Dermatology

A. Salava
Department of Dermatology, University of Helsinki, Meilahdentie 2, 00250 Helsinki, Finland

N. Fyhrquist (✉)
Institute of Environmental Medicine, Karolinska Institutet, Nobels Väg 13, 17177 Stockholm, Sweden
e-mail: Nanna.Fyhrquist@ki.se

Department of Health Sciences, Karlstad University, Universitetsgatan 2, 651 88 Karlstad, Sweden

A. Lauerma et al. (eds.), *The Skin Microbiome Manual*,
https://doi.org/10.1007/978-3-031-82689-4_9

9.1 Clinical Implications

Novel molecular research methods have enabled us a new perspective and different understanding of the cutaneous microbiome in skin diseases and pathologic skin conditions (Fyhrquist et al. 2019). Changes in the microbiome have been to some extend disease specific and we have thus been able to recognize a multitude of disease characteristics in the microbial community of skin disorders (Harris-Tryon and Grice 2022). The rapid development in methodology has progressed hand-in-hand with the aim of finding microbiome-based and microbiome-targeted practical implications in clinical medicine, diagnostic tools and treatments of skin diseases. The continuing increase in knowledge and ongoing intensive research of the skin microbiome with both its dynamics and disease-specificity have particularly in recent years raised an interest in finding microbiome-targeted therapeutics in dermatology (Hou et al. 2022). As the physiological microbiome of healthy human skin and that of several frequent skin diseases and even disease states (e.g. flare of atopic dermatitis) is characterized from the microbiome perspective already quite well, many studies are currently directed to additionally investigate its potential as a supplementary diagnostic tool, e.g. besides traditional histopathology (Salava et al. 2017).

9.2 Microbiome-Based Diagnostics

Microbiome characteristics and disease-state dependent dynamics of the colonizing microbial communities have been so far demonstrated in a variety of frequent skin disorders (Lewis et al. 2019). More recently, there have been efforts to explore these disease-specific microbiome changes as a biomarker in skin diseases. Many inflammatory skin disorders, such as atopic dermatitis, psoriasis, acne, or chronic wounds, have been shown to cause specific changes in the cutaneous microbiome (O'Neill and Gallo 2018). However, it has largely remained unclear if the observed changes are caused by the microbiome itself or if they represent only secondary changes, i.e., an epiphenomenon (Carmona-Cruz et al. 2022).

During and even before disease flares of atopic dermatitis the microbial diversity undergoes substantial alterations. There is robust evidence that when the disease flares in a patient with atopic dermatitis the skin microbiome changes more susceptible towards *Staphylococcus aureus* colonization (decrease in colonization resistance) (Edslev et al. 2020). Additionally, there have been many reports that commensal bacterial communities inhibit the colonization of known pathogens, especially specific strains of *Staphylococcus aureus* and *Streptococcus pyogenes*. Here, the interest has been not only in exploring host-microbiome interactions and immunity but also factors contributing to the dynamics inside the microbial community, e.g. colonization resistance.

Based on observations of in vitro and in vivo microbiome research, an interest has been growing to find microbiome-targeted diagnostic tools. Candidates for possible application fields have been discussed concerning the prevention and diagnosis of specific skin diseases, the characterization of high-risk patients (unfavorable disease course, malignant transformation), and information about microbiome-targeted therapies and prognostic factors concerning treatment responses (Fyhrquist et al. 2016).

However, we still have only a limited understanding about the role of the microbiome in diagnosing and preventing skin disorders (Smythe and Wilkinson 2023; Salava et al. 2016). Although some recent studies have demonstrated a possible association of microbiome changes with skin barrier malfunctions and immunologic dysfunctions, microbiome-targeted diagnostics represent at present only theoretical concepts. We are still far from using the cutaneous microbiome as a diagnostic tool in clinical dermatology and this topic needs to be further investigated and validated in clinical practice. Nevertheless, the strategies presented in this chapter characterize interesting and novel perspectives to the etiological and pathogenetic background of skin diseases and may possibly yield future potential for diagnostic use in clinical dermatology (Niemeyer-van der Kolk et al. 2018).

9.3   Microbiome-Targeted Therapeutics

Microbiome studies in clinical settings have shown that many therapies used standardly in the treatment of skin diseases (e.g., topical corticosteroids, calcineurin inhibitors, acne therapies) have a profound influence on the skin microbiome (Kelhälä et al. 2018). The restoration of a normal diverse microbial community structure after topical and systemic treatments has been demonstrated most apparently in atopic dermatitis and acne (Callewaert et al. 2019; Wongpiyabovorn et al. 2019; Ahluwalia et al. 2019). However, here too, it has remained essentially unclear if the observed microbiome changes have played a pathogenetic role in the particular skin disease or if they have been only a byproduct (epiphenomenon) appearing after treatment response, e.g., the decrease of cutaneous inflammation and restitution of the epidermal skin barrier.

Similarly to microbiome-targeted diagnostics, skin microbiome-targeted therapies have not yet established themselves in routine clinical practice. In recent years however, there has been an increasing amount of in vitro research and clinical studies exploring their potential (Aguwa et al. 2023; Yu et al. 2019). Although we are still far from the point where microbiome-targeted therapies may be used as standard treatment regiments, research data and clinical experience have, nevertheless been growing continuously about their use in the treatment of skin diseases (Notay et al. 2017).

There are different ways to influence or modify the cutaneous microbial community (Table 9.1). So far, we have seen three concepts evolving regarding the use of microbiome-targeted therapies in skin diseases. These are largely based on theoretical models derived from mostly experimental studies and most of the microbiome-targeted therapies have not yet been validated sufficiently in clinical studies or practice (Lopes et al. 2017, Rosignoli 2018).

Firstly, the cutaneous microbiome can be influenced by using methods that affect the skin microbiome directly, e.g. topical pro- and prebiotics, topical synbiotics (i.e. a mixture of the former), bacterial lysates or topical antimicrobial therapies. There have been few studies investigating the use of topical probiotics in atopic dermatitis. As the pathogenesis of atopic dermatitis is known to include changes in the skin microbiome and there have been responses to microbe-targeted treatments (e.g., antibiotics), these results have been encouraging (Salava and Lauerma 2014). There have also been studies on topical probiotics in the treatment of chronic wounds and in improvement of facial wrinkles (dermatocosmetics), with controversial effects and need for further research (Ong et al. 2019, Huang et al. 2017).

Secondly, a healthy or modified microbiome or single microbial strains can be relocated (transplantation or engraftment) onto the patients' skin (Alam et al. 2022). It has been shown that after serial applications of a donor microbiome, the microbiome of the receiver becomes more similar to the donor and is often characterized by the dominance of donor strains (Paetzold et al. 2019). The level of engraftment depends on the composition of the recipient and donor microbiomes (colonization resistance), and the applied bacterial load. The potential role of Gram-negative skin bacteria transplantation in atopic dermatitis has been explored in mouse models and to some amount also on human skin. Experimental studies have revealed that isolates of Gram-negative commensal bacteria from healthy volunteers improved outcomes in mouse and cell culture models of atopic dermatitis (Myles et al. 2016). In contrast, isolates from patients with atopic dermatitis worsened outcomes in these models. The results of open label preclinical studies have been promising and have shown that a treatment with Gram-negative isolates (e.g., *Roseomonas mucosa*) was associated with significant decreases in disease severity, topical steroid requirement, and *S. aureus* burden (Myles et al. 2018). To date no adverse events or treatment complications have been reported from skin microbiome transplantations (McBain et al. 2019).

And thirdly, by using mechanisms that affect the skin microbiome indirectly, e.g., by targeting the gut-skin axis (gastrointestinal probiotics) (Petersen et al. 2019; Codoñer-Cortés 2018; Huang et al. 2017). There is an increasing amount of evidence that supports the theory that an intestinal dysbiosis, i.e. pathologies or imbalances in the composition of microbial community, can almost invariably be observed in common inflammatory skin diseases, such as atopic dermatitis (Kim et al. 2019), psoriasis (Hidalgo-Cantabrana et al. 2019), rosacea (Nam et al. 2018) and acne (Bowe and Logan 2011). This understanding gave rise to the recognition of the gut-skin axis (Szántó et al. 2019; Sinha et al. 2021). There have been many studies investigating the use of oral probiotics in atopic dermatitis and the current consensus is that oral probiotic supplementation (especially *Lactobacilli*) can decrease the risk of atopic dermatitis in high-risk children. The use of oral probiotics in the treatment of already existent skin diseases is still controversial, but there have been some promising results

Table 9.1 Different theoretical and practical concepts of microbiome-targeting therapies

Therapeutic concept	Mechanisms (selected)	Clinical examples	References
Direct targeting of the cutaneous microbiome	• Selection of microbial growth • Bacteriostatic and bactericidal effects of therapies • Utilization of local microbial colonization resistance	• Topical pro- and prebiotics • Topical synbiotics • Bacterial lysates or topical antimicrobial therapies	Herbert et al. (2023), [a] Demessant-Flavigny et al. (2023), [b] Lebeer et al. (2022)[c]
Relocation of normal microbes to the skin	• Microbial transplantation or contamination • Autoinoculation of the microbiome	• Microbiome transplantations • Cutaneous engraftments • Microbial contamination	Bromfield et al. (2023), [d]Myles et al. (2018), Deng et al. (2023)[e]
Indirect targeting of the cutaneous microbiome	• Skin-gut-axis • Influencing gastrointestinal dysbiosis • Neural links to the cutaneous microbiome	• Peroral probiotics or prebiotics • Oral antibiotics or and therapies targeting the microbiome in other locations than the skin	Ha et al. (2023), [f]Stec et al. (2023), [g] Miyauchi et al. (2023)h

[a] Herbert S, Haughton R, Nava J, Ji-Xu A, Le ST, Maverakis E. A review of topical probiotic therapy for atopic dermatitis. Clin Exp Dermatol. 2023 Mar 22;48(4):319–324.

[b] Demessant-Flavigny AL, Connétable S, Kerob D, Moreau M, Aguilar L, Wollenberg A. Skin microbiome dysbiosis and the role of Staphylococcus aureus in atopic dermatitis in adults and children: A narrative review. J Eur Acad Dermatol Venereol. 2023 Jun;37 Suppl 5:3–17.

[c] Lebeer S, Oerlemans EFM, Claes I, Henkens T, Delanghe L, Wuyts S, Spacova I, van den Broek MFL, Tuyaerts I, Wittouck S, De Boeck I, Allonsius CN, Kiekens F, Lambert J. Selective targeting of skin pathobionts and inflammation with topically applied lactobacilli. Cell Rep Med. 2022 Feb 15;3(2):100521.

[d] Bromfield JI, Hugenholtz P, Frazer IH, Khosrotehrani K, Chandra J. Targeting Staphylococcus aureus dominated skin dysbiosis in actinic keratosis to prevent the onset of cutaneous squamous cell carcinoma: Outlook for future therapies? Front Oncol. 2023 Feb 2;13:1091379.

[e] Deng WY, Chen WJ, Zhong HJ, Wu LH, He XX. Washed microbiota transplantation: a case report of clinical success with skin and gut microbiota improvement in an adolescent boy with atopic dermatitis. Front Immunol. 2023 Nov 15;14:1275427.

[f] Ha MV, McCormick TS, Salem I, Al-Shakhshir H, Ghannoum MA, Carroll BT. Skin and gut microbial associations with squamous cell carcinoma in solid organ transplant recipients. Arch Dermatol Res. 2023 Nov;315(9):2709–2713.

[g] Stec A, Sikora M, Maciejewska M, Paralusz-Stec K, Michalska M, Sikorska E, Rudnicka L. Bacterial Metabolites: A Link between Gut Microbiota and Dermatological Diseases. Int J Mol Sci. 2023 Feb 9;24(4):3494.

[h] Miyauchi E, Shimokawa C, Steimle A, Desai MS, Ohno H. The impact of the gut microbiome on extra-intestinal autoimmune diseases. Nat Rev Immunol. 2023 Jan;23(1):9–23.

in atopic dermatitis and acne (Ibáñez et al. 2018; Sánchez-Pellicer et al. 2022). In a recent randomized clinical trial oral supplementation of strains of *Bifidobacterium lactis* decreased the disease severity and the need of topical treatments in young patients with atopic dermatitis (Navarro-López et al. 2018).

There have been studies investigating all of the above-mentioned therapeutic concepts, but until now, skin microbiome-targeted therapies have remained mainly on the experimental level. Few clinical trials exist that explore the utility of probiotics for the prevention and treatment of dermatologic diseases. Most widely they have been investigated atopic dermatitis (Paller et al. 2019). Most studies have investigated the effects of oral probiotics, thus targeting the skin-gut axis (Ibáñez et al. 2018). Here, oral supplementation of probiotics (e.g., *Lactobacilli*) have shown to have some effect in preventing the onset of atopic dermatitis in high-risk children. The role of oral probiotics in the treatment of already existing atopic dermatitis is still debated (Makrgeorgou et al. 2018; Li et al. 2019). A recent study investigated the use of an oral probiotic mixture in the treatment of psoriasis (Navarro-López et al. 2019). The patients showed a lower risk of relapse in the follow up after the intake of the probiotic mixture. In addition, the analysis of gut microbiota confirmed the efficacy of the probiotic in modulation of the gut microbiome composition.

In studies that have used direct topical probiotics, only few have included typical skin commensals. Most studies have used topical probiotic lysates or prebiotics. Topical application of antimicrobial coagulase-negative *Staphylococcus* strains have shown to improve atopic dermatitis and specifically decrease the *S. aureus* burden through antimicrobial peptides (Nakatsuji et al. 2017). Topical lysates (e.g. heat treated probiotics) of *Lactobacillus* strains have shown increase colonization resistance towards pathogenic bacteria (e.g. decrease *Staphylococcus aureus* colonization) and reduce flairs of atopic dermatitis under maintenance treatment (Blanchet-Réthoré et al. 2017). Recently, an open-label trial study investigating the use of commensal skin transplants in atopic dermatitis have produced encouraging results (Myles 2018). Here, topical treatment with the commensal bacterium *Rosemonas mucosa* was associated with significant decreases in disease severity, *S. aureus* colonization and topical corticosteroids.

9.4 Future Perspectives

In summary, skin microbiome-based diagnostic and microbiome-targeting therapies are an interesting and evolving field with potential for future clinical implications. Many questions have remained unclear about the cutaneous microbiome, the host-microbiome relationship and its significance in the treatment of skin diseases. In clinical trials, some positive results have been observed with topical probiotic lysates and oral probiotics. To some extent, also the use of commensal transplants has yielded promising results. These therapies seem to be safe and partly effective in the treatment of specific skin diseases. Additionally skin-microbiome-targeted treatments have shown a promising role in wound healing and skin cancer.

Several experimental and clinical studies have explored the efficacy of microbiome-targeted therapies in the prevention and treatment of atopic dermatitis. Overall, the current evidence suggests that topical and oral probiotics could be an option to improve moderate and severe atopic dermatitis recovery rates in children and adults. Transplantation of a healthy microbiome or single bacterial strains yields also promising results in some subgroups of patients. However, to date, there is no strong experimental evidence supporting the effectiveness and safety of microbiome targeted treatments in clinical practice. Most importantly, evidence and clinical trials demonstrating strain-specific effects and studies considering security issues are still lacking.

The skin microbiome remains an interesting area of research in developing new diagnostic tools and therapeutics in clinical dermatology. In addition, microbiome studies have had a great effect on our understanding of skin diseases.

References

Aguwa C, Enwereji N, Santiago S, Hine A, Kels GG, McGee J, Lu J. Targeting dysbiosis in psoriasis, atopic dermatitis, and hidradenitis suppurativa: the gut-skin axis and microbiome-directed therapy. Clin Dermatol. 2023;41(5):640–9.

Ahluwalia J, Borok J, Haddock ES, Ahluwalia RS, Schwartz EW, Hosseini D, Amini S, Eichenfield LF. The microbiome in preadolescent acne: assessment and prospective analysis of the influence of benzoyl peroxide. Pediatr Dermatol. 2019;36(2):200–6.

Alam MJ, Xie L, Yap YA, Marques FZ, Robert R. Manipulating microbiota to treat atopic dermatitis: functions and therapies. Pathogens. 2022;11(6):642.

Blanchet-Réthoré S, Bourdès V, Mercenier A, Haddar CH, Verhoeven PO, Andres P. Effect of a lotion containing the heat-treated probiotic strain Lactobacillus johnsonii NCC 533 on Staphylococcus aureus colonization in atopic dermatitis. Clin Cosmet Investig Dermatol. 2017;3(10):249–57.

Bowe WP, Logan AC. Acne vulgaris, probiotics and the gut-brain-skin axis—back to the future? Gut Pathog. 2011;3(1):1. https://doi.org/10.1186/1757-4749-3-1.

Bromfield JI, Hugenholtz P, Frazer IH, Khosrotehrani K, Chandra J. Targeting Staphylococcus aureus dominated skin dysbiosis in actinic keratosis to prevent the onset of cutaneous squamous cell carcinoma: outlook for future therapies? Front Oncol. 2023;2(13):1091379.

Callewaert C, Nakatsuji T, Knight R, Kosciolek T, Vrbanac A, Kotol P, Ardeleanu M, Hultsch T, Guttman-Yassky E, Bissonnette R, Silverberg JI, Krueger J, Menter A, Graham NMH, Pirozzi G, Hamilton JD, Gallo RL. IL-4Rα Blockade by Dupilumab Decreases Staphylococcus aureus Colonization and Increases Microbial Diversity in Atopic Dermatitis. J Invest Dermatol. 2019 pii: S0022-202X(19)31789-0. https://doi.org/10.1016/j.jid.2019.05.024. [Epub ahead of print].

Carmona-Cruz S, Orozco-Covarrubias L, Sáez-de-Ocariz M. The human skin microbiome in selected cutaneous diseases. Front Cell Infect Microbiol. 2022;7(12): 834135.

Demessant-Flavigny AL, Connétable S, Kerob D, Moreau M, Aguilar L, Wollenberg A. Skin microbiome dysbiosis and the role of Staphylococcus aureus in atopic dermatitis in adults and children: a narrative review. J Eur Acad Dermatol Venereol. 2023;37(Suppl 5):3–17.

Deng WY, Chen WJ, Zhong HJ, Wu LH, He XX. Washed microbiota transplantation: a case report of clinical success with skin and gut microbiota improvement in an adolescent boy with atopic dermatitis. Front Immunol. 2023;15(14):1275427.

Edslev SM, Agner T, Andersen PS. Skin microbiome in atopic dermatitis. Acta Derm Venereol. 2020;100(12):adv00164.

Fyhrquist N, Salava A, Auvinen P, Lauerma A. Skin biomes. Curr Allergy Asthma Rep. 2016;16(5):40.

Fyhrquist N, Muirhead G, Prast-Nielsen S, Jeanmougin M, Olah P, Skoog T, Jules-Clement G, Feld M, Barrientos-Somarribas M, Sinkko H, van den Bogaard EH, Zeeuwen PLJM, Rikken G, Schalkwijk J, Niehues H, Däubener W, Eller SK, Alexander H, Pennino D, Suomela S, Tessas I, Lybeck E, Baran AM, Darban H, Gangwar RS, Gerstel U, Jahn K, Karisola P, Yan L, Hansmann B, Katayama S, Meller S, Bylesjö M, Hupé P, Levi-Schaffer F, Greco D, Ranki A, Schröder JM, Barker J, Kere J, Tsoka S, Lauerma A, Soumelis V, Nestle FO, Homey B, Andersson B, Alenius H. Microbe-host interplay in atopic dermatitis and psoriasis. Nat Commun. 2019;10(1):4703.

Ha MV, McCormick TS, Salem I, Al-Shakhshir H, Ghannoum MA, Carroll BT. Skin and gut microbial associations with squamous cell carcinoma in solid organ transplant recipients. Arch Dermatol Res. 2023;315(9):2709–13.

Harris-Tryon TA, Grice EA. Microbiota and maintenance of skin barrier function. Science. 2022;376(6596):940–5.

Herbert S, Haughton R, Nava J, Ji-Xu A, Le ST, Maverakis E. A review of topical probiotic therapy for atopic dermatitis. Clin Exp Dermatol. 2023;48(4):319–24.

Hidalgo-Cantabrana C, Gómez J, Delgado S, Requena-López S, Queiro-Silva R, Margolles A, Coto E, Sánchez B, Coto-Segura P. Gut microbiota dysbiosis in a cohort of patients with psoriasis. Br J Dermatol. 2019. https://doi.org/10.1111/bjd.17931.

Hou K, Wu ZX, Chen XY, Wang JQ, Zhang D, Xiao C, Zhu D, Koya JB, Wei L, Li J, Chen ZS. Microbiota in health and diseases. Signal Transduct Target Ther. 2022;7(1):135.

Huang R, Ning H, Shen M, Li J, Zhang J, Chen X. Probiotics for the treatment of atopic dermatitis in children: a systematic review and meta-analysis of randomized controlled trials. Front Cell Infect Microbiol. 2017;7:392.

Ibáñez MD, Rodríguez Del Río P, González-Segura Alsina D, Villegas IV. Effect of synbiotic supplementation on children with atopic dermatitis: an observational prospective study. Eur J Pediatr. 2018;177(12):1851–8.

Kelhälä HL, Aho VTE, Fyhrquist N, Pereira PAB, Kubin ME, Paulin L, Palatsi R, Auvinen P, Tasanen K, Lauerma A. Isotretinoin and lymecycline treatments modify the skin microbiota in acne. Exp Dermatol. 2018;27(1):30–6.

Kim IS, Lee SH, Kwon YM, Adhikari B, Kim JA, Yu DY, Kim GI, Lim JM, Kim SH, Lee SS, Moon YS, Choi IS, Cho KK. Oral administration of β-glucan and lactobacillus plantarum alleviates atopic dermatitis-like symptoms. J Microbiol Biotechnol. 2019. https://doi.org/10.4014/jmb.1907.07011.

Lebeer S, Oerlemans EFM, Claes I, Henkens T, Delanghe L, Wuyts S, Spacova I, van den Broek MFL, Tuyaerts I, Wittouck S, De Boeck I, Allonsius CN, Kiekens F, Lambert J. Selective targeting of skin pathobionts and inflammation with topically applied lactobacilli. Cell Rep Med. 2022;3(2): 100521.

Lewis DJ, Chan WH, Hinojosa T, Hsu S, Feldman SR. Mechanisms of microbial pathogenesis and the role of the skin microbiome in psoriasis: a review. Clin Dermatol. 2019;37(2):160–6.

Li L, Han Z, Niu X, Zhang G, Jia Y, Zhang S, He C. Probiotic supplementation for prevention of atopic dermatitis in infants and children: a systematic review and meta-analysis. Am J Clin Dermatol. 2019;20(3):367–77.

Lopes EG, Moreira DA, Gullón P, Gullón B, Cardelle-Cobas A, Tavaria FK. Topical application of probiotics in skin: adhesion, antimicrobial and antibiofilm in vitro assays. J Appl Microbiol. 2017;122(2):450–61.

Makrgeorgou A, Leonardi-Bee J, Bath-Hextall FJ, Murrell DF, Tang ML, Roberts A, Boyle RJ. Probiotics for treating eczema. Cochrane Database Syst Rev. 2018;11:CD006135.

McBain AJ, O'Neill CA, Amezquita A, Price LJ, Faust K, Tett A, Segata N, Swann JR, Smith AM, Murphy B, Hoptroff M, James G, Reddy Y, Dasgupta A, Ross T, Chapple IL, Wade WG, Fernandez-Piquer J. Consumer safety considerations of skin and oral microbiome perturbation. Clin Microbiol Rev. 2019;2(4).

Miyauchi E, Shimokawa C, Steimle A, Desai MS, Ohno H. The impact of the gut microbiome on extra-intestinal autoimmune diseases. Nat Rev Immunol. 2023;23(1):9–23.

Myles IA, Williams KW, Reckhow JD, Jammeh ML, Pincus NB, Sastalla I, Saleem D, Stone KD, Datta SK. Transplantation of human skin microbiota in models of atopic dermatitis. JCI Insight. 2016;1(10).

Myles IA, Earland NJ, Anderson ED, Moore IN, Kieh MD, Williams KW, Saleem A, Fontecilla NM, Welch PA, Darnell DA, Barnhart LA, Sun AA, Uzel G, Datta SK. First-in-human topical microbiome transplantation with Roseomonas mucosa for atopic dermatitis. JCI Insight. 2018;3(9).

Nakatsuji T, Chen TH, Narala S, Chun KA, Two AM, Yun T, Shafiq F, Kotol PF, Bouslimani A, Melnik AV, Latif H, Kim JN, Lockhart A, Artis K, David G, Taylor P, Streib J, Dorrestein PC, Grier A, Gill SR, Zengler K, Hata TR, Leung DY, Gallo RL. Antimicrobials from human skin commensal bacteria protect against Staphylococcus aureus and are deficient in atopic dermatitis. Sci Transl Med. 2017;9(378).

Nam JH, Yun Y, Kim HS, Kim HN, Jung HJ, Chang Y, Ryu S, Shin H, Kim HL, Kim WS. Rosacea and its association with enteral microbiota in Korean females. Exp Dermatol. 2018;27(1):37–42.

Navarro-López V, Martínez-Andrés A, Ramírez-Boscá A, Ruzafa-Costas B, Núñez-Delegido E, Carrión-Gutiérrez MA, Prieto-Merino D, Codoñer-Cortés F, Ramón-Vidal D, Genovés-Martínez S, Chenoll-Cuadros E, Pérez-Orquín JM, Picó-Monllor JA, Chumillas-Lidón S. Efficacy and safety of oral administration of a mixture of probiotic strains in patients with psoriasis: a randomized controlled clinical trial. Acta Derm Venereol. 2019. https://doi.org/10.2340/00015555-3305.

Navarro-López V, Ramírez-Boscá A, Ramón-Vidal D, Ruzafa-Costas B, Genovés-Martínez S, Chenoll-Cuadros E, Carrión-Gutiérrez M, Horga de la Parte J, Prieto-Merino D, Codoñer-Cortés FM. Effect of oral administration of a mixture of probiotic strains on SCORAD index and use of topical steroids in young patients with moderate atopic dermatitis: a randomized clinical trial. JAMA Dermatol. 2018;154(1):37–43.

Niemeyer-van der Kolk T, van der Wall HEC, Balmforth C, Van Doorn MBA, Rissmann R. A systematic literature review of the human skin microbiome as biomarker for dermatological drug development. Br J Clin Pharmacol. 2018;84(10):2178–93.

Notay M, Foolad N, Vaughn AR, Sivamani RK. Probiotics, prebiotics, and synbiotics for the treatment and prevention of adult dermatological diseases. Am J Clin Dermatol. 2017;18(6):721–32.

Notay M, Saric-Bosanac S, Vaughn AR, Dhaliwal S, Trivedi M, Reiter PN, Rybak I, Li CC, Weiss LB, Ambrogio L, Burney W, Sivamani RK. The use of topical Nitrosomonas eutropha for cosmetic improvement of facial wrinkles. J Cosmet Dermatol. 2019. https://doi.org/10.1111/jocd.13060 [Epub ahead of print].

O'Neill AM, Gallo RL. Host-microbiome interactions and recent progress into understanding the biology of acne vulgaris. Microbiome. 2018;6:177.

Ong JS, Taylor TD, Yong CC, Khoo BY, Sasidharan S, Choi SB, Ohno H, Liong MT. Lactobacillus plantarum USM8613 aids in wound healing and suppresses staphylococcus aureus infection at wound sites. Probiotics Antimicrob Proteins. 2019. https://doi.org/10.1007/s12602-018-9505-9 [Epub ahead of print].

Paetzold B, Willis JR, Pereira de Lima J, Knödlseder N, Brüggemann H, Quist SR, Gabaldón T, Güell M. Skin microbiome modulation induced by probiotic solutions. Microbiome. 2019;7(1):95.

Paller AS, Kong HH, Seed P, Naik S, Scharschmidt TC, Gallo RL, Luger T, Irvine AD. The microbiome in patients with atopic dermatitis. J Allergy Clin Immunol. 2019;143(1):26–35. https://doi.org/10.1016/j.jaci.2018.11.015.

Petersen EBM, Skov L, Thyssen JP, Jensen P. Role of the gut microbiota in atopic dermatitis: a systematic review. Acta Derm Venereol. 2019;99(1):5–11.

Rosignoli C, Thibaut de Ménonville S, Orfila D, Béal M, Bertino B, Aubert J, Mercenier A, Piwnica D. A topical treatment containing heat-treated Lactobacillus johnsonii NCC 533 reduces Staphylococcus aureus adhesion and induces antimicrobial peptide expression in an in vitro reconstructed human epidermis model. Exp Dermatol. 2018;27(4):358–65.

Salava A, Lauerma A. Role of the skin microbiome in atopic dermatitis. Clin Transl Allergy. 2014;17(4):33.

Salava A, Pereira P, Aho V, Väkevä L, Paulin L, Auvinen P, Ranki A, Lauerma A. Skin Microbiome in Small- and Large-plaque Parapsoriasis. Acta Derm Venereol. 2017;97(6):685–91.

Salava A, Aho V, Pereira P, Koskinen K, Paulin L, Auvinen P, Lauerma A. Skin microbiome in melanomas and melanocytic nevi. Eur J Dermatol. 2016;26(1):49–55.

Sánchez-Pellicer P, Navarro-Moratalla L, Núñez-Delegido E, Ruzafa-Costas B, Agüera-Santos J, Navarro-López V. Acne, microbiome, and probiotics: the gut-skin axis. Microorganisms. 2022;10(7):1303.

Sinha S, Lin G, Ferenczi K. The skin microbiome and the gut-skin axis. Clin Dermatol. 2021;39(5):829–39.

Smythe P, Wilkinson HN. The skin microbiome: current landscape and future opportunities. Int J Mol Sci. 2023;24(4):3950.

Stec A, Sikora M, Maciejewska M, Paralusz-Stec K, Michalska M, Sikorska E, Rudnicka L. Bacterial metabolites: a link between gut microbiota and dermatological diseases. Int J Mol Sci. 2023;24(4):3494.

Szántó M, Dózsa A, Antal D, Szabó K, Kemény L, Bai P. Targeting the gut-skin axis—probiotics as new tools for skin disorder management? Exp Dermatol. 2019. https://doi.org/10.1111/exd. 14016.

Wongpiyabovorn J, Soonthornchai W, Wilantho A, Palasuk M, Payungporn S, Sodsai P, Poomipak W, Weschawalit S, Ruchusatsawat K, Baillie GS, Hirankarn N, Somboonna N. Effect of tacrolimus on skin microbiome in atopic dermatitis. Allergy. 2019. https://doi.org/10.1111/all. 13743 [Epub ahead of print] No abstract available.

Yu Y, Dunaway S, Champer J, Kim J, Alikhan A. Changing our microbiome: probiotics in dermatology. Br J Dermatol. 2019. https://doi.org/10.1111/bjd.18088.

Chapter 10
Skin Homeostasis Through AHR-Mediated Interactions Between Host and Microbiome

Jos P. H. Smits, Cristina Gomez Casado, Ellen H. van den Bogaard, and Bernhard Homey

Abstract The microbiome, including the cutaneous microbiome, has been a center of attention since the commencement of the Human Microbiome Project, well over 15 years ago. The goal was to characterize the inhabitants of all body sites and to analyze the microbiome's role in health and disease. Around the same time, the aryl hydrocarbon receptor (AHR) was identified to play an important role in epithelial barrier organogenesis, homeostasis, and maintenance. Evidence is emerging that the cutaneous microbiome can reciprocally interact with keratinocytes in the epidermis through activation of host's AHR. Via host AHR signaling and downstream initiation of host defense mechanisms, the commensal inhabitants of the skin aim to protect their micromilieu and compete for their individual niche. This chapter aims to summarize the current evidence for physiological functions of microbe-driven, canonical AHR signaling in the skin and to set the stage for investigative studies on the AHR-driven molecular mechanisms of dermatological conditions in which microbiome dysbiosis is eminent. We identify opportunities to translate knowledge gained in other epithelial organs to physiological processes important in skin homeostasis.

Keywords Epidermis · Homeostasis · Microbiota · Host-microbe interaction · Aryl hydrocarbon receptor

J. P. H. Smits · C. Gomez Casado · B. Homey (✉)
Department of Dermatology, Medical Faculty, University Hospital Düsseldorf, Heinrich Heine University, Düsseldorf, Germany
e-mail: Bernhard.Homey@med.uni-duesseldorf.de

J. P. H. Smits (✉) · E. H. van den Bogaard
Department of Dermatology, Radboud Research Institute for Medical Innovation, Radboud University Medical Center (Radboudumc), Nijmegen, The Netherlands
e-mail: Jos.PH.Smits@radboudumc.nl

© The Author(s), under exclusive license to Springer Nature Switzerland AG 2025
A. Lauerma et al. (eds.), *The Skin Microbiome Manual*,
https://doi.org/10.1007/978-3-031-82689-4_10

10.1 Aryl Hydrocarbon Receptor

The aryl hydrocarbon receptor (AHR) has long been known in the context of toxicology and pharmacology. As mediator of xenobiotic toxicity, for example by polychlorinated dioxins (2,3,7,8-tetrachlorodibenzo-*p*-dioxin (TCDD)) or polyaromatic hydrocarbons (PAHs), AHR was studied extensively in the twentieth century (Mandal 2005; Okey 2007). AHR is a ligand-activated transcription factor that belongs to the basic helix-loop-helix (bHLH) Per-ARNT-SIM (PAS) family of transcription factors that are evolutionary conserved and characterized by their ability to sense environmental factors, such as pollutants, exhaust particulate matter, and fire smoke (Gu et al. 2000; Hahn et al. 1997).

AHR resides in the cytoplasm in complex with its chaperone proteins heat shock protein 90 (Hsp90), p23, X-associated protein 2 (XAP2), and cellular SRC kinase (c-SRC). Characteristic for the AHR canonical pathway, upon ligand binding the AHR, the chaperone proteins are displaced and AHR translocates to the nucleus where it binds to AHR nuclear translocator (ARNT) (Omiecinski et al. 2011). The AHR/ARNT complex recognizes particular DNA motifs referred to as dioxin-responsive elements (DREs) or xenobiotic response elements (XREs) that consist of a core consensus sequence 5'-GCGTGA-3' (Lusska et al. 1993). Binding of AHR/ARNT to its responsive element can initiate transcription of a wide variety of genes triggering various signaling pathways, including those regulating the clearance of xenobiotics, such as the cytochrome P450 (CYP) superfamily of enzymes (McDonnell and Dang 2013). Studies into toxicological effects of prolonged exposure and accumulation of AHR-activating ligands like TCDD or benzo[a]pyrene (BaP) indicated many adverse effects, ranging from (chlor)acne outbreaks (May 1973)—characterized by follicular plugging, cysts, pustules, and erythema—to liver failure (Randerath et al. 1988), renal failure (Shalat et al. 1989), mutagenicity (Giri 1986), thymic atrophy and suppressed cellular immunity (Vos and Moore 1974), and myocardial degeneration (Kociba et al. 1978). During the last century, several incidents have led to the accidental exposure to TCDD, for example occupational exposure (May 1973) and exposure through contaminated dust or soil (Reggiani 1980), often with detrimental outcome for nature. This led to hesitation of using AHR-activating ligands in biomedical research, especially for development into therapeutics.

Over recent years, the AHR was recognized not solely as an environmental sensor of xenobiotic substances and key component of phase I xenobiotic metabolism via CYP450 enzyme transcription, but as an important regulator of immune cell development (Gutierrez-Vazquez and Quintana 2018) and epithelial barrier organ integrity, development, and homeostasis, i.e., in the gut (Stockinger et al. 2021), the lung (Guerrina et al. 2018), and in the skin (Sutter et al. 2011; Bogaard et al. 2015; Fernandez-Gallego et al. 2021; Haas et al. 2016; Esser and Rannug 2015). Literature suggests that the AHR activated in one organ can influence other organs, for example gut AHR and the brain (as reviewed in Barroso et al. (2021) and (Salminen 2023)) or the lung (Dong et al. 2023). We postulate that from a physiological perspective, cutaneous AHR serves as a communication hub between man and its environment.

Upon sensing of environmental threats, either increased exposure levels or damage to the skin, the AHR quickly acts to eliminate harmful substance by (i) xenobiotic metabolism, (ii) inducing innate host defense responses, and (iii) fortifying the skin barrier through induction of epidermal renewal and *stratum corneum* formation. However, upon loss of physiological signals (e.g., dysbiosis or pollutant exposure), this danger signal is lost or perturbed contributing to disease. In the following paragraph we summarize the current evidence that underpins the therapeutic properties of AHR ligands in the skin, further specifying the role for AHR in skin barrier reinforcement or repair. By identifying the AHR-mediated route of action, we can hypothesize on the potential influence of commensal bacteria on the host, via AHR modulation.

10.2 AHR as a Targetable, Physiologically Important Sensor of Its Surroundings

After being recognized in the context of tissue development and homeostasis, several studies have indicated that activation of the AHR by endogenous and exogenous ligands has beneficial effects on inflammatory diseases of the skin, such as atopic dermatitis (AD) (Bogaard et al. 2013) and psoriasis (PSO) (Meglio et al. 2014). Furthermore, recent findings indicated that downregulation of the endogenous AHR machinery leads to inflammatory adverse events (Hawerkamp et al. 2019). AHR-activating ligands with therapeutic effects are either endogenous and short-lived, like UVB-induced molecules such as the tryptophan (Trp) derivative FICZ (6-formylindolo[3,2-*b*]carbazole), or exogenous ligands with varying half-lives, including polyaromatic hydrocarbons in coal tar (Bogaard et al. 2013; Smits et al. 2020) and soybean tar (glyteer) (Takeuchi et al. 1985), carboxamide derivatives from laquinimod, tasquinimod, and roquinimex (Rikken et al. 2022), selective AHR modulators (SAhRMs) (Rikken et al. 2023), and the recently FDA-approved tapinarof (Smith et al. 2017; Peppers et al. 2019; Robbins et al. 2019). Activation of the AHR by endogenous and exogenous ligands during non-inflammatory conditions instigates the development of the skin barrier by initializing keratinocyte proliferation and regulating keratinocyte terminal differentiation. However, under inflammatory conditions, such as AD and PSO, dampening of the immune response is an important therapeutic effect adding to the reinstation of homeostatic keratinocyte differentiation and normalizing the inflammation-induced keratinocyte hyperproliferative state. This nowadays accepted therapeutic potential of AHR targeting, yet also recognizing the detrimental effects of AHR activation in the context of environmental pollutants, renders the question whether activation of keratinocyte AHR by microbiome-derived ligands can shape the epidermal niche in favor of host health but also favoring the microbiota themselves. To appreciate the potential impact of bacteria-induced AHR activation in the host, it is crucial to understand the physiological role of AHR in skin barrier homeostasis and function.

10.3 Physiological Role of AHR in Skin Barrier Homeostasis and Function

As the largest organ of the human body, the skin has the irreplaceable task to continuously protect us against our daily environment. Keratinocytes of the epidermis live in a sensitive balance between proliferation and (terminal) differentiation to assure timely renewal of the epidermis and proper skin barrier formation, respectively. Zooming in on the skin barrier, distinction can be made between outside-in barrier functionality—to prevent environmental factors to penetrate the body—and inside-out barrier functionality—that protects our body from extensive water loss and nutrient deprivation. The skin is harnessed with a variety of (sub)cellular mechanisms that together form a distinct physical, immunological, chemical, and microbial barrier.

The **physical barrier** is characterized by adhesive (tight) junction connections between keratinocytes in the epidermis, and strongly crosslinked corneocytes in the *stratum corneum*. The cornified envelope is complemented by a lipid matrix of ceramides and fatty acids that provide the *stratum corneum* with its hydrophobic and thus water repellent character. Driving epidermal differentiation, the AHR plays an important role in the overall process of terminal stratification and barrier formation (Sutter et al. 2011; Bogaard et al. 2015). *In silico* predictionary analysis of AHR and ARNT binding sites identified thousands of AHR- and ARNT-(co)bound regions (Lo and Matthews 2012), in accordance with TCDD-treated mouse liver experiments (Cholico et al. 2022). Nevertheless, our recent chromatin immunoprecipitation experiments in primary epidermal keratinocytes have indicated far less and highly transient AHR/ARNT binding sites (Smits et al. 2023). Following AHR activation, a battery of transcription factors known to induce epidermal differentiation is upregulated, e.g., AP-1 and AP-2 (*TFAP2A*) (Smits et al. 2023), OVO-like 1 (*OVOL1*) (Tsuji et al. 2017), and Sirtuin1 (*SIRT1*) (Sutter et al. 2019). Knockdown of *SIRT1* was shown to downregulate filaggrin and thus impair skin barrier integrity in mice (Ming et al. 2015). Tight junction protein claudin-1 (*CLDN1*) was induced by AHR activation in keratinocytes and AHR signaling enhanced the function of the tight junctions (Lin et al. 2013). Studies using intestinal Caco-2 cells have furthermore shown that AHR activation increases the expression of zonula occludens 1 protein (ZO-1) (Yu et al. 2018), occludin (*OCLN*) (Yu et al. 2018), *CLDN1* (Yu et al. 2018), and *CLDN3* (Ganapathy et al. 2023), while decreasing *CLDN2* expression (Ganapathy et al. 2023), altogether decreasing paracellular permeability. It is not unlikely that epidermal AHR signaling results in similar skin barrier modulation via tight junction protein expression. In addition, AHR signaling appears involved in ceramide processing, as *Arnt* knockout mice indicated a deficiency of dihydroceramide desaturases leading to replacement of 4-sphinganine by sphinganine and a reduction of 4-hydroxysphingenine (Takagi et al. 2003). TCDD treatment of human keratinocytes furthermore increased the expression of ceramide metabolism and transport genes (i.e., UGCG, ABCA12, GBA1, and SMPD1), and in addition, *Ahr* knockout mice showed decreased expression of forementioned genes (Sutter 2023), adding to the body of evidence that AHR activation can influence ceramide processing and might be crucial for correct barrier formation. Yet, which specific ceramides, their chain length, exact composition, and effect on lamellar organization remains to be explored.

The **immunological barrier** is provided by vigilant innate and adaptive immune cells that respectively reside in the epidermis (keratinocytes, Langerhans cells, intraepidermal dendritic cells, innate lymphoid cells in the dermis, mast cells, dermal macrophages, and tissue-resident memory T cells) or guard the periphery by continuously be attentive for danger signals and antigens to become activated. Work in immunodeficient mice showed that AHR signaling is needed for antigen presentation by Langerhans cells and that *Ahr*-deficient mice lack dendritic epidermal T cells (Jux et al. 2009). In addition, resident memory T cells move out of the epidermis after infection in these *Ahr*-deficient mice (Zaid et al. 2014). Moreover, using full and conditional *Ahr*-deficient mice, it was discovered that AHR signaling is required for the development and homeostasis of variant and invariant mucosal tissue-specific gamma delta T cells, via active regulation of tryptophan uptake (Li et al. 2011; Kadow et al. 2011; Martin et al. 2009). This ultimately impacts IL-22 secretion (Cibrian et al. 2016). AHR is therefore decisive for optimal differentiation of Th17 cells (Veldhoen et al. 2009) and, in particular, IL-22 production (Zelante et al. 2013; Veldhoen et al. 2008). Th17 cells are key players for anti-bacterial immune responses, but detrimental for inflammatory diseases such as psoriasis (Mills 2008). However, AHR is not only implicated in the differentiation of Th17 cells. It is interesting to note that three independent *Ahr*-deficient mouse strains were generated almost simultaneously (Mimura et al. 1997; Schmidt et al. 1996; Fernandez-Salguero et al. 1995), but only one presented an immune phenotype of skin inflammation, among other features (Fernandez-Salguero et al. 1997), presumably due to different microbial statuses in the animal facilities. One pivotal immune function of AHR signaling is the control of regulatory helper T cells (Treg) and cytotoxic T cells (Marshall and Kerkvliet 2010). Several Treg subsets such as FoxP3$^+$ Treg or Tr1 cells are responsive to AHR signaling, either directly or indirectly via tolerogenic dendritic cells (DC)(Gandhi et al. 2010; Navid et al. 2013; Hauben et al. 2008). This may underlie a novel strategy to expand Tregs with therapeutic potential (Wu et al. 2011). These findings point to an important role for AHR in the maturation of the innate and adaptive immune cells and in maintaining the immunological barrier of the skin.

The **chemical barrier** composes of antimicrobial peptides (AMPs) that are expressed by terminally differentiating keratinocytes of the epidermis, oriented to localize to the apical side of the keratinocyte, and eventually loaded into cornified physical skin barrier—the *stratum corneum*. In this way, AMPs are optimally primed to defend the host against potentially harmful, penetrating microbes. For some AMPs, interaction with damage-associated molecules (DAMPs), like host DNA (Lande et al. 2007), increases antimicrobial efficiency to seize control of rampant microbial over-colonization or impending tissue infection after breach of the skin barrier. AHR signaling was shown to induce the expression of a range of AMPs (Smits et al. 2020) and signal blockage was accompanied by bacterial outgrowth, possibly via reduced human beta-defensin 3 (hBD3) expression (Rademacher et al. 2019). In addition to

AMPs, the chemical skin barrier entails the ability of keratinocytes to express reactive oxygen species (ROS) as a defense mechanism upon breach of the skin barrier or to overcome DNA damage, e.g., after UVB exposure (Dunaway et al. 2018). The production of ROS is increased upon AHR mediated CYP1A1 expression which drives epidermal differentiation and barrier formation (Kennedy et al. 2013; Kopf and Walker 2010; Sutter et al. 2020). At the same time, AHR signaling initiates the expression of nuclear factor erythroid 2-related factor-2 (NRF2, *NFE2L2*), an important molecule in the antioxidative response, effectively fine-tuning ROS production and limiting potential harmful effects in damaged tissues (Furue et al. 2017; Miao et al. 2005; Kohle and Bock 2007). As reviewed, NRF2 is considered not only as a regulator of damage-induced stress response, but might also serve as a therapeutic target for initiating epithelial repair in case of tissue injury (Hiebert and Werner 2023) and in reinforcement of the skin barrier as a protective measure, for example in solar UVB-induced tissue damage (Hiebert and Werner 2023).

The **microbial barrier** is composed of all commensal microbiota that live in symbiosis with our skin. The skin microbiome varies greatly between body sites and shows temporal changes during our lifetime (Grice et al. 2009; Grice and Segre 2011). By residing on the skin's outer layer, the *stratum corneum*, or within the pilosebaceous unit, they populate the niche that is often overgrown by pathogenic bacteria during cutaneous inflammation, leading to dysbiosis and skin infections, e.g., in atopic dermatitis (Kong et al. 2012). Actually, several publications have indicated that commensal bacteria not only reside on the skin, but produce factors to fend off pathogenic or opportunistic microbes, protecting and competing for their own niche. The next examples are focused on non-AHR-mediated microbe-host interaction. For example, coagulase-negative *Staphylococcus* species (CoNS) were found to produce several bacteriocins inhibiting growth of *Cutibacterium acnes*, *Staphylococcus epidermidis*, and *Staphylococcus aureus* (O'Sullivan et al. 2019, 2020). Other studies showed *S. aureus* colonization inhibited by *Staphylococcus hominis* through expression of autoinducing peptides that inhibit *S. aureus agr* quorum sensing. In turn, increasingly abundant *S. aureus* was able to lower CoNS-derived peptides and restore their toxin production (Williams et al. 2019). In addition, *S. epidermidis* inhibits *S. aureus* biofilm formation through production of serine proteases (Iwase et al. 2010; Sugimoto et al. 2013), while *C. acnes* was shown to block *S. epidermidis* biofilm formation through production of short-chain fatty acids (Nakamura et al. 2020). *Corynebacterium accolens* releases short-chain fatty acids to halt the growth of *Streptococcus pneumoniae* (Bomar et al. 2016). Moreover, *C. acnes* was revealed to secrete cutimycin, a new antibiotic/lantibiotic that protects the pilosebaceous unit against colonization by several *Staphylococcus* species (Claesen et al. 2020). Additional microbe-host interactions in context of AHR signaling will be discussed later in this chapter.

After introducing the overarching physiological roles of the AHR in skin homeostasis and barrier formation, we can address the few studies that indicated microbiota- and yeast-derived components to activate the host AHR.

10.4 Microbiota and AHR-Dependent Host-Microbe Interactions

The cutaneous microbiome is well known to interact with epidermal keratinocytes and immune cells as reviewed extensively (Flowers and Grice 2020; Chen et al. 2018). Yet, the molecular mechanisms, at least in keratinocytes, remain often unexplored and mostly focused on the downstream cellular effects. Recently, a few studies have emerged indicating that microbiota-derived metabolites are capable of activating the AHR in the skin (Rademacher et al. 2019; Bogaard et al. 2021; Krieken et al. 2023; Uberoi et al. 2021). Yet, much is to learn from a decade of research into the influence of commensal bacteria on the barrier function in the gut. Many studies have illustrated host AHR activation by a wide range of bacteria and yeasts, indicating how omnipresent this mechanism of microbe-initiated AHR activation is. For example, microbiota-derived Trp metabolites, e.g., kynurenines, indoles, and their derivatives, can directly activate AHR in the gut (Agus et al. 2018; Jin et al. 2014; Hubbard et al. 2015a; Shimada et al. 2013). Interestingly, compared to murine *Ahr*, the human AHR has adapted to be more sensitive to microbe-derived Trp metabolites like indoles (Hubbard et al. 2015b), underlining the importance to identify and characterize the physiological implications that cutaneous microbes can have on the host. In addition to local effects of gut microbiota-induced AHR activation, cross-organ effects have been identified between the gut and the lung (Dong et al. 2023), and the gut and the brain (Barroso et al. 2021). Dietary intake of AHR-ligand rich food sources like cruciferous vegetables (containing indole-3-carbinol (I3C) that is processed into indolo[3,2-b]carbazol (ICZ) can be linked to gut immunity and peripheral effects (Li et al. 2011). It is now speculated that the rise in allergic and cutaneous diseases in the Western population may be due to a lack of cruciferous food intake, potentially through an AHR-mediated gut-skin axis (Perdew et al. 2022). Given the beneficial effects of AHR activation in AD and PSO skin, the gut-skin axis implicates an interesting therapeutic avenue apart from the usual topical AHR-activating treatments such as coal tar or tapinarof cream (Bogaard et al. 2013; Smits et al. 2020; Smith et al. 2017). Although non-AHR-mediated gut-skin axis is studied quite well (as reviewed by Pessemier et al. (2021)), evidence for an AHR-mediated gut-skin axis in which production of AHR ligands in the gut that have peripheral effects in the skin through systemic circulation remains to be identified. Interestingly, environmental pollution (Fouladi et al. 2020) and UVB exposure (Bosman et al. 2019; Conteville and Vicente 2020) were shown to affect the gut microbiome in an AHR-dependent fashion, substantiating the cross-organ communication along a lung-gut and skin-gut axis, respectively. This potentially has far-reaching implications for the development of disease therapeutics and our basic understanding of disease mechanisms.

Similar to the gut microbiome, the skin microbiome is a direct source of AHR ligands. Tryptophan metabolites and catabolites are amongst the identified ligands derived from the skin microbes and yeasts (summarized in Table 10.1). *Malassezia* yeasts have been known for over 20 years to produce AHR ligands. For example, indirubin (Magiatis et al. 2013), pityriacitrin (Gaitanis et al. 2008), malassezin

(Magiatis et al. 2013; Gaitanis et al. 2008; Wille et al. 2001), 6-formylindolo[3,2-b]carbazole (FICZ) (Magiatis et al. 2013; Gaitanis et al. 2008; Wille et al. 2001), and several indoles (Krieken et al. 2023; Yu et al. 2019), are all products of *Malassezia* species.

Commensal cutaneous bacteria, however, were only recently identified and verified to be producing AHR-activating ligands. The first study dates from 2019, where Rademacher and colleagues from Jürgen Harder' group used human primary keratinocytes transfected with an AHR firefly plasmid to measure AHR activity after co-transfection with *Staphylococcus epidermidis* (Rademacher et al. 2019). Using *S. epidermidis* culture supernatant, the authors showed that S. epidermidis produces AHR activating ligands, although they did not analyze the exact ligands produced. In addition to reporter assay analysis, expression of *CYP1A1* and *CYP1B1* verified the activation of host AHR as well. Co-cultured keratinocytes responded to bacterial presence by activating IL-1 signaling and induction of IL-1β which was mediated through activation of AHR as well. More recent work from 2021 by Uberoi and Elizabeth Grice's laboratory, indicated that the mixture of commensal microbes *S. epidermidis, S. hemolyticus, S. warneri, Corynebacterium aurimucosum*, and *Micrococcus luteus* was able to induce AHR activation in mice keratinocytes (Uberoi et al. 2021). Germ-free mice presented a diminished skin barrier function that was improved by inoculation of the skin with the mixture of the aforementioned bacteria for two weeks. In HaCaT keratinocytes, a *CYP1A1* luciferase reporter assay was used to verify the activation of host AHR by each of the commensal microbes used. Quantitative PCR on murine skin samples further verified the expression of *Ahr*, its downstream genes *Cyp1a1*, and *Cyp1b1*, and keratinocyte differentiation genes *Cdsn, Ivl*, and *Krt14*. The induction of AHR by *S. epidermidis* is in line with the earlier study from Rademacher in 2019, although also here, the exact microbial AHR ligands produced are unknown. Studies from Van der Krieken and Ellen van den Bogaard's group very recently analyzed the activation of host AHR by addition of either live bacteria, heat-killed bacteria, or supernatants of *S. epidermidis* and *S. aureus* to primary human keratinocytes (Krieken et al. 2023). In discordance with previous studies, our results did not indicate host AHR activation by *Staphylococci*. In contrary to both *Staphylococcus* strains, several commensal gram-positive anaerobic cocci (GPAC), i.e. *Finegoldia nericia, Anaerococcus prevotii*, and *Peptoniphilus asaccharolyticus*, known to be less abundant on skin of ichthyosis vulgaris and atopic dermatitis patients (Fyhrquist et al. 2019; Zeeuwen et al. 2017), were shown to activate epidermal AHR in organotypic human models (Krieken et al. 2023). Studies with *Pseudomonas aeruginosa*, a common opportunistic pathogen in skin infections, showed that host AHR can be activated by a range of microbe-derived phenazines (pigments) (Moura-Alves et al. 2014). Pathogenic *Mycobacterium tuberculosis* was shown to produce napthoquinone phthiocol, another bacterial pigment that is able to activate the AHR (Moura-Alves et al. 2014). It is proposed that AHR is a sensor for these specific bacterial virulence factors, thus playing a role in the innate protection of the tissue as well. Although these findings were reported in peripheral blood monocytes, lung cells, and in pulmonary infection models of WT and *Ahr*-deficient mice, the production of bacterial, pigmented virulence factors that serve as AHR

Table 10.1 Overview of AHR-activating ligands produced by skin microbiota

AHR ligand	Bacterial/yeast strain(s)	Reference
L-Tryptophan (Trp) metabolites		
2,3-Benzopyrrole (indole)	*Peptoniphilus asaccharolyticus*	Krieken et al. (2023)
Indole-3-carboxaldehyde (IAld)	*Lactobacillus bulgaricus, L. acidophilus, L. reuteri, L. johnsonii*	Zelante et al. (2013), Yu et al. (2019)
1,4-dihydroxy-2-naphthoic acid (DHNA)	*Propionibacterium freudenrichi*	Fukumoto et al. (2014)
Indirubin	*Malassezia furfur, M. obtusa, M. globose, M. japonica, M. yamatoensis*	Magiatis et al. (2013)
2-(1H-indol-3-ylmethyl)-1H-indole-3-carbaldehyde (malassezin)	*M. furfur, M. pachydermatitis, M. japonica, M. nana, M. yamatoensis*	Magiatis et al. (2013), Gaitanis et al. (2008), Wille et al. (2001)
6-formylindolo[3,2-b]carbazole (FICZ)	*M. furfur*	Magiatis et al. (2013)
Indolo[3,2-b]carbazole (ICZ)	*M. furfur*	Magiatis et al. (2013), Gaitanis et al. (2008), Wille et al. (2001)
Pityriacitrin	*M. furfur, M. japonica, M. yamatoensis*	Magiatis et al. (2013)
Tryptanthrin	*M. furfur, M. globose, M. japonica*	Magiatis et al. (2013)
Bacterial pigments		
1-hydroxyphenazine (1-HP)	*Pseudomonas aeruginosa*	Moura-Alves et al. (2014)
Phenazine-1-carboxylic acid (PCA)	*P. aeruginosa*	Moura-Alves et al. (2014)
Phenazine-1-carboxamide (PCN)	*P. aeruginosa*	Moura-Alves et al. (2014)
Pyocyanin (Pyo)	*P. aeruginosa*	Moura-Alves et al. (2014)

(continued)

Table 10.1 (continued)

AHR ligand	Bacterial/yeast strain(s)	Reference
Naphthoquinone phthiocol (Pht)	*Mycobacterium tuberculosis*	Moura-Alves et al. (2014)
Unknown ligands (at time of publication)	*L. bulgaricus, Staphylococcus epidermidis, S. hemolyticus, S. warneri, S. aureus, Corynebacterium aurimucosum, C. amycolatum, Finegoldia nericia, Anaerococcus prevotii,*	Rademacher et al. (2019) Krieken et al. (2023), Uberoi et al. (2021), Takamura et al. (2011)

ligands might hold true in the skin as well. More research is needed towards these types of AHR ligands in the cutaneous context.

The contradictory results with *Staphylococcus* species summarized above leads to the question whether strain-dependent variation, the combination of bacteria, separate or combined culture conditions, or environmental factors, are decisive in the production or secretion of microbe-derived AHR ligands. Secretion of the Trp metabolite indole-3-aldehyde (Iald), for example, was induced when bacteria used for inoculation were cultured in tryptophan-rich medium allowing the highly adaptive bacterial strains (i.e., *lactobacilli*) to switch from sugar metabolism to tryptophan metabolism (Zelante et al. 2013). Through AHR-mediated activation of interleukin-22 (IL-22), the survival of a mixed microbial community was shown providing resistance against *Candida albicans* colonization and mucosal inflammation (Zelante et al. 2013). Interestingly, an altered microbial Trp metabolism was suggested in AD and PSO microbiomes (Yu et al. 2019; Fyhrquist et al. 2019; Chng et al. 2016). The altered metabolism results in accumulation of 3-hydroxyanthranilic acid (3-HAA) (Fyhrquist et al. 2019) which was identified as an inflammatory mediator (Bohar et al. 2015). However, a study from Krause et al. indicates that 3-HAA can also dampen inflammation (Krause et al. 2011). These discrepancies are most likely explained by the step-wise, complex Trp metabolism, meaning that alteration of the metabolism can yield differences in Trp metabolites and catabolites produced. Dependent on the precise alteration, AHR-activating metabolites can accumulate. Those metabolites able to activate the AHR might attenuate the inflammation as shown in the intestines (Schiering et al. 2017), or in AD (Yu et al. 2019).

In summary, we propose the following concept: through activation of keratinocyte AHR, and thereby induction of epidermal differentiation and skin barrier function, the microbiota are thought to play a significant role in maintenance of the skin barrier (Alwan and Meglio 2021; Harris-Tryon and Grice 2022; Belkaid and Segre 2014). Activation of AHR and subsequent upregulation of cutaneous AMPs is thought to affect and restore the microbiome in atopic dermatitis (Smits et al. 2020), although elevated AMP expression following GPAC stimulation is not completely

AHR-dependent (Krieken et al. 2023). The activation of AHR by microbial components implicates that the microbiota themselves can play an active role in sculpting and securing their own favorable micromilieu (Rademacher et al. 2021).

Although recent findings suggest that many more cutaneous bacteria and yeasts might produce AHR ligands that help the organism to sense and respond to their environment, much has to be explored (Fig. 10.1). Our community would benefit from methods for systematic identification of ligand-producing bacteria and yeasts, starting with whole genome analysis, automated gene annotation, and subsequently classifying bacteria on their (theoretical) abilities to metabolize and produce AHR ligands. Follow-up experiments would entail validation of these bacteria to produce AHR ligands, e.g., through genome-wide or microbiome-wide transcription analysis and by precise identification of the produced AHR ligands. Next, research in human experimental cutaneous research models would help to better estimate the bacterial and yeast contribution to host epithelial barrier reinforcement and repair. For example, by studying the prerequisites for microbial and yeast AHR ligand production, we can better understand how and when AHR ligands are produced and use this information in (personalized) therapeutical settings.

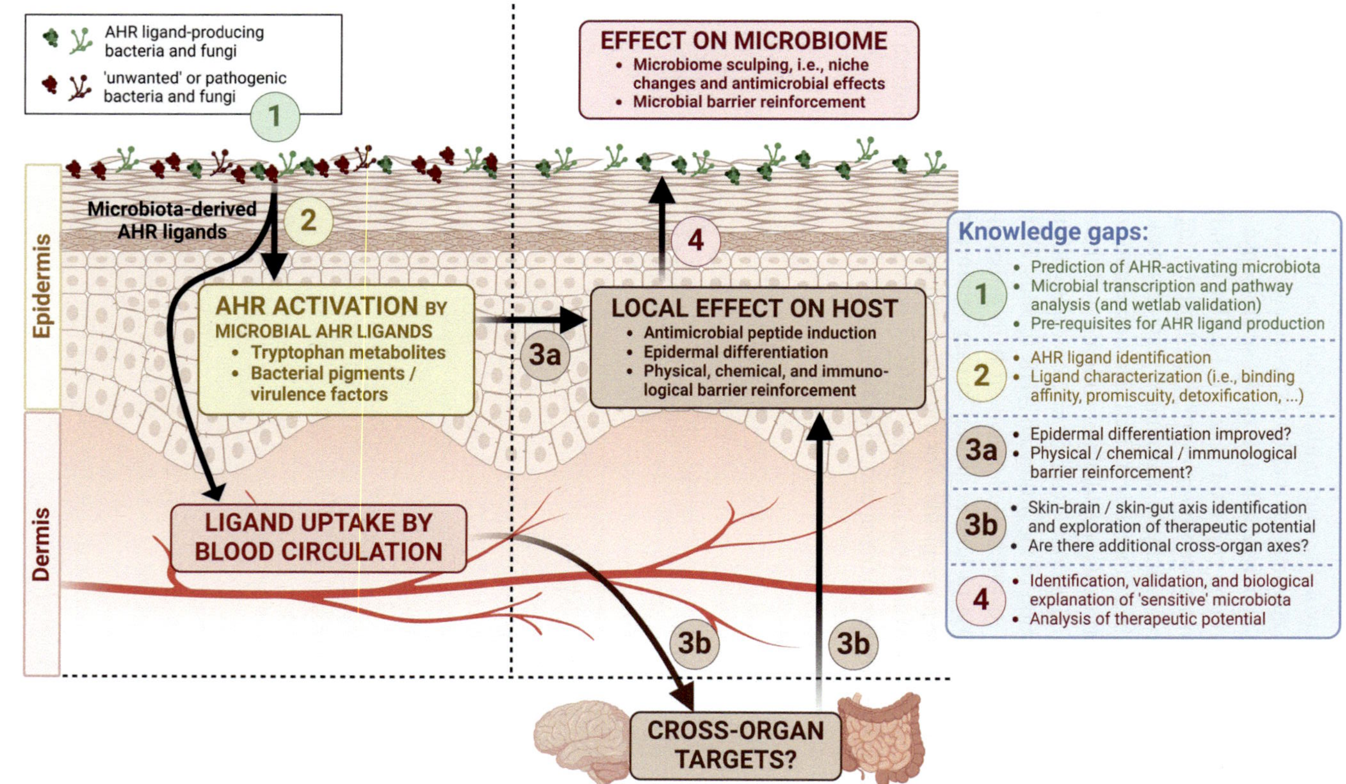

Fig. 10.1 Knowledge gaps and opportunities for further investigation. Created in BioRender.com

Acknowledgments This collaborative work was supported by LEO Foundation grant LF-OC-22-001056 (JS and EB), European Innovation Council under grant agreement number 101098826 ("SKINDEV"; EB and BH), Deutsche Forschungsgemeinschaft grants HO 2092/8-1 (BH) and HO 2092/9-1 (BH).

References

Agus A, Planchais J, Sokol H. Gut microbiota regulation of tryptophan metabolism in health and disease. Cell Host Microbe. 2018;23(6):716–24.

Alwan W, Di Meglio P. Guardians of the barrier: microbiota engage AHR in keratinocytes to mantain skin homeostasis. Cell Host Microbe. 2021;29(8):1213–6.

Barroso A, et al. The aryl hydrocarbon receptor and the gut-brain axis. Cell Mol Immunol. 2021;18(2):259–68.

Belkaid Y, Segre JA. Dialogue between skin microbiota and immunity. Science. 2014;346(6212):954–9.

Bohar Z, et al. Changing the face of kynurenines and neurotoxicity: therapeutic considerations. Int J Mol Sci. 2015;16(5):9772–93.

Bomar L, et al. Corynebacterium accolens Releases Antipneumococcal free fatty acids from human nostril and skin surface triacylglycerols. mBio. 2016;7(1):e01725–15.

Bosman ES, et al. Skin exposure to narrow band ultraviolet (UVB) light modulates the human intestinal microbiome. Front Microbiol. 2019;10:2410.

Chen YE, Fischbach MA, Belkaid Y. Skin microbiota-host interactions. Nature. 2018;553(7689):427–36.

Chng KR, et al. Whole metagenome profiling reveals skin microbiome-dependent susceptibility to atopic dermatitis flare. Nat Microbiol. 2016;1(9):16106.

Cholico GN, Nault R, Zacharewski TR. Genome-wide ChIPseq analysis of AhR, COUP-TF, and HNF4 enrichment in TCDD-treated mouse liver. Int J Mol Sci. 2022;23(3):1558.

Cibrian D, et al. CD69 controls the uptake of L-tryptophan through LAT1-CD98 and AhR-dependent secretion of IL-22 in psoriasis. Nat Immunol. 2016;17(8):985–96.

Claesen J, et al. A Cutibacterium acnes antibiotic modulates human skin microbiota composition in hair follicles. Sci Transl Med. 2020;12(570).

Conteville LC, Vicente ACP. Skin exposure to sunlight: a factor modulating the human gut microbiome composition. Gut Microbes. 2020;11(5):1135–8.

De Pessemier B, et al. Gut-skin axis: current knowledge of the interrelationship between microbial dysbiosis and skin conditions. Microorganisms. 2021;9(2):353.

Di Meglio P, et al. Activation of the aryl hydrocarbon receptor dampens the severity of inflammatory skin conditions. Immunity. 2014;40(6):989–1001.

Dong F, et al. Complex chemical signals dictate Ah receptor activation through the gut-lung axis. FASEB J. 2023;37(7): e23010.

Dunaway S, et al. Natural antioxidants: multiple mechanisms to protect skin from solar radiation. Front Pharmacol. 2018;9:392.

Esser C, Rannug A. The aryl hydrocarbon receptor in barrier organ physiology, immunology, and toxicology. Pharmacol Rev. 2015;67(2):259–79.

Fernandez-Gallego N, Sanchez-Madrid F, Cibrian D. Role of AHR Ligands in skin homeostasis and cutaneous inflammation. Cells. 2021;10(11):3176.

Fernandez-Salguero P, et al. Immune system impairment and hepatic fibrosis in mice lacking the dioxin-binding Ah receptor. Science. 1995;268(5211):722–6.

Fernandez-Salguero PM, et al. Lesions of aryl-hydrocarbon receptor-deficient mice. Vet Pathol. 1997;34(6):605–14.

Flowers L, Grice EA. The skin microbiota: balancing risk and reward. Cell Host Microbe. 2020;28(2):190–200.

Fouladi F, et al. Air pollution exposure is associated with the gut microbiome as revealed by shotgun metagenomic sequencing. Environ Int. 2020;138: 105604.

Fukumoto S, et al. Identification of a probiotic bacteria-derived activator of the aryl hydrocarbon receptor that inhibits colitis. Immunol Cell Biol. 2014;92(5):460–5.

Furue M, et al. Antioxidants for healthy skin: the emerging role of aryl hydrocarbon receptors and nuclear factor-erythroid 2-related factor-2. Nutrients. 2017;9(3):223.

Fyhrquist N, et al. Microbe-host interplay in atopic dermatitis and psoriasis. Nat Commun. 2019;10(1):4703.

Gaitanis G, et al. AhR ligands, malassezin, and indolo[3,2-b]carbazole are selectively produced by Malassezia furfur strains isolated from seborrheic dermatitis. J Invest Dermatol. 2008;128(7):1620–5.

Ganapathy AS, et al. Alpha-tocopherylquinone differentially modulates claudins to enhance intestinal epithelial tight junction barrier via AhR and Nrf2 pathways. Cell Rep. 2023;42(7): 112705.

Gandhi R, et al. Activation of the aryl hydrocarbon receptor induces human type 1 regulatory T cell-like and Foxp3(+) regulatory T cells. Nat Immunol. 2010;11(9):846–53.

Giri AK. Mutagenic and genotoxic effects of 2,3,7,8-tetrachlorodibenzo-p-dioxin: a review. Mutat Res. 1986;168(3):241–8.

Grice EA, Segre JA. The skin microbiome. Nat Rev Microbiol. 2011;9(4):244–53.

Grice EA, et al. Topographical and temporal diversity of the human skin microbiome. Science. 2009;324(5931):1190–2.

Gu YZ, Hogenesch JB, Bradfield CA. The PAS superfamily: sensors of environmental and developmental signals. Annu Rev Pharmacol Toxicol. 2000;40:519–61.

Guerrina N, et al. The Aryl hydrocarbon receptor and the maintenance of lung health. Int J Mol Sci. 2018;19(12):3882.

Gutierrez-Vazquez C, Quintana FJ. Regulation of the immune response by the aryl hydrocarbon receptor. Immunity. 2018;48(1):19–33.

Haas K, et al. Aryl hydrocarbon receptor in keratinocytes is essential for murine skin barrier integrity. J Invest Dermatol. 2016;136(11):2260–9.

Hahn ME, et al. Molecular evolution of two vertebrate aryl hydrocarbon (dioxin) receptors (AHR1 and AHR2) and the PAS family. Proc Natl Acad Sci. 1997;94(25):13743–8.

Harris-Tryon TA, Grice EA. Microbiota and maintenance of skin barrier function. Science. 2022;376(6596):940–5.

Hauben E, et al. Activation of the aryl hydrocarbon receptor promotes allograft-specific tolerance through direct and dendritic cell-mediated effects on regulatory T cells. Blood. 2008;112(4):1214–22.

Hawerkamp HC, et al. Vemurafenib acts as an aryl hydrocarbon receptor antagonist: implications for inflammatory cutaneous adverse events. Allergy. 2019;74(12):2437–48.

Hiebert P, Werner S. Targeting NRF2 to promote epithelial repair. Biochem Soc Trans. 2023;51(1):101–11.

Hubbard TD, Murray IA, Perdew GH. Indole and tryptophan metabolism: endogenous and dietary routes to Ah receptor activation. Drug Metab Dispos. 2015a;43(10):1522–35.

Hubbard TD, et al. Adaptation of the human aryl hydrocarbon receptor to sense microbiota-derived indoles. Sci Rep. 2015b;5:12689.

Iwase T, et al. Staphylococcus epidermidis Esp inhibits Staphylococcus aureus biofilm formation and nasal colonization. Nature. 2010;465(7296):346–9.

Jin UH, et al. Microbiome-derived tryptophan metabolites and their aryl hydrocarbon receptor-dependent agonist and antagonist activities. Mol Pharmacol. 2014;85(5):777–88.

Jux B, Kadow S, Esser C. Langerhans cell maturation and contact hypersensitivity are impaired in aryl hydrocarbon receptor-null mice. J Immunol. 2009;182(11):6709–17.

Kadow S, et al. Aryl hydrocarbon receptor is critical for homeostasis of invariant gammadelta T cells in the murine epidermis. J Immunol. 2011;187(6):3104–10.

Kennedy LH, et al. 2,3,7,8-Tetrachlorodibenzo-p-dioxin-mediated production of reactive oxygen species is an essential step in the mechanism of action to accelerate human keratinocyte differentiation. Toxicol Sci. 2013;132(1):235–49.

Kociba RJ, et al. Results of a two-year chronic toxicity and oncogenicity study of 2,3,7,8-tetrachlorodibenzo-p-dioxin in rats. Toxicol Appl Pharmacol. 1978;46(2):279–303.

Kohle C, Bock KW. Coordinate regulation of Phase I and II xenobiotic metabolisms by the Ah receptor and Nrf2. Biochem Pharmacol. 2007;73(12):1853–62.

Kong HH, et al. Temporal shifts in the skin microbiome associated with disease flares and treatment in children with atopic dermatitis. Genome Res. 2012;22(5):850–9.

Kopf PG, Walker MK. 2,3,7,8-tetrachlorodibenzo-p-dioxin increases reactive oxygen species production in human endothelial cells via induction of cytochrome P4501A1. Toxicol Appl Pharmacol. 2010;245(1):91–9.

Krause D, et al. The tryptophan metabolite 3-hydroxyanthranilic acid plays anti-inflammatory and neuroprotective roles during inflammation: role of hemeoxygenase-1. Am J Pathol. 2011;179(3):1360–72.

van der Krieken DA, et al. Gram-positive anaerobic cocci guard skin homeostasis by regulating host-defense mechanisms. iScience. 2023;26(4):106483.

Lande R, et al. Plasmacytoid dendritic cells sense self-DNA coupled with antimicrobial peptide. Nature. 2007;449(7162):564–9.

Li Y, et al. Exogenous stimuli maintain intraepithelial lymphocytes via aryl hydrocarbon receptor activation. Cell. 2011;147(3):629–40.

Lin YK, et al. Indigo naturalis upregulates claudin-1 expression in human keratinocytes and psoriatic lesions. J Ethnopharmacol. 2013;145(2):614–20.

Lo R, Matthews J. High-resolution genome-wide mapping of AHR and ARNT binding sites by ChIP-Seq. Toxicol Sci. 2012;130(2):349–61.

Lusska A, Shen E, Whitlock JP. Protein-DNA interactions at a dioxin-responsive enhancer. Analysis of six bona fide DNA-binding sites for the liganded Ah receptor. J Biol Chem 1993;268(9):6575–80.

Magiatis P, et al. Malassezia yeasts produce a collection of exceptionally potent activators of the Ah (dioxin) receptor detected in diseased human skin. J Invest Dermatol. 2013;133(8):2023–30.

Mandal PK. Dioxin: a review of its environmental effects and its aryl hydrocarbon receptor biology. J Comp Physiol B. 2005;175(4):221–30.

Marshall NB, Kerkvliet NI. Dioxin and immune regulation: emerging role of aryl hydrocarbon receptor in the generation of regulatory T cells. Ann N Y Acad Sci. 2010;1183:25–37.

Martin B, et al. Interleukin-17-producing gammadelta T cells selectively expand in response to pathogen products and environmental signals. Immunity. 2009;31(2):321–30.

May G. Chloracne from the accidental production of tetrachlorodibenzodioxin. Br J Ind Med. 1973;30(3):276–83.

McDonnell AM, Dang CH. Basic review of the cytochrome p450 system. J Adv Pract Oncol. 2013;4(4):263–8.

Miao W, et al. Transcriptional regulation of NF-E2 p45-related factor (NRF2) expression by the aryl hydrocarbon receptor-xenobiotic response element signaling pathway: direct cross-talk between phase I and II drug-metabolizing enzymes. J Biol Chem. 2005;280(21):20340–8.

Mills KH. Induction, function and regulation of IL-17-producing T cells. Eur J Immunol. 2008;38(10):2636–49.

Mimura J, et al. Loss of teratogenic response to 2,3,7,8-tetrachlorodibenzo-p-dioxin (TCDD) in mice lacking the Ah (dioxin) receptor. Genes Cells. 1997;2(10):645–54.

Ming M, et al. Loss of sirtuin 1 (SIRT1) disrupts skin barrier integrity and sensitizes mice to epicutaneous allergen challenge. J Allergy Clin Immunol. 2015;135(4):936–45.

Moura-Alves P, et al. AhR sensing of bacterial pigments regulates antibacterial defence. Nature. 2014;512(7515):387–92.

Nakamura K, et al. Short chain fatty acids produced by Cutibacterium acnes inhibit biofilm formation by Staphylococcus epidermidis. Sci Rep. 2020;10(1):21237.

Navid F, et al. The Aryl hydrocarbon receptor is involved in UVR-induced immunosuppression. J Invest Dermatol. 2013;133(12):2763–70.

Okey AB. An aryl hydrocarbon receptor odyssey to the shores of toxicology: the deichmann lecture, international congress of toxicology-XI. Toxicol Sci. 2007;98(1):5–38.

Omiecinski CJ, et al. Xenobiotic metabolism, disposition, and regulation by receptors: from biochemical phenomenon to predictors of major toxicities. Toxicol Sci. 2011;120 Suppl (Suppl 1):S49–75.

O'Sullivan JN, et al. Nisin J, a novel natural nisin variant, is produced by staphylococcus capitis sourced from the human skin microbiota. J Bacteriol. 2020;202(3):10–1128.

O'Sullivan JN, et al. Human skin microbiota is a rich source of bacteriocin-producing staphylococci that kill human pathogens. FEMS Microbiol Ecol. 2019;95(2).

Peppers J, et al. A phase 2, randomized dose-finding study of tapinarof (GSK2894512 cream) for the treatment of atopic dermatitis. J Am Acad Dermatol. 2019;80(1):89–98.

Perdew GH, et al. The Ah receptor from toxicity to therapeutics: report from the 5th AHR meeting at Penn State University, USA, 2022. Int J Mol Sci. 2023;24(6).

Rademacher F, et al. Staphylococcus epidermidis activates aryl hydrocarbon receptor signaling in human keratinocytes: implications for cutaneous defense. J Innate Immun. 2019;11(2):125–35.

Rademacher F, Glaser R, Harder J. Antimicrobial peptides and proteins: interaction with the skin microbiota. Exp Dermatol. 2021;30(10):1496–508.

Randerath K, et al. Organ-specific effects of long term feeding of 2,3,7,8-tetrachlorodibenzo-p-dioxin and 1,2,3,7,8-pentachlorodibenzo-p-dioxin on I-compounds in hepatic and renal DNA of female Sprague-Dawley rats. Carcinogenesis. 1988;9(12):2285–9.

Reggiani G. Acute human exposure to TCDD in Seveso Italy. J Toxicol Environ Health. 1980;6(1):27–43.

Rikken G, et al. Carboxamide derivatives are potential therapeutic AHR ligands for restoring IL-4 mediated repression of epidermal differentiation proteins. Int J Mol Sci. 2022;23(3):1773.

Rikken G, et al. Lead optimization of aryl hydrocarbon receptor ligands for treatment of inflammatory skin disorders. Biochem Pharmacol. 2023;208: 115400.

Robbins K, et al. Phase 2, randomized dose-finding study of tapinarof (GSK2894512 cream) for the treatment of plaque psoriasis. J Am Acad Dermatol. 2019;80(3):714–21.

Salminen A. Activation of aryl hydrocarbon receptor (AHR) in Alzheimer's disease: role of tryptophan metabolites generated by gut host-microbiota. J Mol Med (Berl). 2023;101(3):201–22.

Schiering C, et al. Feedback control of AHR signalling regulates intestinal immunity. Nature. 2017;542(7640):242–5.

Schmidt JV, et al. Characterization of a murine Ahr null allele: involvement of the Ah receptor in hepatic growth and development. Proc Natl Acad Sci. 1996;93(13):6731–6.

Shalat SL, et al. Kidney cancer in utility workers exposed to polychlorinated biphenyls (PCBs). Br J Ind Med. 1989;46(11):823–4.

Shimada Y, et al. Commensal bacteria-dependent indole production enhances epithelial barrier function in the colon. PLoS ONE. 2013;8(11): e80604.

Smith SH, et al. Tapinarof Is a natural AHR agonist that resolves skin inflammation in mice and humans. J Invest Dermatol. 2017;137(10):2110–9.

Smits JPH, et al. Targeting the cutaneous microbiota in atopic dermatitis by coal tar via AHR-dependent induction of antimicrobial peptides. J Invest Dermatol. 2020;140(2):415–24.

Smits JPH, et al. The aryl hydrocarbon receptor regulates epidermal differentiation through transient activation of TFAP2A. bioRxiv 2023.

Stockinger B, Shah K, Wincent E. AHR in the intestinal microenvironment: safeguarding barrier function. Nat Rev Gastroenterol Hepatol. 2021;18(8):559–70.

Sugimoto S, et al. Staphylococcus epidermidis Esp degrades specific proteins associated with Staphylococcus aureus biofilm formation and host-pathogen interaction. J Bacteriol. 2013;195(8):1645–55.

Sutter CH, et al. 2,3,7,8-Tetrachlorodibenzo-p-dioxin increases the expression of genes in the human epidermal differentiation complex and accelerates epidermal barrier formation. Toxicol Sci. 2011;124(1):128–37.

Sutter CH, et al. AHR regulates metabolic reprogramming to promote SIRT1-dependent keratinocyte differentiation. J Invest Dermatol. 2019;139(4):818–26.

Sutter CH, Rainwater HM, Sutter TR. Contributions of Nitric Oxide to AHR-ligand-mediated keratinocyte differentiation. Int J Mol Sci. 2020;21(16):5680.

Sutter CH, et al. Ligand activation of the aryl hydrocarbon receptor upregulates epidermal uridine diphosphate glucose ceramide glucosyltransferase and glucosylceramides. J Invest Dermatol. 2023;143:1964–72.

Takagi S, et al. Alteration of the 4-sphingenine scaffolds of ceramides in keratinocyte-specific Arnt-deficient mice affects skin barrier function. J Clin Invest. 2003;112(9):1372–82.

Takamura T, et al. Lactobacillus bulgaricus OLL1181 activates the aryl hydrocarbon receptor pathway and inhibits colitis. Immunol Cell Biol. 2011;89(7):817–22.

Takeuchi K, et al. Anti-inflammatory activity of the dry distillation tar of delipidated soybean (Glyteer) (1). Nihon Yakurigaku Zasshi. 1985;85(5):397–406.

Tsuji G, et al. Aryl hydrocarbon receptor activation restores filaggrin expression via OVOL1 in atopic dermatitis. Cell Death Dis. 2017;8(7): e2931.

Uberoi A, et al. Commensal microbiota regulates skin barrier function and repair via signaling through the aryl hydrocarbon receptor. Cell Host Microbe. 2021;29(8):1235–1248 e8.

van den Bogaard EH, et al. Coal tar induces AHR-dependent skin barrier repair in atopic dermatitis. J Clin Invest. 2013;123(2):917–27.

van den Bogaard EH, et al. Genetic and pharmacological analysis identifies a physiological role for the AHR in epidermal differentiation. J Invest Dermatol. 2015;135(5):1320–8.

van den Bogaard EH, Esser C, Perdew GH. The aryl hydrocarbon receptor at the forefront of host-microbe interactions in the skin: a perspective on current knowledge gaps and directions for future research and therapeutic applications. Exp Dermatol. 2021;30(10):1477–83.

Veldhoen M, et al. The aryl hydrocarbon receptor links TH17-cell-mediated autoimmunity to environmental toxins. Nature. 2008;453(7191):106–9.

Veldhoen M, et al. Natural agonists for aryl hydrocarbon receptor in culture medium are essential for optimal differentiation of Th17 T cells. J Exp Med. 2009;206(1):43–9.

Vos JG, Moore JA. Suppression of cellular immunity in rats and mice by maternal treatment with 2,3,7,8-tetrachlorodibenzo-p-dioxin. Int Arch Allergy Appl Immunol. 1974;47(5):777–94.

Wille G, et al. Malassezin–a novel agonist of the arylhydrocarbon receptor from the yeast Malassezia furfur. Bioorg Med Chem. 2001;9(4):955–60.

Williams MR, et al. Quorum sensing between bacterial species on the skin protects against epidermal injury in atopic dermatitis. Sci Transl Med. 2019;11(490).

Wu HY, et al. In vivo induction of Tr1 cells via mucosal dendritic cells and AHR signaling. PLoS ONE. 2011;6(8): e23618.

Yu M, et al. Aryl hydrocarbon receptor activation modulates intestinal epithelial barrier function by maintaining tight junction integrity. Int J Biol Sci. 2018;14(1):69–77.

Yu J, et al. A tryptophan metabolite of the skin microbiota attenuates inflammation in patients with atopic dermatitis through the aryl hydrocarbon receptor. J Allergy Clin Immunol. 2019;143(6):2108–2119 e12.

Zaid A, et al. Persistence of skin-resident memory T cells within an epidermal niche. Proc Natl Acad Sci. 2014;111(14):5307–12.

Zeeuwen PL, et al. Gram-positive anaerobe cocci are underrepresented in the microbiome of filaggrin-deficient human skin. J Allergy Clin Immunol. 2017;139(4):1368–71.

Zelante T, et al. Tryptophan catabolites from microbiota engage aryl hydrocarbon receptor and balance mucosal reactivity via interleukin-22. Immunity. 2013;39(2):372–85.

Chapter 11
Effect of Gut Microbiome on Skin Microbiome

Inge Kortekaas Krohn, Britta De Pessemier, and Chris Callewaert

Abstract The microbiome is part of a complex ecosystem of the human body. The skin is not only influenced by commensal microbes that colonize the skin, but it is also affected by the gastrointestinal microbiome. An interactive relationship and communication between the gastrointestinal tract, skin and immune system is called the gut-skin axis. This interplay is mediated through inflammatory mediators, metabolites and the intestinal or skin barrier. The human microbiome functions also as a regulator of the innate and adaptive immune system with a profound impact on the host homeostasis. The gut and skin microbiome composition and diversity is influenced by the host exposome throughout life, including but not limited to the route of delivery, diet, climate and many other factors. A dysbiosis of the microbiome can therefore have significant consequences for the development of diseases affecting the skin and or the intestines. The skin–gut axis is an area of emerging research. Gaining a deeper understanding of the bidirectional relationship between the gut and skin microbiome will reveal the role of an altered microbiome in gastrointestinal and/or skin pathologies. We may unlock novel therapeutic approaches for managing diseases by restoring a healthy microbiome and improve well-being and quality of life.

Keywords Diversity · Dysbiosis · Exposome · Gut microbiome · Gut-skin axis · Homeostasis · Metabolites · Skin diseases · Skin microbiome · Therapeutic approaches

I. Kortekaas Krohn (✉)
Skin Immunology & Immune Tolerance (SKIN) Research Group, Vrije Universiteit Brussel (VUB), Laarbeeklaan 103, 1090 Brussels, Belgium
e-mail: Inge.kortekaas@vub.be

Department of Dermatology, Vrije Universiteit Brussel (VUB), Universitair Ziekenhuis Brussel (UZ Brussel), Universitair Ziekenhuis Brussel, Laarbeeklaan 101, 1090 Brussels, Belgium

B. De Pessemier · C. Callewaert
Center for Microbial Ecology and Technology (CMET), Faculty of Bioscience Engineering, Ghent University, Ghent University, Coupure Links 653, 9000 Gent, Belgium
e-mail: Britta.depessemier@ugent.be

C. Callewaert
e-mail: Chris.callewaert@ugent.be

© The Author(s), under exclusive license to Springer Nature Switzerland AG 2025
A. Lauerma et al. (eds.), *The Skin Microbiome Manual*,
https://doi.org/10.1007/978-3-031-82689-4_11

11.1   Exploring Parallels Between Gut and Skin

The gut and skin barriers exhibit numerous similarities. They both serve essential roles in immunity and neuroendocrine function (O'Neill et al. 2016), sharing a resemblance referred to as the gut-skin axis (O'Neill et al. 2016). These barriers consist of epithelial cells on the inner gut surface and outer skin surface, forming the first line of defense against external elements (Shaykhiev and Bals 2007). Epithelial cells play a vital role in distinguishing harmful from beneficial substances, a process that begins early in life and underlies the concept of tolerance (Bach 2002). They prevent microorganism entry, with skin's keratin offering a physical barrier (Madison 2003). Mucous membranes also serve as mechanical barriers, housing commensal bacteria (Pelaseyed et al. 2014). Both tissues produce protective chemicals (Janeway 2001) and maintain unfavorable conditions for pathogens, like the skin's acidity and sebum production (Schmid-Wendtner and Korting 2006).

In the immune system, antimicrobial peptides (AMPs), phagocytes, and innate lymphoid cells form the first line of defense (Spits and Cupedo 2012). AMPs like cathelicidin and psorasin, produced by keratinocytes, bolster skin defense (Braff et al. 2005). The gut's epithelial barrier differs along the digestive tract, with varying cell types (Johansson et al. 2013). Paneth cells in the small intestine secrete AMPs. Communication between the host and microbiome is enabled via signaling through microbial-associated molecular patterns (MAMPs), for instance ligand expression of the Toll-like receptor (TLR) on gut and skin epithelial cells or on innate immune cells. MAMPs are sensed by innate lymphoid cells, triggering immune responses (Sonnenberg et al. 2011). Especially after birth, the gut microbiome contributes to the development of the immune system by the formation of tertiary lymphoid structures (e.g. Peyer's patches) in the intestines for the development of T cells and IgA-producing plasma cells (Ohnmacht et al. 2011). Epithelial cells and dendritic cells play crucial roles in antigen sensing, and Langerhans cells are unique to the skin (Shaykhiev and Bals 2007).

Both gut and skin tissues experience high cellular turnover, preventing microbiome adherence and infection (Barker 2014). They host symbiotic microorganisms, yet imbalances contribute to diseases like inflammatory bowel disease (IBD) and psoriasis, which involve immune responses and dysbiosis (Vlachos 2016). The gut microbiome acts as an endocrine organ, producing hormone-like compounds influencing distant organs, including the skin (Clarke et al. 2014). The gut-skin axis plays a pivotal role in the maintenance of human health and involves a link with the brain as well (Bowe and Logan 2011; Clarke et al. 2014; Ferraretto et al. 2023). The involvement of the brain in the gut-skin axis is mainly facilitated via the neuroendocrine system. The neurotransmitters (e.g. norepinephrine, serotonin, acetylcholine) produced by the gut microbiota lead to activation of neural pathways. This stimulates enteroendocrine cells to produce and release hormones with systemic effects. There's a bidirectional link between gastrointestinal and skin health through the immune system (Fig. 11.1), primarily modulated by gut microbiota (Benyacoub et al. 2014). Commensal skin microbiota also contribute to skin immune homeostasis. Both systems host various microbial species, and disrupting this balance impairs barrier function, affecting innate and adaptive immunity (Kortekaas Krohn et al. 2024).

11.2   Impact of Gut Microbiome on Skin Diseases and Microbiome

The commensals in the gut and skin play an important role in various physiological processes, including digestion, nutrient absorption, and metabolism with effects on the immune function, maintenance of regulatory signaling pathways and training of the immune system to induce immune tolerance (Belkaid and Hand 2014). In recent years it has become clear that skin health is not only influenced by its own microbiome, but also by the gastrointestinal microbiome (Bowe and Logan 2011). In the gut–skin axis, the gut microbiota plays an essential role which can affect skin health via the bacterial metabolites and modulation of the immune response.

It is well known that dietary components (e.g. gluten, catechins and polyphenols) modulate the gut microbiota. Conversely, bacterial metabolism of dietary nutrients results in metabolites. Gut microbiota actively produce metabolites that affect the immune system and human health in general. Short-chain fatty acids (SCFAs), including butyrate, propionate, and acetate, as well as branched-chain fatty acids and polyphenols are important microbial metabolites with anti-inflammatory properties. They function as signaling molecules that engage in crosstalk with the host, exerting direct or indirect modulatory effects on gut and skin cells by inhibiting inflammatory cell proliferation, migration, cytokine production, histone deacetylase and NF-κB signaling (Krautkramer et al. 2021; De Pessemier et al. 2021). Retinoic acid was found to control the development of the anti-inflammatory regulatory T cells (Tregs) and to impede the IL-6–dependent induction of proinflammatory T helper (Th)17 cells (Mucida et al. 2007). Proliferation of Tregs is also stimulated by the family of bacteria belonging to the *Clostridium* cluster IV and XIVa, by polysaccharide A of *Bacteroides fragilis* and by *Faecalibacterium prausnitzii* (Atarashi et al. 2013). These findings indicate that the gut microbiota modulates the Th1, Th2, Th17 and Treg-mediated immune responses as well as the intestinal barrier function via interactions with the epithelial cells (Kosiewicz et al. 2014). In this manner, the gut microbiome contributes to the maintenance of homeostatic conditions (Kosiewicz et al. 2014).

The presence of a highly diverse gut microbiome is associated with overall human health and homeostasis including reduced inflammatory status, enhanced immune tolerance and protection against autoimmune and inflammatory diseases (reviewed by Belkaid and Hand 2014; Byrd et al. 2018; De Pessemier et al. 2021). Recent advancements in research have unveiled the consequences of dysbiosis and its potential to promote the development of both skin and intestinal diseases. A gut microbial dysbiosis may trigger immune activity and is linked with a low gut microbiome

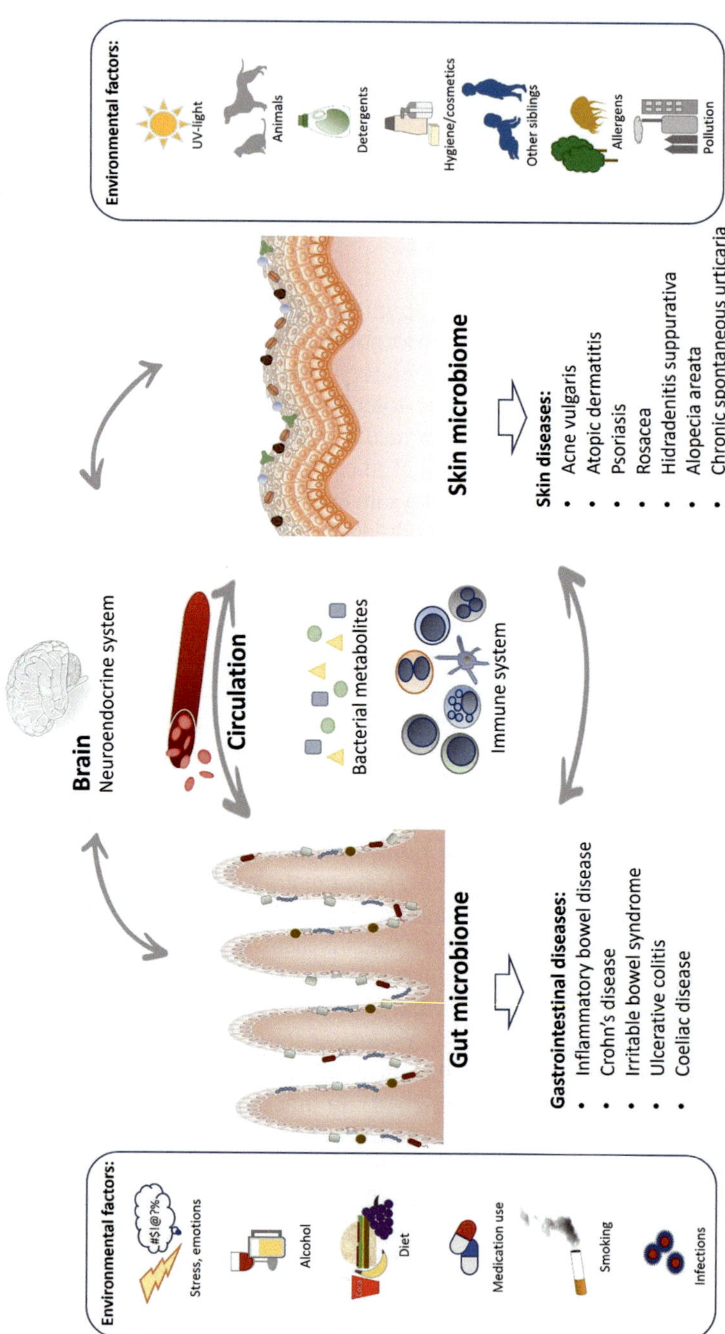

Fig. 11.1 Gut-skin axis. The gut and skin microbiome are influenced by the exposome. The bacterial metabolites produced by the microbiome on the intestinal mucosa and skin depend on the composition and diversity of the bacterial colonization, which subsequently affect the function of the immune system

diversity, high-fat diet and the presence of inflammatory mediators as the result of continuous immunological triggering in the intestinal lamina propria leading to impaired gut barrier function. A low diversity of commensals in the gut leads to a decreased function of the microbiota, for instance the inability to degrade nutrients in short chain fatty acids (Louis et al. 2010) or competition for colonization with pathogens. This can result in an increased intestinal permeability ("leaky gut") and further progress into a systemic inflammation and the prevalence of pathologies, such as acne, eczema, psoriasis, rosacea or IBD or irritable bowel syndrome (IBS) (Le Chatelier et al. 2013; Muszer et al. 2015; Sun et al. 2021). IBD often co-occurs with other inflammatory diseases, such as asthma, psoriasis, rheumatoid arthritis, multiple sclerosis (Weng et al. 2007). Several studies have investigated gut dysbiosis in relation to inflammatory skin diseases, which will be discussed in further detail in this chapter.

11.2.1 Acne Vulgaris

Acne vulgaris involves inflammation of the hair follicles and sebaceous gland (pilosebaceous units) due to blockage. Acne commonly affects the face, back and chest. In the development of acne, an increased sebum production, which is under the control of androgen hormones and testosterone, plays a distinct role. It is assumed that the gut microbiome is involved in the pathophysiology of acne due to the Western-diet intake and stress, which disturbs the production of SCFAs by the intestinal microbiota. Evidence was found for a link between high-glycaemic food, milk (or other dairy products) consumption and the presence of acne (Melnik 2011). *Cutibacterium acnes* species in the skin have been associated with acne (Fitz-Gibbon et al. 2013). The presence of several *Cutibacterium acnes* species in the skin of patients with acne have been linked with disease severity (Lomholt et al. 2017). Also in patients with acne, decreased gut microbiome diversity and reduced numbers of *Firmicutes* and increase in *Bacteroides* were found (Smith et al. 2007). Another study demonstrated a decrease in *Bifidobacterium, Lactobacillus, Coprobacillus, Butyricicoccus*, and *Allobusulum* in acne patients (Deng et al. 2018). In acne patients, *Bacteroides* spp. have been identified (Yan et al. 2018).

Modulation of the gut microbiome as therapeutic strategy in patients with acne can be effective to modulate the skin microbiota to restore the skin homeostasis.

11.2.2 Atopic Dermatitis

Atopic dermatitis (AD), a type of eczema, is a common acute or chronic skin disease usually with a very early disease onset (before the age of 2 years), but can also be (continued) in adulthood. AD is characterized by dryness of the skin, itchiness and rashes leading to skin lesions, infections and T cell mediated inflammation. AD is associated with *Staphylococcus aureus* skin colonization, but also gastrointestinal microbiota composition has been linked to the presence of AD. The role of microbial composition in the pathogenesis of AD is not fully understood. It is well-known that delivery via cesarean section leads to skin colonization by bacteria from the hospital and delayed maternal bacteria colonization resulting in a different bacterial composition than vaginally delivered newborn children (Grönlund et al. 1999; Dominguez-Bello et al. 2010). C-section delivery can decrease the numbers of *Bifidobacterium* and *Bacteroides* strains and increase the risk for colonization with *Clostridium difficile* (Grönlund et al. 1999; Penders et al. 2006). Additionally, evidence was found for the mode and place of delivery (at home versus hospital) and differences in the gut microbiota composition with consequences for the development of AD and asthma (Van Nimwegen et al. 2011).

The association between the skin microbiome composition and AD flares and progression was analyzed using skin samples from children with active AD (Kong et al. 2012). In AD patients, the microbial composition differed from the controls, depending on the recently used treatment. The abundance of *Staphylococcus* species, in particular *S. aureus*, increased during active disease, while *Streptococcus*, *Cutibacterium*, and *Corynebacterium* species were enriched following therapy (Kong et al. 2012). Investigation of the skin microbiome composition in 59 children, 13 adolescents and 56 adults with AD and 68 age-matched controls, demonstrated remarkable differences in the skin microbiome between young children and adults-teenagers with AD. The microbiome of the lesional skin correlated with clinical parameters, disease history, and medication use and disease severity (Shi et al. 2016). A study on the interplay between the skin microbiome, the skin surface microenvironment and the immune response investigated 80 skin microbiome samples (Chng et al. 2016). Non-flare, baseline skin microbiome samples were more abundant for *Streptococcus* and *Gemella*, whereas *Dermacoccus* was depleted in AD-prone compared to healthy skin. IL-1-mediated, and Th1-mediated immune responses with *S. aureus* and *S. epidermidis* were observed using bacterial challenge assays with keratinocytes and monocyte-derived dendritic cells. This highlights the interactive relationship between the microbiome, skin and immune cells that drives the disease (Chng et al. 2016).

In the gut of children with AD, the relative abundance of *Clostridia* was associated with the age of AD onset and inversely correlated with eosinophilic inflammation in the blood compared to healthy children (Lee et al. 2016). In a birth cohort, 298 fecal samples from infants were collected for the investigation of the gut microbiome composition and the risk for development of childhood atopy and asthma. A decreased relative abundance of *Bifidobacterium, Akkermansia* and *Faecalibacterium* was found in the highest risk group in parallel with increased relative abundance of the fungi *Candida* and *Rhodotorula* as well as a distinct fecal metabolome enriched for pro-inflammatory metabolites (Fujimura et al. 2016). A profound relationship between increased numbers of *F. prausnitzii* in the intestines and the chronic course of the disease was found most likely as a consequence of an impaired gut epithelial barrier, resulting in the induction of a Th2 immune response to allergens in the skin (Song et al. 2016). Under normal conditions, butyrate and propionate have anti-inflammatory properties, but stool samples from patients with AD were found to have reduced levels of butyrate and propionate possibly due to a shift in the composition within the family of *F. prausnitzii* (Song et al. 2016).

11.2.3 Psoriasis

Psoriasis is a skin disease with raised, scaly patches on the skin due to systemic inflammation. The patches are often seen on the outside of the flexures (knees, elbows), the trunk and scalp. Damaged keratinocytes of affected skin release the antimicrobial peptide LL-37 which subsequently forms complexes with DNA or RNA leading to activation of dendritic cells of the innate immune system. While the exact pathophysiology of psoriasis remains unclear, emerging evidence suggests a major contribution of the gut microbiota in contributing to disease development via modulation of the immune responses. Psoriasis is associated with concomitant gut disorders, such as IBD and Crohn's disease. Several studies have demonstrated differences in the gut microbiota composition in patients with psoriasis compared to healthy controls (Hidalgo-Cantabrana et al. 2019; Huang et al. 2019). Alterations are characterized by reduced bacterial diversity, the presence of pro-inflammatory bacteria (e.g. *E. coli* and *Streptococcus* spp.), and decreased levels of beneficial commensal bacteria (e.g. *Bifidobacterium* and *Akkermansia muciniphila*). This can lead to decreased levels of SCFAs and contribute to the production of pro-inflammatory cytokines.

A recent update on the gut microbiome in psoriasis included the analysis of 10 studies published between 2000 and 2020. Of those, all studies confirmed changes in beta-diversity, but there was no consensus on the alpha-diversity. Also, a lower relative abundance of *Bacteroidetes*, and higher *Firmicutes* were reported in psoriasis patients versus healthy individuals. Despite a clear relationship between dysbiosis in the gut microbiome and psoriasis, the composition of the intestinal microbiota varies. A study on the involvement of the gut microbiota in psoriasis development demonstrated increased gastrointestinal discomfort in patients with psoriasis (85.5%) compared to healthy control subjects (58.1%) and an increased variation of gut microbiota was accompanied with an improvement of psoriasis symptoms (Sun et al. 2021). Further, the authors found evidence for sustained levels of IL-17A in mice that were transplanted with fecal microbiota from psoriasis patients compared to mice that received fecal microbiota from matched non-psoriatic control subjects (Sun et al. 2021).

Untreated patients with psoriatic arthritis or patients with skin psoriasis had a decreased variety of gut microbiota compared to healthy controls, including a relative reduction of *Coprococcus* species and several beneficial commensals. Additionally, psoriatic arthritis patients had also reduced numbers of *Akkermansia*, *Ruminococcus* and *Pseudobutyrivibrio*, which resembles dysbiosis in IBD, supporting the involvement of gut microbiota (Scher et al. 2015). Also, the gut-brain axis and stress can contribute to this process as well via activation of the neurons of the enteric nerve plexus and increasing intestinal permeability (Vanuytsel et al. 2014). Analysis of fecal microbiota samples of 30 patients with psoriasis and 15 healthy individuals revealed that the gut microbiota of psoriatic patients showed an alteration in microbial taxa distribution, but not a difference in microbial diversity (Xiao et al. 2021). The investigators found a distinct composition of the gut microbiome in psoriasis patients, including an elevated presence of the phyla *Firmicutes*, *Actinobacteria* and *Verrucomicrobia* and genera *Faecalibacterium*, *Bacteroides*, *Bifidobacterium*, *Megamonas* and *Roseburia* and a decreased abundance of the phyla *Bacteroidetes*, *Euryarchaeota* and *Proteobacteria* and genera *Prevotella*, *Alistipes*, and *Eubacterium*. In these patients, lipopolysaccharide biosynthesis, WNT signaling, apoptosis, bacterial secretion system, and phosphotransferase system, were elevated. Additionally, five metabolites (hydrogen sulfide, isovalerate, isobutyrate, hyaluronan and hemicellulose) were dysregulated. These results suggest that dysbiosis of the intestinal microbiota is associated with genetic and metabolic dysregulation (Xiao et al. 2021).

Fecal samples from 33 healthy controls with samples from 29 patients with psoriasis, 31 patients with IBD, and 13 patients with concomitant IBD and psoriasis were analyzed for the abundance of *F. prausnitzii* and *E. coli*. Like patients with IBD, psoriasis patients the presence of *F. prausnitzii* was decreased compared to healthy individuals. Additionally, an increased abundance of *E. coli* was found in the samples of patients with psoriasis. Interestingly, patients with concomitant IBD and psoriasis had the most profound decrease of *F. prausnitzii* and increase of *E. coli* in their samples (Eppinga et al. 2016).

Further, a murine study showed that gut microbiome dysbiosis can induce psoriasis by alterations in fatty acid metabolism (Zhao et al. 2023). Transfer of gut microbiota from mice with severe psoriasis-like skin phenotype exacerbated mild psoriasis symptoms in K14-VEGF transgenic mice with increased infiltration and differentiation of Th17 cells. The authors found elevated numbers of *Prevotella* as well as reduction of *Parabacteroides distasonis* in the colon. The fatty acid metabolism was altered and the levels of oleic and stearic acids were elevated. Additionally, administration of oleic and stearic acids exacerbated psoriasis-like symptoms, including increased Th17 and monocyte-derived dendritic cell infiltration in the skin lesions (Zhao et al. 2023).

Secukinumab (anti-IL-17), used for the treatment of psoriasis, can cause modifications in the gut microbiome (Yeh et al. 2019). Following secukinumab therapy, an increased relative abundance was identified of phylum Proteobacteria, Pseudomonadaceae family, Enterobacteriaceae family and Pseudomonadales as well as decreases in Bacteroidetes and Firmicutes. Interestingly, the gut microbiome may act as a biomarker to predict the response to secukinumab therapy, because differences were found in the gut microbiome between responders and non-responders to the treatment (Yeh et al. 2019). The inability of ustekinumab (anti-IL-12/IL-23) therapy to change the gut microbiome (Yeh et al. 2019) suggests that IL-17 may be more involved in gut microbiome alterations than IL-12 and/or IL-23.

These studies have highlighted that gut dysbiosis in psoriasis patients may contribute to metabolic dysregulation and an imbalance of Th17 cells including IL-17 production. A dysregulated Treg/Th17 axis can promote pro-inflammatory cytokines, leading to skin inflammation, gut microbiome alterations and exacerbating psoriatic lesions.

11.2.4 Rosacea

Rosacea is an inflammatory skin condition characterized by facial redness, small red bumps and visible small blood vessels. The cheeks, forehead, nose and chin are commonly affected. An impaired barrier function may underlie the disorder. Factors that can trigger the symptoms are changes in temperature, stress, alcohol consumption, exercise and UV-light.

Microbes that are known to contribute to the development of rosacea belong to the symbiotic microbiota, such as *Demodex folliculorum* and *Staphylococcus epidermidis*, or to the pathogens, e.g. *Bacillus oleronius, Cutibacterium acnes, Helicobacter pylori* and *Chlamydia pneumoniae* (summarized by Holmes 2013; Kim 2020). A study on the bacterial microbiome on the cheeks of 60 twin pairs with or without rosacea demonstrated that the four most abundant phyla were *Firmicutes* (43.0%), *Proteobacteria* (39.3%), *Actinobacteria* (15.9%) and *Bacteroidetes* (1.0%) (Zaidi et al. 2018). The relative percentage abundance of *Gordonia* positively correlated with rosacea severity, while *Geobacillus* was negatively associated. Interestingly, the overall microbiome composition was largely unchanged because no differences in facial microbiome alpha and beta diversity were found (Zaidi et al. 2018). A case–control study including 19 individuals with rosacea (erythematotelangiectatic, papulopustular, or both) and 19 matched controls without rosacea also characterized skin microbiota composition on the cheeks (Rainer et al. 2020). This study showed that *Roseomonas mucosa* was depleted in patients with erythematotelangiectatic rosacea as compared to the controls, while in papulopustular rosacea the skin microbiota was enriched with *Campylobacter ureolyticus, Corynebacterium kroppenstedtii*, and *Prevotella intermedia*. In individuals with both erythematotelangiectatic and papulopustular rosacea the highest relative abundance of *C. kroppenstedtii* was found (19.2%), which was associated with a more comprehensive disease course (Rainer et al. 2020).

A case–control study with 65 rosacea patients and 65 controls demonstrated that rosacea is associated with several systemic comorbidities in a rosacea severity-dependent manner (Rainer et al. 2015). Gastrointestinal diseases, such as coeliac disease, Crohn disease, ulcerative colitis, *Helicobacter pylori* infection, small intestinal bacterial overgrowth and IBS, are often present as comorbid diseases in individuals with rosacea (Egeberg et al. 2017). This suggests a relation between the gastrointestinal diseases and the pathophysiology of rosacea. The role of the gut microbiota remains unclear and more research in large-scale studies is warranted. It can be assumed that the brain also is implicated in the development of rosacea, because it is persuaded or provoked by emotions and increased levels of stress (Lee et al. 2018), which highlights the relation of the gut-brain-skin axis.

11.2.5 Hidradenitis Suppurativa

Hidradenitis suppurativa (HS) is a chronic inflammation of the skin causing painful nodules, abscesses and fibrotic scars. The scarring lesions are usually deep in the skin at intertriginous areas and skin rich in apocrine glands (axillae, inner thighs, and groin area). Genetic predisposition in combination with hormones, smoking, obesity and diet (dairy, sugar-rich foods, and brewer's yeast) can play a role in the pathophysiology. Patients with HS often share common activated inflammatory pathways that often occur in intestinal disorders. Crohn's disease and IBD are typical comorbidities, which supports the role of the gut microbiota in HS. Differences in skin and gut microbiome composition between HS patients and healthy controls can relate to a decrease in the diversity of the microbiome in HS patients (Schneider et al. 2020) or increase in anaerobic infections in the lesional skin (Guet-Revillet et al. 2017). The skin and gut microbiome in HS was summarized in a systematic review (Lelonek et al. 2023).

A case–control study including 30 patients with HS and 24 control subjects investigated skin biopsies (Ring et al. 2017). Five microbiome types were identified: *Corynebacterium* species (type I), *Acinetobacter* and *Moraxella* species (type II), *Staphylococcus epidermidis* (type III), *Porphyromonas* and *Peptoniphilus* species (type IV), and *Cutibacteriumm acnes* (type V). Affected skin was dominated by the microbiome types I or IV, while type IV was not found in healthy control skin. A more abundant presence of *Cutibacterium* in the skin of healthy controls than from HS patients suggests that a loss of *Cutibacterium* can be involved in the development of HS (Ring et al. 2017). In a study with 12 adult HS patients and matched healthy controls, differences in relative abundances of the skin microbiota were examined (Naik 2020). A decreased abundance of *Cutibacterium* spp. was found in HS skin, while *Porphyromonadeacea*, *Prevotellaceae*, *Fusobacteria* and *Clostridales* were increased compared to healthy skin (Naik 2020). Another recent study investigated the microbiome at armpits, inguinal folds, and gluteal clefts of 60 HS patients and 17 healthy individuals (Riverain-Gillet et al. 2020). An elevated presence of anaerobes, especially *Prevotella*, as well as *Actinomyces*, *Campylobacter ureolyticus*, and *Mobiluncus* were identified in the HS skinfolds. On the other hand, *Staphylococcus epidermidis*, *Kocuria* and *Micrococcus luteus* were decreased. These findings suggest that microbiome dysbiosis in HS lesions can drive the inflammatory response and can exacerbate the formation of lesions (Riverain-Gillet et al et al. 2020).

While most of the studies focused on the skin microbiome, the gut microbiome was evaluated in only a few studies. One study investigated nasal and skin swabs as well as fecal samples in 59 HS patients and 30 healthy participants. The alpha diversity was decreased in the fecal, skin, and nasal samples of HS patients. A higher abundance of *Ruminococcus gnavus* was found in the fecal samples of HS patients. *Finegoldia magna* was increased in swabs from HS skin compared to the samples from healthy skin (McCarthy et al. 2022). A study including only three HS patients and three healthy subjects demonstrated a difference in biodiversity and the gut microbial alpha diversity in HS patients (Kam et al. 2021). The relative abundance of the phylum *Firmicutes* was decreased compared to healthy individuals. Also, the *Lachnobacterium* and *Veillonella* genera were less abundant in HS patients compared with healthy controls, while the abundance of *Bilophila* and *Holdemania* genera were overrepresented (Kam et al. 2021). A fecal microbiome study explored the gut-skin axis in 17 HS and 20 healthy controls. The results of this study showed that the biodiversity and the relative abundance of species found in HS patients and controls were comparable. However, *Robinsoniella* was found in the majority of fecal samples of HS patients (59%), whereas this was absent in the controls. Additionally, the presence of *Sellimonas* was more frequent in HS patients (76%) compared to healthy subjects (25%). On the other hand, the fecal samples of HS patients showed a decrease of a member of the *Christensenellaceae* family, but not those of the healthy individuals (Lam et al. 2021).

The results of these studies underline an association of HS with changed gut microbiota composition, including decreases in specific species and the microbial diversity in general.

11.2.6 Alopecia Areata

Alopecia areata (AA) is a T cell mediated autoimmune disease, characterized by the loss of hair resulting in patchy baldness. The exact pathomechanism of AA is unclear, but research supports a role of the gut or skin microbiota dysbiosis in the development of AA. The human scalp hair, hair shaft and follicles are colonized by bacterial communities that can reach to the subepidermal layers. Bacterial colonization of the hair roots may give challenges for swab sampling of the scalp. Investigation of the bacterial colonies of scalp hair shafts and roots from participants with different hair lengths, ages, and gender, demonstrated that the majority of the bacterial colonies were equal, including two species of *Pseudomonas* (phylum *Proteobacteria*), *Cutibacterium* and *Lawsonella* (phylum *Actinobacteria*), and *Staphylococcus* (phylum *Firmicutes*) (Watanabe et al. 2019). In healthy conditions, the microbiota of the hair follicles is relatively comparable to that of the skin (Byrd et al. 2018). In patients with AA, a higher prevalence of eczema has been found (Mohan and Silverberg 2015), suggesting that an impaired skin barrier function might provide access to bacteria or bacterial products that could play a role in the development of AA. The first study on the microbiota of the scalp at the site of the affected skin included 15 patients with AA and 15 healthy individuals. At the genus level, *Cutibacterium* dominated in AA subjects, while a decrease of *Staphylococcus* was found. Analysis of the main bacterial species on the scalp, showed higher relative abundance of *Cutibacterium acnes* in patients with AA than in healthy controls. On the other hand, decreased relative abundance of *Staphylococcus epidermidis* was found in AA lesions, but no changes in *Staphylococcus aureus* colonization (Pinto et al. 2019). The same research group performed another study including 47 patients with AA and 47 healthy subjects to study the microbiota of the affected skin using skin swabs and the microbial colonization of different layers of the skin using skin biopsies from

4 AA patients (Pinto et al. 2020). Analysis of the skin swabs showed higher proportions of *Anaerococcus* and *Neisseria* in AA patients, together with an absence of SMB53 genus (*Clostridiacea*) and lower proportion of *Staphylococcus*. The dermis layer of the skin biopsies showed a lower abundance of *Candidatus Aquiluna*, *Staphylococcus* and increased levels of *Acinetobacter* in AA patients (Pinto et al. 2020). Another study investigating the microbiome of the scalp using skin swabs included 33 AA patients (26 mild and 7 severe AA) and 12 control subjects (Won et al. 2022). An increased abundance of *Corynebacterium* species and lower levels of *Staphylococcus caprae* were found in severe AA patients compared with mild AA or healthy controls. Interestingly, a higher *Cutibacterium* species/*S. caprae* ratio was observed in severe AA (Won et al. 2022). These research data support a different microbial composition of the normal or AA affected scalp.

Investigation of the gut microbiome in fecal samples from 25 patients with active AA, revealed that the four major genera consist of *Lachnoclostridium*, *Bifidobacterium*, *Streptococcus*, and *Eubacterium*, and the three major phyla are: *Firmicutes*, *Proteobacteria*, and *Actinobacteria*. The composition of the fecal microbiome showed a decrease in microbial richness and diversity in general. Further an increased abundance of *Firmicutes* and *Proteobacteria* were identified (Brzychcy et al. 2022). Another gut microbiome study, including 15 patients with alopecia universalis and 15 control subjects found no differences in alpha or beta diversity between alopecea patients and controls. However, increased abundance of *Holdemania filiformis*, *Erysipelotrichacea*, *Lachnospiraceae*, *Parabacteroides johnsonii*, *Clostridiales vadin* BB60 group, *Bacteroides eggerthii* and *Parabacteroides distasonis* were identified in patients with alopecia. Interestingly, bacterial counts of *Parabacteroides distasonis* and *Clostridiales vadin* BB60 group could be used as biomarkers, as 80% correctly predicted the disease status (Moreno-Arrones et al. 2020).

These findings also indicate that AA is associated with a disturbed intestinal microflora. The gut microbiota composition could be of interest for future investigation, because of their involvement in the pathophysiology of AA. Also, their potential as biomarkers could be investigated in future studies.

11.2.7 Chronic Spontaneous Urticaria

Chronic spontaneous urticaria (CSU) is characterized by raised hives or bumps on the skin that causes an itchy skin (pruritis) leading to swelling (angioedema), redness and pain. In patients with CSU, several studies have identified a possible role for dysbiosis in the gut microbiota composition to the pathophysiology of the disease.

A study on the fecal microbial composition including 20 CSU patients and 20 normal controls, demonstrated an increased relative abundance of *Firmicutes*, *Bacteroidetes*, *Proteobacteria*, and *Verrucomicrobia* in CSU patients (Zhang et al. 2021). The differential analysis identified an increase of the *Proteobacteria*,

Bacilli, Enterobacterales and *Enterobacteriaceae* in CSU patients, while *Megamonas, Megasphaera,* and *Dialister* were decreased compared to healthy subjects (Zhang et al. 2021). A study including 25 chronic symptomatic dermographism patients and 25 healthy control subjects, found that the intestinal alpha diversity was decreased in CSD patients. *Subdoligranulum* and *Ruminococcus bromii* decreased in CSD patients compared to the healthy controls. Further analysis revealed that *Enterobacteriaceae* and *Klebsiella* positively correlated with the duration of CSD, and *Clostridium disporicum* was positively linked with the dermatology life quality index (Liu et al. 2021). Also, the fecal microbial composition was investigated in 25 CSU patients with non-sedative antihistamine resistance, 19 CSU patients without non-sedative antihistamine resistance and 19 healthy individuals (Song et al. 2022). A lower alpha-diversity was found in CSU patients with antihistamine resistance compared to those without resistance. In addition, genera *Prevotella, Megamonas,* and *Escherichia* were dominant, but a decrease in *Blautia, Alistipes, Anaerostipes,* and *Lachnospira* in antihistamine resistant CSU patients (Song et al. 2022). Finally, fecal samples of responders and non-responders to non-sedative antihistamine as monotherapy with CSU were analyzed (Liu et al. 2022). The presence of *Lachnospira* was increased, especially in responders compared to non-responders and the main difference in gut microbiota between these groups. This suggests a possible prediction of the response to antihistamines in patients with CSU (Liu et al. 2022).

In line with the above described skin diseases, CSU is also associated with gut microbiota dysbiosis. In conclusion, different intestinal microbial composition negatively influences the gastrointestinal function, leading to skewed immune pathways and an impaired metabolism. Most likely this affects the pathogenesis and the gut microbiome composition might provide insights in the therapeutic response.

11.3 Preventive Measures and Therapeutic Interventions

A healthy lifestyle, diet and avoidance of exogenous triggers is of utmost importance to maintain a healthy and diverse microbiome. Dietary changes can therefore be implicated to improve the skin and gut homeostasis. Modified intermittent fasting (restricted calorie intake for 2 non-consecutive days per week) has been proposed as a potential therapeutic strategy to improve the skin condition in individuals with psoriasis. However, the results could not yet confirm this, due to the co-founding factors (Grine et al. 2022). High-stress conditions and decreased physiological well-being have been associated with changed gut microbiome activity. Evidence was found for a reduction in beneficial fecal lactic acid bacterial levels during academic exams in 23 healthy undergraduate students (Knowles et al. 2008). Therefore, to avoid or reduce alterations in bacterial flora activity, the management of stress management is an important factor in prevention and treatment. Further, exposure to UV radiation contributes to skin dryness, pro-inflammatory cytokine production and reduced levels of type I collagen leading to skin-aging (Chen et al. 2015). These changes can affect the skin microbiome composition. Excessive UV light should be avoided to prevent these effects.

It is assumed that modulation of the gut microbiota by the use of probiotics (beneficial live microflora) or prebiotics (beneficial components for the microflora, e.g. high-fiber food) are effective to improve skin conditions or to prevent the development of allergic diseases. A double-blind, placebo-controlled study showed that modulation of the gut microbiome, using oral supplementation of *L. plantarum* HY7714, reversed the effects of UV radiation including cutaneous elasticity and skin hydration (Lee et al. 2015). Also, *Lactobacillus sakei* LTA was shown to neutralize UV-mediated skin aging via modulation of monocytes (You et al. 2013). In a large population-based pregnancy cohort, prenatal and postnatal probiotic milk supplements were provided to women and their infants. Probiotic milk products reduced the development of AD and rhinoconjunctivitis, but not the incidence of asthma at 36 months (Bertelsen et al. 2014). For the use of probiotics in pregnant women, the WAO guideline indicates the lack of clear scientific evidence of efficacy of probiotic supplementation as a preventive strategy for allergy development. Therefore, the WAO panel makes a suggestion to use probiotics during pregnancy by women at high risk for allergic diseases in their children based on a "net benefit" resulting primarily from prevention of AD (Ricci et al. 2016). For the use of prebiotics, the WAO guidelines suggest the use of prebiotic supplements in not-exclusively breastfed infants, but not in exclusively breastfed infants. Importantly, these recommendations are also conditional and based on very low certainty of the evidence due to the lack of studies on this topic (Cuello-Garcia et al. 2016).

In patients with acne vulgaris, application of oral pre or probiotic supplements can result in improved skin condition and tolerance, while the inflammatory status (IL-1alpha) and systemic oxidative stress levels are reduced (Bowe and Logan 2011).

Evidence for the beneficial effects of probiotic supplements in psoriasis was demonstrated in several studies using probiotic interventions. The effect of oral application of *Bifidobacterium infantis* 35624 was investigated in patients with ulcerative colitis (n = 22), chronic fatigue syndrome (n = 48), psoriasis (n = 26) and healthy subjects (n = 22) in separated placebo-controlled interventions (Groeger et al. 2013). After 8 weeks, *B. infantis* 35624 intake showed decreased levels of TNF-α and IL-6 compared to placebo controls. Also, peripheral blood mononuclear cells from healthy subjects stimulated with lipopolysaccharide produced lower levels of TNF-α and IL-6 in presence of *B. infantis* 35624 (Groeger et al. 2013). Another placebo-controlled trial also explored the efficacy and safety of a probiotic mixture in 90 adult patients with plaque psoriasis. After 12-weeks, both the probiotic group (66.7%) and the placebo group (41.9%) demonstrated reduced disease severity. At 6 months after termination of the study, a lower risk of relapse was found in the group with probiotics application (Navarro-López et al. 2019). These data suggest the potential treatment strategy of probiotics for patients with psoriasis on the modulation of gut microbiota and also at systemic inflammation levels.

Finally, fecal microbiota transplantation (FMT) is also a potential strategy to restore the homeostatic conditions of the gut microbiome. The efficacy of FMT might depend on the inflammatory condition and diversity of the gut microbiome as well as the bacterial load and route of delivery (Allegretti et al. 2019; Chen et al. 2020). Collection of stool samples from healthy donors is a crucial aspect, but factors that decrease the motivation of the donors are the invasive and unpleasant conditions for the collection of the samples (McSweeney et al. 2020). Receiving beneficial microflora from donors may gain interest among the patients because of the high efficacy and safety as well as the mode of the transfer or convenience (Ramai et al. 2019). FMT might be explored as a potential treatment strategy for psoriasis patients with severe gut dysbiosis. Until date, this has mainly been investigated in murine studies (Chen et al. 2020). Successful restoration of the gut microbiome by FMT and improvement of AD symptoms was proven in mice, suggesting FMT as a potential therapy in AD (Kim et al. 2021). Transplantation of the beneficial strains of *C. acnes* to the skin of patients with acne has shown promise and is safe, however, further studies in larger cohorts are needed (Karoglan et al. 2019).

Therapeutic strategies with focus on restoring the balance of the gastrointestinal microbiome have the potential to improve the skin conditions despite the long distance from the gut to the skin. This highlights the important aspects of the gut-skin axis. The efficacy of pre and probiotic supplements or FMT as novel therapeutic modalities in patients with inflammatory skin diseases is a clear research gap, but hold great promise and should be further explored in future human studies.

11.4 Conclusions

The complexity of skin diseases stems from interactions among genetic factors, lifestyle, and the immune system, closely intertwined with the nervous and endocrine systems. This interplay is particularly evident in organs like the skin and gut, richly populated with microbiota and immune regulators. The interactive relationship between gut microbes and the host immune system highlights the importance of the gut-skin axis in understanding skin diseases pathogenesis. Research suggests a link between skin diseases and the gastrointestinal system, primarily influenced by gut health, dietary factors, the intestinal microbiome, and the immune system, which collectively affect overall skin health. An impaired intestinal barrier, often debated as a "leaky gut," plays a pivotal role.

Exploring the potential of pre- and probiotics for the gut microbiome reveals positive effects on skin health. Studies in mice and humans show improved skin conditions with probiotic consumption, offering hope for managing skin diseases like acne, dermatitis, and psoriasis. Similarly, diets like caloric restriction and low fat diets exhibit benefits for intestinal and cutaneous health, including acne, dermatitis, psoriasis, wound healing, skin cancer, and skin aging.

Targeting the gut microbiome orally to influence the gut-skin axis is promising but complex. Properly designed clinical trials are needed to evaluate microbiome-targeted treatments, aided by advanced sequencing technologies and biomarker analyses. While viral microbiota are part of the microbiome, their role in skin diseases and intestinal health remains underexplored, awaiting insights from whole-genome sequencing.

Measuring skin health outcomes and optimizing study protocols are crucial. Noninvasive methods like skin tape stripping can aid in data collection, although limited compared to skin biopsies. Dietary habits, sampling moments, and circadian rhythms must be considered in study designs, as they can influence the gut microbiome and overall health.

In conclusion, the gut-skin axis, governed by our microbiota, presents a promising avenue for research and potential therapeutic and cosmetic applications. Increased knowledge on the gut and skin microbiota and their role in the pathophysiology of skin diseases may help to better understand the microbiome-host-interactions and to improve targeted therapies. Understanding the intricate interactions between the microbiome and host tissues holds the key to advancing our knowledge of health and disease, necessitating well-designed multidisciplinary trials to explore this fascinating frontier.

References

Allegretti JR, Fischer M, Sagi SV, Bohm ME, Fadda HM, Ranmal SR, Budree S, Basit AW, Glettig DL, de la Serna EL, Gentile A, Gerardin Y, Timberlake S, Sadovsky R, Smith M, Kassam Z. Fecal microbiota transplantation capsules with targeted colonic versus gastric delivery in recurrent clostridium difficile infection: a comparative cohort analysis of high and lose dose. Dig Dis Sci. 2019;64(6):1672–8 PMID: 30519847.

Atarashi K, Tanoue T, Oshima K, Suda W, Nagano Y, Nishikawa H, Fukuda S, Saito T, Narushima S, Hase K, Kim S, Fritz JV, Wilmes P, Ueha S, Matsushima K, Ohno H, Olle B, Sakaguchi S, Taniguchi T, Morita H, Hattori M, Honda K. Treg induction by a rationally selected mixture of Clostridia strains from the human microbiota. Nature. 2013;500(7461):232–6 PMID: 23842501.

Bach JF. The effect of infections on susceptibility to autoimmune and allergic diseases. N Engl J Med. 2002;347:911–20.

Barker N. Adult intestinal stem cells: critical drivers of epithelial homeostasis and regeneration. Nat Rev Mol Cell Biol. 2014;15:19–33.

Belkaid Y, Hand TW. Role of the microbiota in immunity and inflammation. Cell. 2014;157(1):121–41 PMID: 24679531.

Benyacoub J, Bosco N, Blanchard C, Demont A, Philippe D, Castiel-Higounenc I, Guéniche A. Immune modulation property of Lactobacillus paracasei NCC2461 (ST11) strain and impact on skin defences. Benef Microbes. 2014;5(2):129–36 PMID: 24322880.

Bertelsen RJ, Brantsæter AL, Magnus MC, Haugen M, Myhre R, Jacobsson B, Longnecker MP, Meltzer HM, London SJ. Probiotic milk consumption in pregnancy and infancy and subsequent childhood allergic diseases. J Allergy Clin Immunol. 2014;133(1):165–71.e1-8 PMID: 24034345.

Bowe WP, Logan AC. Acne vulgaris, probiotics and the gut-brain-skin axis—back to the future? Gut Pathog. 2011;3(1):1 PMID: 21281494.

Braff MH, Zaiou M, Fierer J, Nizet V, Gallo RL. Keratinocyte production of cathelicidin provides direct activity against bacterial skin pathogens. Infect Immun. 2005;73:6771–81.

Brzychcy K, Dróżdż I, Skoczylas S, Płoszaj T, Sobolewska-Sztychny D, Skibińska M, Narbutt J, Lesiak A. Gut microbiota in alopecia areata. Postepy Dermatol Alergol. 2022;39(6):1162–70 PMID: 36686014.

Byrd AL, Belkaid Y, Segre JA. The human skin microbiome. Nat Rev Microbiol. 2018;16(3):143–55 PMID: 29332945.

Chen B, Li R, Yan N, Chen G, Qian W, Jiang HL, Ji C, Bi ZG. Astragaloside IV controls collagen reduction in photoaging skin by improving transforming growth factor-β/Smad signaling suppression and inhibiting matrix metalloproteinase-1. Mol Med Rep. 2015;11(5):3344–8 PMID: 25591734.

Chen L, Li J, Zhu W, Kuang Y, Liu T, Zhang W, Chen X, Peng C. Skin and gut microbiome in psoriasis: gaining insight into the pathophysiology of it and finding novel therapeutic strategies. Front Microbiol. 2020;11: 589726 PMID: 33384669.

Chng KR, Tay ASL, Li C, Ng AHQ, Wang J, Suri BK, Matta SA, McGovern N, Janela B, Wong XFCC, et al. Whole metagenome profiling reveals skin microbiome-dependent susceptibility to atopic dermatitis flare. Nat Microbiol. 2016;1:1–10.

Clarke G, Stilling RM, Kennedy PJ, Stanton C, Cryan JF, Dinan TG. Minireview: gut microbiota: the neglected endocrine organ. Mol Endocrinol. 2014;28:1221–38.

Cuello-Garcia CA, Fiocchi A, Pawankar R, et al. World allergy organization-mcmaster university guidelines for allergic disease prevention (GLAD-P): prebiotics. World Allergy Organ J. 2016;9:10 PMID: 26962387.

De Pessemier B, Grine L, Debaere M, Maes A, Paetzold B, Callewaert C. Gut-skin axis: current knowledge of the interrelationship between microbial dysbiosis and skin conditions. Microorganisms. 2021;9(2):353 PMID: 33670115.

Deng Y, Wang H, Zhou J, Mou Y, Wang G, Xiong X. Patients with acne vulgaris have a distinct gut microbiota in comparison with healthy controls. Acta Derm Venereol. 2018;98:783–90.

Dominguez-Bello MG, Costello EK, Contreras M, Magris M, Hidalgo G, Fierer N, Knight R. Delivery mode shapes the acquisition and structure of the initial microbiota across multiple body habitats in newborns. Proc Natl Acad Sci. 2010;107(26):11971–5 PMID: 20566857.

Egeberg A, Weinstock LB, Thyssen EP, Gislason GH, Thyssen JP. Rosacea and gastrointestinal disorders: a population-based cohort study. Br J Dermatol. 2017;176(1):100–6 PMID: 27501017.

Eppinga H, Sperna Weiland CJ, Thio HB, van der Woude CJ, Nijsten TE, Peppelenbosch MP, Konstantinov SR. Similar depletion of protective faecalibacterium prausnitzii in psoriasis and inflammatory bowel disease, but not in hidradenitis suppurativa. J Crohns Colitis. 2016;10(9):1067–75 PMID: 26971052.

Ferraretto A, Donetti E, García-Mena J, Pacheco-López G. Editorial: the gut-skin-brain axis in human health and disease. Front Nutr. 2023;10:1155614 PMID: 36875850.

Fitz-Gibbon S, Tomida S, et al. Propionibacterium acnes strain populations in the human skin microbiome associated with acne. J Invest Dermatol. 2013;133(9):2152–60 PMID: 23337890.

Fujimura KE, Sitarik AR, Havstad S, et al. Neonatal gut microbiota associates with childhood multisensitized atopy and T cell differentiation. Nat Med. 2016;22(10):1187–91 PMID: 27618652.

Grine L, Hilhorst N, Michels N, Abbeddou S, De Henauw S, Lambert J. The effects of modified intermittent fasting in psoriasis (MANGO): protocol for a two-arm pilot randomized controlled open cross-over study. JMIR Res Protoc. 2022;11(2): e26405 PMID: 35195533.

Groeger D, O'Mahony L, Murphy EF, Bourke JF, Dinan TG, Kiely B, Shanahan F, Quigley EM. Bifidobacterium infantis 35624 modulates host inflammatory processes beyond the gut. Gut Microbes. 2013;4(4):325–39 PMID: 23842110.

Grönlund MM, Lehtonen OP, Eerola E, Kero P. Fecal microflora in healthy infants born by different methods of delivery: permanent changes in intestinal flora after cesarean delivery. J Pediatr Gastroenterol Nutr. 1999;28(1):19–25.

Guet-Revillet H, Jais J-P, Ungeheuer M-N, Coignard-Biehler H, Duchatelet S, Delage M, Lam T, Hovnanian A, Lortholary O, Nassif X, et al. The microbiological landscape of anaerobic infections in hidradenitis suppurativa: a prospective metagenomic study. Clin Infect Dis. 2017;65:282–91.

Hidalgo-Cantabrana C, Gómez J, Delgado S, Requena-López S, Queiro-Silva R, Margolles A, Coto E, Sánchez B, Coto-Segura P. Gut microbiota dysbiosis in a cohort of patients with psoriasis. Br J Dermatol. 2019;181(6):1287–95 PMID: 30920647.

Holmes AD. Potential role of microorganisms in the pathogenesis of rosacea. J Am Acad Dermatol. 2013;69(6):1025–32 PMID: 24011460.

Huang L, Xiao X, Zhao G. Microbes: the hidden giant behind the biogeochemical cycling of elements in the hydrosphere. Sci China Life Sci. 2019;62(10):1271–4 PMID: 31578664.

Janeway CA Jr, Travers P, Walport M, Shlomchik MJ. The front line of host defense. Immunobiology: the immune system in health and disease. 5th ed. New York: Garland Science, NY, USA, 2001.

Johansson ME, Sjövall H, Hansson GC. The gastrointestinal mucus system in health and disease. Nat Rev Gastroenterol Hepatol. 2013;10(6):352–61 PMID: 23478383.

Kam S, Collard M, Lam J, Alani RM. Gut microbiome perturbations in patients with hidradenitis suppurativa: a case series. J Invest Dermatol. 2021;141(1):225-228.e2 PMID: 32422215.

Karoglan A, Paetzold B, et al. Safety and efficacy of topically applied selected cutibacterium acnes strains over five weeks in patients with acne vulgaris: an open-label pilot study. Acta Derm Venereol. 2019;99(13):1253–7 PMID: 31573666.

Kim HS. Microbiota in Rosacea. Am J Clin Dermatol. 2020;21(Suppl 1):25–35 PMID: 32914214p

Kim JH, Kim K, Kim W. Gut microbiota restoration through fecal microbiota transplantation: a new atopic dermatitis therapy. Exp Mol Med. 2021;53(5):907–16 PMID: 34017060.

Knowles SR, Nelson EA, Palombo EA. Investigating the role of perceived stress on bacterial flora activity and salivary cortisol secretion: a possible mechanism underlying susceptibility to illness. Biol Psychol. 2008;77:132–7.

Kong HH, Oh J, Deming C, Conlan S, Grice EA, Beatson MA, Nomicos E, Polley EC, Komarow HD, Murray PR, Turner ML, Segre JA. Temporal shifts in the skin microbiome associated with disease flares and treatment in children with atopic dermatitis. Genome Res. 2012;22(5):850–9 PMID: 22310478

Kortekaas Krohn I, Callewaert C, Belasri H, De Pessemier B, Diez Lopez C, Mortz CG, O'Mahony L, Pérez-Gordo M, Sokolowska M, Unger Z, Untersmayr E, Homey B, Gomez-Casado C. The influence of lifestyle and environmental factors on host resilience through a homeostatic skin microbiota: an EAACI task force report. Allergy 2024;79(12):3269–84. https://doi.org/10.1111/all.16378. Epub 2024 Nov 1. PMID: 39485000; PMCID: PMC11657040

Kosiewicz MM, Dryden GW, Chhabra A, Alard P. Relationship between gut microbiota and development of T cell associated disease. FEBS Lett. 2014;588(22):4195–206 PMID: 24681103.

Krautkramer KA, Fan J, Bäckhed F. Gut microbial metabolites as multi-kingdom intermediates. Nat Rev Microbiol. 2021;19(2):77–94 PMID: 32968241.

Lam SY, Radjabzadeh D, Eppinga H, Nossent YRA, van der Zee HH, Kraaij R, Konstantinov SR, Fuhler GM, Prens EP, Thio HB, et al. A microbiome study to explore the gut-skin axis in hidradenitis suppurativa. J Dermatol Sci. 2021;101:218–20.

Le Chatelier E, Nielsen T, Qin J, Prifti E, Hildebrand F, Falony G, Almeida M, Arumugam M, Batto JM, Kennedy S, Leonard P, Li J, Burgdorf K, et al. Richness of human gut microbiome correlates with metabolic markers. Nature. 2013;500(7464):541–6 PMID: 23985870.

Lee DE, Huh CS, Ra J, Choi ID, Jeong JW, Kim SH, Ryu JH, Seo YK, Koh JS, Lee JH, Sim JH, Ahn YT. Clinical evidence of effects of lactobacillus plantarum HY7714 on skin aging: a randomized double blind placebo-controlled study. J Microbiol Biotechnol. 2015;25(12):2160–8 PMID: 26428734.

Lee E, Lee SY, Kang MJ, Kim K, Won S, Kim BJ, Choi KY, Kim BS, Cho HJ, Kim Y, Yang SI, Hong SJ. Clostridia in the gut and onset of atopic dermatitis via eosinophilic inflammation. Ann Allergy Asthma Immunol. 2016;117(1):91-92.e1 PMID: 27179583.

Lee JB, Moon J, Moon KR, Yang JH, Kye YC, Kim KJ, Kim NI, Ro YS, Park KY, Park MY, Song M, Ahn KJ, Ahn HH, Lee MW, Lee WJ, Choi YS, Choi YW, Kwon HH, Suh DH. Epidemiological and clinical features of rosacea in Korea: a multicenter cross-sectional study. J Dermatol. 2018;45(5):546–53 PMID: 29574999.

Lelonek E, Bouazzi D, Jemec GBE, Szepietowski JC. Skin and gut microbiome in hidradenitis suppurativa: a systematic review. Biomedicines. 2023;11(8):2277 PMID: 37626773.

Liu R, Peng C, Jing D, Xiao Y, Zhu W, Zhao S, Zhang J, Chen X, Li J. Biomarkers of gut microbiota in chronic spontaneous urticaria and symptomatic dermographism. Front Cell Infect Microbiol. 2021;11: 703126 PMID: 34858864.

Liu R, Peng C, Jing D, Xiao Y, Zhu W, Zhao S, Zhang J, Chen X, Li J. Lachnospira is a signature of antihistamine efficacy in chronic spontaneous urticaria. Exp Dermatol. 2022;31(2):242–7 PMID: 34558729.

Lomholt HB, Scholz CFP, et al. A comparative study of Cutibacterium (Propionibacterium) acnes clones from acne patients and healthy controls. Anaerobe. 2017;47:57–63.

Louis P, Young P, Holtrop G, Flint HJ. Diversity of human colonic butyrate-producing bacteria revealed by analysis of the butyryl-CoA:acetate CoA-transferase gene. Environ Microbiol. 2010;12(2):304–14 PMID: 19807780.

Madison KC. Barrier function of the skin: "la raison d'être" of the epidermis. J Invest Dermatol. 2003;121(2):231–41 PMID: 12880413.

McCarthy S, Barrett M, Kirthi S, Pellanda P, Vlckova K, Tobin AM, Murphy M, Shanahan F, O'Toole PW. Altered skin and gut microbiome in hidradenitis suppurativa. J Invest Dermatol. 2022;142(2):459-468.e15 PMID: 34364884.

McSweeney B, Allegretti JR, Fischer M, Xu H, Goodman KJ, Monaghan T, McLeod C, Mullish BH, Petrof EO, Phelps EL, Chis R, Edmison A, Juby A, Ennis-Davis R, Roach B, Wong K, Kao D. In search of stool donors: a multicenter study of prior knowledge, perceptions, motivators, and deterrents among potential donors for fecal microbiota transplantation. Gut Microbes. 2020;11(1):51–62 PMID: 31122134.

Melnik BC. Evidence for acne-promoting effects of milk and other insulinotropic dairy products. Nestlé Nutr Workshop Ser Pediatric Program. 2011;67:131–45.

Mohan GC, Silverberg JI. Association of vitiligo and alopecia areata with atopic dermatitis: a systematic review and meta-analysis. JAMA Dermatol. 2015;151:522–8.

Moreno-Arrones OM, Serrano-Villar S, Perez-Brocal V, Saceda-Corralo D, Morales-Raya C, Rodrigues-Barata R, Moya A, Jaen-Olasolo P, Vano-Galvan S. Analysis of the gut microbiota in alopecia areata: identification of bacterial biomarkers. J Eur Acad Dermatol Venereol. 2020;34(2):400–5 PMID: 31419351.

Mucida D, Park Y, Kim G, Turovskaya O, Scott I, Kronenberg M, Cheroutre H. Reciprocal TH17 and regulatory T cell differentiation mediated by retinoic acid. Science. 2007;317(5835):256–60 PMID: 17569825.

Muszer M, Noszczyńska M, Kasperkiewicz K, Skurnik M. Human microbiome: when a friend becomes an enemy. Arch Immunol Ther Exp (Warsz). 2015;63(4):287–98 PMID: 25682593.

Navarro-López V, Martínez-Andrés A, Ramírez-Boscá A, Ruzafa-Costas B, Núñez-Delegido E, Carrión-Gutiérrez MA, Prieto-Merino D, Codoñer-Cortés F, Ramón-Vidal D, Genovés-Martínez S, Chenoll-Cuadros E, Pérez-Orquín JM, Picó-Monllor JA, Chumillas-Lidón S. Efficacy and safety of oral administration of a mixture of probiotic strains in patients with psoriasis: a randomized controlled clinical trial. Acta Derm Venereol. 2019;99(12):1078–84.

van Nimwegen FA, Penders J, Stobberingh EE, Postma DS, Koppelman GH, Kerkhof M, Reijmerink NE, Dompeling E, van den Brandt PA, Ferreira I, Mommers M, Thijs C. Mode and place of delivery, gastrointestinal microbiota, and their influence on asthma and atopy. J Allergy Clin Immunol. 2011;128(5):948–55.e1-3 PMID: 21872915.

Ohnmacht C, Marques R, Presley L, Sawa S, Lochner M, Eberl G. Intestinal microbiota, evolution of the immune system and the bad reputation of pro-inflammatory immunity. Cell Microbiol. 2011;13(5):653–9 PMID: 21338464.

O'Neill CA, Monteleone G, McLaughlin JT, Paus R. The gut-skin axis in health and disease: a paradigm with therapeutic implications. BioEssays. 2016;38(11):1167–76 PMID: 27554239.

Pelaseyed T, Bergström JH, Gustafsson JK, Ermund A, Birchenough GM, Schütte A, van der Post S, Svensson F, Rodríguez-Piñeiro AM, Nyström EE, Wising C, Johansson ME, Hansson GC. The mucus and mucins of the goblet cells and enterocytes provide the first defense line of the gastrointestinal tract and interact with the immune system. Immunol Rev. 2014;260(1):8–20 PMID: 24942678.

Penders J, Thijs C, Vink C, Stelma FF, Snijders B, Kummeling I, van den Brandt PA, Stobberingh EE. Factors influencing the composition of the intestinal microbiota in early infancy. Pediatrics. 2006;118(2):511–21 PMID: 16882802.

Penders J, Thijs C, van den Brandt PA, Kummeling I, Snijders B, Stelma F, Adams H, van Ree R, Stobberingh EE. Gut microbiota composition and development of atopic manifestations in infancy: the KOALA birth cohort study. Gut. 2007;56(5):661–7 PMID: 17047098.

Pinto D, Sorbellini E, Marzani B, Rucco M, Giuliani G, Rinaldi F. Scalp bacterial shift in Alopecia areata. PLoS ONE. 2019;14(4): e0215206 PMID: 30973913.

Pinto D, Calabrese FM, De Angelis M, Celano G, Giuliani G, Gobbetti M, Rinaldi F. Predictive metagenomic profiling, urine metabolomics, and human marker gene expression as an integrated approach to study alopecia areata. Front Cell Infect Microbiol. 2020;10:146.

Rainer BM, Thompson KG, Antonescu C, Florea L, Mongodin EF, Bui J, Fischer AH, Pasieka HB, Garza LA, Kang S, Chien AL. Characterization and analysis of the skin microbiota in rosacea: a case-control study. Am J Clin Dermatol. 2020;21(1):139–47 PMID: 31502207.

Rainer BM, Fischer AH, Luz Felipe da Silva D, Kang S, Chien AL. Rosacea is associated with chronic systemic diseases in a skin severity-dependent manner: results of a case-control study. J Am Acad Dermatol. 2015;73(4):604–8 PMID: 26256428.

Ramai D, Zakhia K, Ofosu A, Ofori E, Reddy M. Fecal microbiota transplantation: donor relation, fresh or frozen, delivery methods, cost-effectiveness. Ann Gastroenterol. 2019;32(1):30–8 PMID: 30598589.

Ricci G, Cipriani F, Cuello-Garcia CA, Brożek JL, Fiocchi A, Pawankar R, Yepes-Nuñes JJ, Terraciano L, Gandhi S, Agarwal A, Zhang Y, Schünemann HJ. A clinical reading on "world allergy organization-mcmaster university guidelines for allergic disease prevention (GLAD-P): probiotics." World Allergy Organ J. 2016;9:9 PMID: 26998191.

Ring HC, Thorsen J, Saunte DM, Lilje B, Bay L, Riis PT, Larsen N, Andersen LO, Nielsen HV, Miller IM, Bjarnsholt T, Fuursted K, Jemec GB. The follicular skin microbiome in patients with hidradenitis suppurativa and healthy controls. JAMA Dermatol. 2017;153(9):897–905 PMID: 28538949.

Riverain-Gillet É, Guet-Revillet H, Jais JP, Ungeheuer MN, Duchatelet S, Delage M, Lam T, Hovnanian A, Nassif A, Join-Lambert O. The surface microbiome of clinically unaffected skinfolds in hidradenitis suppurativa: a cross-sectional culture-based and 16S rRNA gene amplicon sequencing study in 60 patients. J Invest Dermatol. 2020;140(9):1847-1855.e6 PMID: 32339539.

Scher JU, Ubeda C, Artacho A, et al. Decreased bacterial diversity characterizes the altered gut microbiota in patients with psoriatic arthritis, resembling dysbiosis in inflammatory bowel disease. Arthritis Rheumatol. 2015;67(1):128–39 PMID: 25319745.

Schmid-Wendtner MH, Korting HC. The pH of the skin surface and its impact on the barrier function. Skin Pharmacol Physiol. 2006;19(6):296–302. https://doi.org/10.1159/000094670. PMID: 16864974.

Schneider AM, Cook LC, Zhan X, Banerjee K, Cong Z, Imamura-Kawasawa Y, Gettle SL, Longenecker AL, Kirby JS, Nelson AM. Loss of skin microbial diversity and alteration of bacterial metabolic function in hidradenitis suppurativa. J Invest Dermatol. 2020;140(3):716–20 PMID: 31465743.

Shaykhiev R, Bals R. Interactions between epithelial cells and leukocytes in immunity and tissue homeostasis. J Leukoc Biol. 2007;82(1):1–15 PMID: 17452476.

Shi B, Bangayan NJ, Curd E, Taylor PA, Gallo RL, Leung DYM, Li H. The skin microbiome is different in pediatric versus adult atopic dermatitis. J Allergy Clin Immunol. 2016;138(4):1233–6.

Smith RN, Mann NJ, Braue A, Mäkeläinen H, Varigos GA. A low-glycemic-load diet improves symptoms in acne vulgaris patients: a randomized controlled trial. Am J Clin Nutr. 2007;86(1):107–15. https://doi.org/10.1093/ajcn/86.1.107. PMID: 17616769.

Song H, Yoo Y, Hwang J, Na YC, Kim HS. Faecalibacterium prausnitzii subspecies-level dysbiosis in the human gut microbiome underlying atopic dermatitis. J Allergy Clin Immunol. 2016;137(3):852–60 PMID: 26431583.

Song Y, Dan K, Yao Z, Yang X, Chen B, Hao F. Altered gut microbiota in H1-antihistamine-resistant chronic spontaneous urticaria associates with systemic inflammation. Front Cell Infect Microbiol. 2022;12: 831489 PMID: 35372130.

Sonnenberg GF, Monticelli LA, Elloso MM, Fouser LA, Artis D. CD4(+) lymphoid tissue-inducer cells promote innate immunity in the gut. Immunity. 2011;34(1):122–34 PMID: 21194981.

Spits H, Cupedo T. Innate lymphoid cells: emerging insights in development, lineage relationships, and function. Annu Rev Immunol. 2012;30:647–75 PMID: 22224763.

Sun C, Chen L, Yang H, Sun H, Xie Z, Zhao B, Jiang X, Qin B, Shen Z. Involvement of gut microbiota in the development of psoriasis vulgaris. Front Nutr. 2021;22(8): 761978 PMID: 34881280.

Vanuytsel T, van Wanrooy S, Vanheel H, Vanormelingen C, Verschueren S, Houben E, Salim Rasoel S, Tóth J, Holvoet L, Farré R, Van Oudenhove L, Boeckxstaens G, Verbeke K, Tack J. Psychological stress and corticotropin-releasing hormone increase intestinal permeability in humans by a mast cell-dependent mechanism. Gut. 2014;63(8):1293–9 PMID: 24153250.

Vlachos C, Gaitanis G, Katsanos KH, Christodoulou DK, Tsianos E, Bassukas ID. Psoriasis and inflammatory bowel disease: links and risks. Psoriasis (Auckl). 2016;6:73–92 PMID: 29387596.

Watanabe K, Nishi E, Tashiro Y, Sakai K. Mode and structure of the bacterial community on human scalp hair. Microbes Environ. 2019;34(3):252–9 PMID: 31217363.

Weng X, Liu L, Barcellos LF, Allison JE, Herrinton LJ. Clustering of inflammatory bowel disease with immune mediated diseases among members of a northern california-managed care organization. Am J Gastroenterol. 2007;102(7):1429–35. https://doi.org/10.1111/j.1572-0241.2007.01215.x. PMID: 17437504.

Won EJ, Jang HH, Park H, Kim SJ. A potential predictive role of the scalp microbiome profiling in patients with alopecia areata: staphylococcus caprae, corynebacterium, and cutibacterium species. Microorganisms. 2022;10(5):864 PMID: 35630309.

Xiao S, Zhang G, Jiang C, Liu X, Wang X, et al. Deciphering gut microbiota dysbiosis and corresponding genetic and metabolic dysregulation in psoriasis patients using metagenomics sequencing. Front Cell Infect Microbiol. 2021;11: 605825 PMID: 33869074.

Yan HM, Zhao HJ, Guo DY, Zhu PQ, Zhang CL, Jiang W. Gut microbiota alterations in moderate to severe acne vulgaris patients. J Dermatol. 2018;45(10):1166–71 PMID: 30101990.

Yeh NL, Hsu CY, Tsai TF, Chiu HY. Gut microbiome in psoriasis is perturbed differently during secukinumab and ustekinumab therapy and associated with response to treatment. Clin Drug Investig. 2019;39(12):1195–203 PMID: 31549347.

You GE, Jung BJ, Kim HR, Kim HG, Kim TR, Chung DK. Lactobacillus sakei lipoteichoic acid inhibits MMP-1 induced by UVA in normal dermal fibroblasts of human. J Microbiol Biotechnol. 2013;23(10):1357–64 PMID: 23851272.

Zaidi AK, Spaunhurst K, Sprockett D, Thomason Y, Mann MW, Fu P, Ammons C, Gerstenblith M, Tuttle MS, Popkin DL. Characterization of the facial microbiome in twins discordant for rosacea. Exp Dermatol. 2018;27(3):295–8 PMID: 29283459.

Zhang X, Zhang J, Chu Z, Shi L, Geng S, Guo K. Gut microbiome alterations and functional prediction in chronic spontaneous urticaria patients. J Microbiol Biotechnol 2021;31(5):747–55. https://doi.org/10.4014/jmb.2012.12022. PMID: 33746191; PMCID: PMC9723274

Zhao Q, Yu J, Zhou H, Wang X, Zhang C, Hu J, Hu Y, Zheng H, Zeng F, Yue C, Gu L, Wang Z, Zhao F, Zhou P, Zhang H, Huang N, Wu W, Zhou Y, Li J. Intestinal dysbiosis exacerbates the pathogenesis of psoriasis-like phenotype through changes in fatty acid metabolism. Signal Transduct Target Ther. 2023;8(1):40 PMID: 36710269.

Chapter 12
Effect of Fibers on Microbiome, Health and Allergy

Antti Lauerma, Giulia Costanzo, and Stefano Del Giacco

Abstract Allergy, atopic diseases, and chronic inflammatory conditions like ulcerative colitis have significantly increased over the past 60 years. This rise has occurred alongside improvements in quality of life but also shifts in lifestyle and environmental factors. Many hypotheses have been proposed to explain this increase, including the hygiene hypothesis, the biodiversity hypothesis, and the epithelial barrier hypothesis. These theories suggest that inhabitants in modern, Westernized societies are exposed to declining environmental biodiversity, excess lifestyle chemicals and air pollution, antibiotics, and highly processed foods, as well as decreased dietary fiber intake. The absence of fiber prompts bacteria to target the topmost layer of the gut mucosal barrier, known as mucus, for sustenance, contrary to their typical reliance on fiber. Various factors, including short-chain fatty acids, play a role in this process. The lack of fiber and dysfunction of the mucous barrier, often termed "leaky gut", have profound impications for overall human health and well-being.

Keywords Microbiome · Microbiota · Fiber · Starch · Diet · Health · Allergy · Gut · Skin · Short-chain fatty acid · Butyrate · Propionate · Acetate

12.1 Introduction

Over the past 70 years there has been a significant shift in the lifestyles of human populations worldwide. Initially, improvements in living standards were observed primarily in Western countries, followed by similar trends in emerging nations with large populations. This rise in living standards has had a profound impact on morbidity and mortality rates, with many serious diseases now being treatable or preventable. However, alongside this progress, there has been a notable increase

A. Lauerma (✉)
Department of Dermatology, University of Helsinki, Helsinki, Finland
e-mail: antti.lauerma@helsinki.fi

G. Costanzo · S. Del Giacco
Department of Medical Sciences and Public Health, University of Cagliari, University Hospital, uilio Casula", Cagliari, Sardinia, Italy

© The Author(s), under exclusive license to Springer Nature Switzerland AG 2025
A. Lauerma et al. (eds.), *The Skin Microbiome Manual*,
https://doi.org/10.1007/978-3-031-82689-4_12

in chronic inflammatory disorders, such as ulcerative colitis, multiple sclerosis, diabetes, allergies and atopic diseases.

The reasons behind this increase have been the subject of intense debate and study, ranging from factors such as air pollution and the hygiene hypothesis to nutrition and environmental pollutants (Haahtela et al. 2023). Given the significant impact of these diseases on the lives of a large portion of the global population, billions of people are exposed to these conditions or at risk for developing them. The objective of this chapter is to examine the rise in allergies and skin diseases, with a focus on the microbiome as a potential mediator, and to explore the possible causes underlying this trend.

12.2 Atopic March

The term "atopic march" describes a series of diseases related to atopy and allergy that span from pregnancy and birth through childhood to adulthood. Atopic diseases first manifest as food allergies in breastfed or young children under one year of age, often presenting as atopic dermatitis-like flares. These symptoms usually subside by the age of two as the gastrointestinal tract matures and tolerance to foods develops.

During childhood, many of these children also develop asthma, and later on, allergic rhinoconjunctivitis may emerge. While atopic dermatitis is usually mild during school years, it often worsens during puberty. Rhinoconjunctivitis occurs due to IgE responses to pollens or animals, which can subsequently lead to secondary cross-reactions to vegetables and other plant foods. Anaphylactic reactions may occur during early childhood and later due to cross-reactions from pollens. Primary sensitizations to foods like peanuts and Hymenoptera are the most common causes of anaphylaxis (Kortekaas Krohn et al. 2023).

Despite the apparent chronological appearance of atopic and allergic diseases, there is no consistent cause-and-effect between these disorders. However, one study found that aggressive treatment of atopic dermatitis with calcineurin inhibitors reduced bronchial hyperreactivity (Virtanen et al. 2007). The prevailing viewpoint suggests that maintaining healthy skin to prevent percutaneous sensitization, preserving a normal skin microbiome, and adhering to a diverse diet with early controlled introduction to allergenic foods may be beneficial (Brough et al. 2022).

While there is a significant co-occurrence between asthma, atopic dermatitis, rhinoconjunctivitis, anaphylaxis, and specific IgE-mediated allergies, many patients experience only some of these diseases, not all. Genetics likely play a role (Holloway et al. 2010), but this explanation is complicated by the fact that atopic and allergic diseases have greatly increased over one to two generations, suggesting that Mendelian selection alone cannot account for the rise.

12.3 Allergy Epidemics

Allergic diseases now affect approximately 30% of the global population, indicating an epidemic. While initially affecting Western populations, today, low- and middle-income countries experience the most significant growth trends. Despite advances in research, the burden of allergies continues to increase in both prevalence and severity (Pawankar et al. 2012). The rapid rise in allergy disorders suggests environmental or lifestyle changes rather than genetic modifications. Increased exposure to allergens, such as house dust mites, does not fully account for the increase, as some allergens may actually prevent allergy development (such as early-life exposure to home pets, especially dogs) (Indolfi et al. 2023). The lack of an identifiable cause has prompted the search for other factors to explain the growing prevalence and evolving phenotypes of allergy diseases among genetically predisposed individuals.

The first theory was the Hygiene Hypothesis. David P. Strachan, an epidemiologist, proposed the hygiene hypothesis in 1989, while reporting an inverse link between family size and allergy illness development. Research suggests that decreasing infection rates in early childhood may contribute to an increase in allergy disorders. The hypothesis has expanded to suggest that decreased microbial exposure significantly contributes to the rise in allergy disorders (Strachan 1989; Rachid et al. 2021). Clean food, water, sanitation, antibiotic use, birth delivery procedures, and geographical migration all impact microbial exposure. The hygiene hypothesis is supported by research on the Amish and Hutterites in the United States, of which the latter have higher allergy prevalence. The Hutterites use sophisticated farming equipment. Bacteria activate pattern recognition receptors on innate immune cells, directing adaptive immunity toward pathogen-protective TH cells and regulatory T cells. Dust samples from the Amish population have greater endotoxin levels and protect mice from allergies. Individuals with allergies have a less diversified gut commensal flora, which may not train the immune system to become tolerant of foreign allergens (Stein et al. 2016).

The hygiene theory has drawbacks since it focuses on cleanliness rather than host-microbe interactions, which are believed to contribute to allergy development. There is minimal evidence that cleaning the local or personal environment helps against allergies. Improved cleanliness over the last half-century has been linked to increased allergy disorders and other chronic immunologic diseases (not just Th2 diseases but also Th1, Th17, and/or Th23). (Bloomfield et al. 2016).

Climate change refers to human-induced global warming and its effects on weather patterns. Expanding populations necessitate increased energy consumption to meet food and energy demands. Climate change has significant impact on human health, leading to the deaths of millions each year from cardiovascular, infectious, and mental health illnesses. Climate change can contribute to allergy disorders through various pathways. Global warming alters pollination, affecting factors like seasonality and distribution, and extreme weather events such as flooding, wildfires, thunderstorms and dust storms, all of which exacerbate asthma. Additionally, climate change is associated with the increased growth of allergenic microorganisms, such as mold, and altered spread of allergies. It may also influence housing patterns, leading to factors like crowding, increased time spent indoors, and urbanization, all of which can impact allergy prevalence. Furthermore, climate change contributes to increased air pollution. Overall, climate change is a significant driver of the allergy epidemic, resulting in high global incidence rates and substantial healthcare costs (exceeding $100 billion annually).

12.4 Air Pollution

Air pollution consists of particles and gases released into the atmosphere or generated by chemical or photochemical reactions, including tropospheric or ground-level ozone (O3). Climate change affects local weather and meteorological variables such as temperature, precipitation, and wind patterns, which in turn influence the dispersion of air pollution. Climate-driven changes, such as wildfires, storms, and increasing electricity demand, contribute to air pollution from both biological and anthropogenic sources, perpetuating a cycle of pollution and poor air quality (US Environmental Protection Agency 2021) (US Environmental Protection Agency. Global Greenhouse Emissions 2014).

Air pollution, especially O3 and PM2.5, significantly impact human health, with 90% of the world's population residing in environments with substandard air quality. Approximately 40% of the population in the United States lives in such areas. PM2.5 causes 4.2 million premature deaths annually, with 92% occurring in low- and middle-income nations. The most severe health conditions attributed to air pollution include COPD, lung cancer, and cardiovascular events, with COPD being the leading cause of death (Landrigan et al. 2018; World Health Organization. Air pollution 2021; Cohen et al. 2015).

Air pollution has been associated with TH2 spectrum of diseases such as asthma, atopic dermatitis, and food allergies. It is strongly correlated with the development, exacerbations, and mortality of asthma (Liu et al. 2019; Stefanovic et al. 2021). Air pollutants like volatile organic compounds, particulate matter, traffic pollution, and tobacco smoke can impair the epidermal barrier by generating reactive oxygen species and altering the immune system through epigenetic mechanisms. These processes predispose children to developing atopic dermatitis, thereby increasing the risk of future allergy diseases through the atopic march (Paller et al. 2019). Air pollution triggers an oxidative stress response, leading to epigenetic modifications that regulate gene expression in immune cells, including FOXP3 and other immunoregulatory genes. Increased FOXP3 methylation resulting from air pollution exposure has been linked to an elevated risk and severity of asthma. This interplay between air pollution and climate change forms a feedback loop that contributes to the escalation in the incidence and prevalence of atopic diseases (Prunicki et al. 2021, Nadeau et al. 2010, Gruzieva et al. 2017, Brunst et al. 2013).

12.5 Loss of Biodiversity

Dietary changes, increasing water supply, antibiotic overprescription, obesity, infant formula feeding, and caesarean section births are all likely to have contributed to a rise in allergy disorders over the last 70 years. These alterations have had a significant impact on our commensal microbiomes and may be contributing to the increase in allergy disorders. Changes in the lifestyle of Western civilizations have led to a concerning increase in the frequency and severity of food allergies. Epidemiological research confirms a link between alterations in gut microbial communities and childhood food allergies (Thompson-Chagoyan et al. 2011; Ling et al. 2014; Azad et al. 2015).

Researchers have identified a microbiome signature that distinguishes patients with cow milk's allergy from healthy populations in human fecal donors and colonized mice. They found that a Clostridial species, Anaerostipes caccae, mimics the benefits of a healthy microbiota, indicating that bacteria and their byproducts play a protective role against food allergies (FA). In recent years, there has been a decline in fiber consumption, which has been linked to reduced microbial diversity in mouse models. Certain Clostridia species metabolize dietary fiber to short-chain fatty acids, promoting the differentiation of regulatory T cells (Tregs) and immunological tolerance. These short-chain fatty acids also stimulate the release of IL-22, which enhances gut barrier integrity. Dietary fiber may therefore help maintain a diversified microbiota composition, optimal epithelial barrier function, and immunological tolerance (Chinthrajah et al. 2016).

12.6 Change in Diet Towards "Western" Food During Allergy Epidemics

The diet worldwide has undergone changes during the allergy epidemic. So-called western diets have been introduced to other countries as well. However, the term "Western diet" is not clearly defined, and many studies have either been difficult to conduct or they are purely observational. A focused review published in 2015 assessed all available literature on the matter from 1980 to 2014. In this review, 10 studies from North America, Europe and Asia were identified, involving samples sizes ranging from 153 to 70,000 individuals. These studies did not find evidence supporting a link between the Western diet and an increase in asthma, a major atopic disease.

A recent study from Singapore and Malaysia studied the effect of fast foods, such as burgers, in a prospective study of 11,494 individuals with Chinese ethnicity. The study used an index of glycemic properties of the food the studied individuals ate. The study showed that eating foods with high glycemic index results in greater risk for atopic dermatitis, when compared to individuals eating foods with medium or low glycemic index (Lim et al. 2024).

12.7 Food Processing

Ultra-processed foods and food additives have become more common in recent decades. There is increasing evidence that they contribute to epidemics of gastrointestinal diseases, including irritable bowel syndrome, inflammatory bowel disease and colorectal cancer. The rise in these diseases has parallelled the allergy epidemics, and there is evidence that autoimmune and allergy epidemics have similar underlying factors (Zysk et al. 2024).

A normal gut possesses a healthy microbiome, a protective mucus layer, and an intact epithelium. Emulsifiers increase the levels of proinflammatory bacteria, reduce microbiome diversity, decrease mucus production, and inflames epithelial cells. On the other hand, artificial sweeteners decrease microbial diversity, reduce levels of the anti-inflammatory compound butyrate, and inflame epithelial cells, although they do not affect mucus production. Food colors may directly induce systemic inflammation by compromising the gut barrier. Nanoparticles reduce bacterial diversity in the gut microbiome and activate innate immunity in the epithelium via the NLRP3 inflammasome (Whelan et al. 2024).

12.8 Dietary Fiber

Dietary fiber has garnered interest in recent years, leading to several studies assessing its role in immune health. Increased fiber intake from plant-derived foods has been shown to improve gastrointestinal, cardiovascular, and metabolic health. Recommendations for fiber intake typically range from 25 to 38 g per day. A recent review evaluataed the effect of fiber on human atopic diseases (Venter et al. 2022). Seven studies on asthma demonstrated some beneficial effects, but results were heterogenous. In one study on allergic rhinitis, Iranian barley-based traditional medicine had a similar effect to antihistamine. However, in one study on urticaria, no effect was observed, and in another study in atopic dermatitis, maternal fiber intake increased the risk of atopic dermatitis in children. No clinical studies are available on food allergy (Venter et al. 2022).

Inulin, a fiber rich in, for example, artichokes, was studied in a murine model of psoriasis like dermatitis. An inulin-enriched high-fiber diet reduced dermatitis symptoms while also decreasing the production of proinflammatory cytokines such as IL-17A. Inulin increased the amount of Bacteroides in the gut, along with both serum and fecal concentrations of the short-chain fatty acid (SCFA) propionate. Administration of propionate itself yielded similar results (Yoshida et al. 2023). Other fibers that have been more intensively studied include resistant starch, fructo-oligosaccharides, galacto-oligosaccharides, polydextrose, maltodextrin, and arabinoxylan (Graf et al. 2015).

12.9   Gut Microbiome and Metabolome

In the human gut, millions of bacteria contribute to the gut microbiome, with its composition being highly individual. Diet is a significant factor influencing the content of gut and its associated disorders. The diversity of the microbiome was only revealed after the emergence of next-generation metagenomics (Grice et al. 2009). Key aspects of diet and its relationship to the microbiome include vegetarian diets, Western diets, whole grain products, fruits and nuts, as well as vegetables and legumes (Graf et al. 2015). The gut microbiome also impacts skin health and various skin disorders, including psoriasis, atopic dermatitis, acne vulgaris, rosacea, alopecia areata, and hidradenitis suppurativa (Mahmud et al. 2022). Of recent interest in gut-skin-axis is the role of microRNAs in mediating the effects of gut microbiome on the skin in atopic dermatitis (Pessoa et al. 2023).

12.10   Short Chain Fatty Acids (SCFAs)

The metabolism of fibers results in short-chain fatty acids (SCFAs) including butyrate, propionate and acetate. In a study on a contact hypersensitivity mouse model, it was demonstrated intradermal injection or topical application of butyrate reduced the intensity of skin inflammation (Schwarz et al. 2017). A similar outcome was observed in a psoriasis mouse model with topical butyrate treatment (Schwartz et al. 2021). Psoriasis is a complex disease, and recent advances suggest the potential of dietary interventions in managing this chronic inflammatory skin condition (Komine 2020). Additionally, butyrate inhibits *Staphylococcus aureus*-aggravated atopic dermatitis and IL-33 activation in an atopic dermatitis mouse model (Luo et al. 2023).

SCFAs, metabolic products of fiber degradation in the gut, have also been been suggested to play a role in reducing food allergy. Additionally, SCFAs have been associated with non-atopic diseases such as type I diabetes, multiple sclerosis, rheumatoid arthritis and lupus. They exert broad effects on lymphocyte development, tissue barriers, host metabolism, immunity and inflammation. Decreased SCFAs may lead to dysbiosis and a leaky gut (Kim 2023). In a recent systematic review, 37 studies on SCFAs and allergic diseases were identified. Some evidence suggests that acetate, butyrate, and propionate may have a beneficial effect in early childhood atopic dermatitis, asthma, and food allergy. However, the field is evolving rapidly, and new studies are needed to fully understand the role of SCFAs in allergic diseases (Sasaki et al. 2024).

12.11   Mucous Barrier in Gut

Fiber serves as a vital source of nutrition for numerous gut microbes. Intermittent fasting leads to the enrichment of bacteria capable of utilizing the top layer of gut epithelium mucus as an alternative food source. The absence of fiber consequently leads to the degradation of gut mucus, resulting in a leaky gut and increased susceptibility to pathogens, including lethal colitis from *Citrobacter rodentium* (Desai et al. 2016). Changes in the environment, including diet, as well as the loss of biodiversity, air pollution, and other factors, may collectively disrupt epithelia in the skin, gut, and respiratory tract (Celebi Sozener et al. 2022).

Recently, a mouse study assessed the effect of fiber and the microbiome on food allergy. A lack of dietary fiber increases the amount of mucin-degrading *Akkermansia municiphila* in the gut. This increase in bacteria enhances the expression of type 1 and 2 cytokines, as well as IgE-coated commensals in the colon, leading to a loss of tolerance to food allergens such as ovalbumin and peanuts (Parrish et al. 2023). There is growing evidence suggesting that SCFAs may not be the sole link between fiber-poor diet and disease. It is possible that fiber-poor diet alters bacterial B vitamin synthesis, resulting in a net decrease in locally produced B vitamin content, which subsequently triggers immune activation. The fiber component inulin may restore the availability of microbially produced B vitamins and thereby restore immune homeostasis (Parrish et al. 2022a, 2022b).

12.12   Topical Fiber Materials and Their Effect on Skin Microbiome

The skin, the body's primary interface with the environment, harbors millions of bacteria collectively known as the skin microbiota. Healthy skin relies on the balance of microorganisms, including bacteria, fungi, and viruses. Dysbiosis occurs when this equilibrium is disrupted, leading to changes in skin microbial communities and, in many cases, dermatological diseases due to competition among pathogens for resources. (Byrd et al. 2018; Boxberger et al. 2021). The skin microbiota varies and can be influenced by factors such as age, gender, body region, health conditions, genetics, hygiene practices, cosmetics, and medications. While serving as a barrier against infection, external factors like temperature, humidity, UV radiation, climate, and geographical location can also impact its composition. Textile fibers have been found to affect the composition and diversity of the skin microbiota. (Messager et al. 2004; Teufel et al. 2010). Certain fibers may create a more favorable environment for the growth of specific bacteria or fungi, while others may inhibit microbial growth.

The intimate contact between textile materials and skin encourages germs to spread, resulting in biological degradation, strength loss, discoloration, and an unpleasant odor. Clothing materials can also disseminate these bacteria, potentially resulting in cross-infection, disease transmission, allergic reactions, and odor in people. To solve these concerns, the textile industry focuses on discovering novel bioactive compounds with antibacterial capabilities, which can help prevent these problems. (Zostak-Kotowa 2004; Van Herreweghen et al. 2020; Gulati et al. 2022). On the other hand, in the case of skin dysbiosis, the choice of certain kinds of textile fibers could act as a modulation of the skin microbiota, and it could help mitigate the symptoms of some dermatological conditions (Hofer 2018).

The relationship between textile fibers and the skin microbiota is complex and multifaceted, with implications for both textile design and skin health. Research indicates that natural fibers such as cotton and wool tend to interact more positively with the skin microbiota compared to synthetic fibers like polyester. Natural fibers often exhibit superior moisture absorption and breathability properties, fostering a more balanced environment for the skin microbiota. Some textiles undergo antimicrobial treatment during manufacturing to curb microbial growth and odors. However, these treatments can disrupt the natural balance of skin microbiota, potentially leading to skin irritation or other issues.

Efforts are underway to develop "probiotic textiles" designed to promote the growth of beneficial bacteria on the skin. These textiles may incorporate probiotics or prebiotics to support a healthy skin microbiome. Imbalances in the skin microbiota have been associated with various skin conditions such as acne, eczema, and psoriasis. Understanding the interaction between textiles and the skin microbiota could pave the way for the development of textiles that help manage or prevent these conditions. With advancements in microbiome research, there is potential for personalized textiles tailored to an individual's unique skin microbiota. These textiles could aid in maintaining a healthy skin environment and preventing skin disorders.

Ongoing research seeks to further elucidate these interactions and develop innovative textile solutions that promote skin health (Suellen et al. 2023).

12.13 Conclusions

The ongoing advancements in disease models and research techniques have underscored the significance of dietary fiber in human health. Future human studies are necessary to fully assess its importance, which may initially prompts improvements in dietary guidelines. Furthermore, topical fibers play a distinct role in maintaining the skin microbiome. In the years ahead, we will determine whether the potential of fiber holds true in real-life scenarios for preventing and treating chronic diseases such as asthma, allergies, and other inflammatory disorders.

References

Azad MB, Konya T, Guttman DS, Field CJ, Sears MR, HayGlass KT, Mandhane PJ, Turvey SE, Subbarao P, Becker AB, Scott JA, Kozyrskyj AL. CHILD Study Investigators. Infant gut microbiota and food sensitization: associations in the first year of life. Clin Exp Allergy. 2015;45(3):632–43. https://doi.org/10.1111/cea.12487 PMID: 25599982.

Boxberger M, Cenizo V, Cassir N, La Scola B. Challenges in exploring and manipulating the human skin microbiome. Microbiome. 2021;9(1):125. https://doi.org/10.1186/s40168-021-01062-5. PMID:34053468;PMCID:PMC8166136.

Brough HA, Lanser BJ, Sindher SB, Teng JMC, Leung DYM, Venter C, Chan SM, Santos AF, Bahnson HT, Guttman-Yassky E, Gupta RS, Lack G, Ciaccio CE, Sampath V, Nadeau KC, Nagler CR. Early intervention and prevention of allergic diseases. Allergy. 2022;77(2):416–41.

Brunst KJ, Leung YK, Ryan PH, Khurana Hershey GK, Levin L, Ji H, Lemasters GK, Ho SM. Forkhead box protein 3 (FOXP3) hypermethylation is associated with diesel exhaust exposure and risk for childhood asthma. J Allergy Clin Immunol. 2013;131(2):592–4.e1-3. https://doi. org/10.1016/j.jaci.2012.10.042. Epub 2012 Dec 20. PMID: 23260754; PMCID: PMC3563724.

Byrd AL, Belkaid Y, Segre JA. The human skin microbiome. Nat Rev Microbiol. 2018;16(3):143–155. https://doi.org/10.1038/nrmicro.2017.157. Epub 2018. PMID: 29332945.C.

Celebi Sozener Z, Ozdel Ozturk B, Cerci P, Turk M, Gorgulu Akin B, Akdis M, Altiner S, Ozbey U, Ogulur I, Mitamura Y, Yilmaz I, Nadeau K, Ozdemir C, Mungan D, Akdis CA. Epithelial barrier hypothesis: effect of the external exposome on the microbiome and epithelial barriers in allergic disease. Allergy. 2022;77(5):1418–49.

Chinthrajah RS, Hernandez JD, Boyd SD, Galli SJ, Nadeau KC. Molecular and cellular mechanisms of food allergy and food tolerance. J Allergy Clin Immunol. 2016;137(4):984–97. https://doi. org/10.1016/j.jaci.2016.02.004.PMID:27059726;PMCID:PMC5030841.

Cohen AJ, Brauer M, Burnett R, Anderson HR, Frostad J, Estep K, Balakrishnan K, Brunekreef B, Dandona L, Dandona R, Feigin V, Freedman G, Hubbell B, Jobling A, Kan H, Knibbs L, Liu Y, Martin R, Morawska L, Pope CA 3rd, Shin H, Straif K, Shaddick G, Thomas M, van Dingenen R, van Donkelaar A, Vos T, Murray CJL, Forouzanfar MH. Estimates and 25-year trends of the global burden of disease attributable to ambient air pollution: an analysis of data from the Global Burden of Diseases Study 2015. Lancet. 2017 May 13;389(10082):1907–1918. https://doi.org/10.1016/S0140-6736(17)30505-6. Epub 2017 Apr 10. Erratum in: Lancet. 2017 Jun 17;389(10087):e15. Erratum in: Lancet. 2018 Apr 21;391(10130):1576. PMID: 28408086; PMCID: PMC5439030.

Desai MS, Seekatz AM, Koropatkin NM, Kamada N, Hickey CA, Wolter M, Pudlo NA, Kitamoto S, Terrapon N, Muller A, Young VB, Henrissat B, Wilmes P, Stappenbeck TS, Núñez G, Martens EC. A Dietary fiber-deprived gut microbiota degrades the colonic mucus barrier and enhances pathogen susceptibility. Cell. 2016;167(5):1339-1353.e21.

Graf D, Di Cagno R, Fåk F, Flint HJ, Nyman M, Saarela M, Watzl B. Contribution of diet to the composition of the human gut microbiota. Microb Ecol Health Dis. 2015;4(26):26164.

Grice EA, Kong HH, Conlan S, Deming CB, Davis J, Young AC, Bouffard GG, Blakesley RW, Murray PR, Green ED, Turner ML, Segre JA. Topographical and temporal diversity of the human skin microbiome. Science. 2009 May 29;324(5931):1190–2

Gruzieva O, Xu CJ, Breton CV, Annesi-Maesano I, Antó JM, Auffray C, Ballereau S, Bellander T, Bousquet J, Bustamante M, Charles MA, de Kluizenaar Y, den Dekker HT, Duijts L, Felix JF, Gehring U, Guxens M, Jaddoe VV, Jankipersadsing SA, Merid SK, Kere J, Kumar A, Lemonnier N, Lepeule J, Nystad W, Page CM, Panasevich S, Postma D, Slama R, Sunyer J, Söderhäll C, Yao J, London SJ, Pershagen G, Koppelman GH, Melén E. Epigenome-wide meta-analysis of methylation in children related to prenatal NO2 air pollution exposure. Environ Health Perspect. 2017;125(1):104–110. https://doi.org/10.1289/EHP36. Epub 2016 Jul 22. PMID: 27448387; PMCID: PMC5226705.

Gulati R, Sharma S, Sharma RK. Antimicrobial textile: recent developments and functional perspective. Polym Bull. 2022;79(8):5747–71.

Haahtela T, Alenius H, Auvinen P, Fyhrquist N, von Hertzen L, Jousilahti P, Karisola P, Laatikainen T, Lehtimäki J, Paalanen L, Ruokolainen L, Saarinen K, Valovirta E, Vasankari T, Vlasoff T, Erhola M, Bousquet J, Vartiainen E, Mäkelä MJ. A short history from Karelia study to biodiversity and public health interventions. Front Allergy. 2023;14(4):1152927.

Hofer D. A real-life based evaluation of the effectiveness of antibacterial fabrics in treating atopic dermatitis. Dermatol Res Pract. 2018;2018:7043438.

Holloway JW, Yang IA, Holgate ST. Genetics of allergic disease. J Allergy Clin Immunol. 2010;125(2 Suppl 2):S81-94.

Indolfi C, D'Addio E, Bencivenga CL, Rivetti G, Bettini I, Licari A, Manti S, Mori F, Miraglia del Giudice M, Klain A. The primary prevention of atopy: does early exposure to cats and dogs prevent the development of allergy and asthma in children? a comprehensive analysis of the literature. Life. 2023;13(9):1859. https://doi.org/10.3390/life13091859

Kim CH. Complex regulatory effects of gut microbial short-chain fatty acids on immune tolerance and autoimmunity. Cell Mol Immunol. 2023;20(4):341–50.

Komine M. Recent advances in psoriasis research; the clue to mysterious relation to gut microbiome. Int J Mol Sci. 2020;21(7):2582.

Kortekaas Krohn I, Badloe FMS, Herrmann N, Maintz L, De Vriese S, Ring J, Bieber T, Gutermuth J. Immunoglobulin E autoantibodies in atopic dermatitis associate with Type-2 comorbidities and the atopic march. Allergy. 2023;78(12):3178–92.

Landrigan PJ, Fuller R, Acosta NJR, Adeyi O, Arnold R, Basu NN, Baldé AB, Bertollini R, Bose-O'Reilly S, Boufford JI, Breysse PN, Chiles T, Mahidol C, Coll-Seck AM, Cropper ML, Fobil J, Fuster V, Greenstone M, Haines A, Hanrahan D, Hunter D, Khare M, Krupnick A, Lanphear B, Lohani B, Martin K, Mathiasen KV, McTeer MA, Murray CJL, Ndahimananjara JD, Perera F, Potočnik J, Preker AS, Ramesh J, Rockström J, Salinas C, Samson LD, Sandilya K, Sly PD, Smith KR, Steiner A, Stewart RB, Suk WA, van Schayck OCP, Yadama GN, Yumkella K, Zhong M. The lancet commission on pollution and health. lancet. 2018;391(10119):462–512. https://doi.org/10.1016/S0140-6736(17)32345-0. Epub 2017 Oct 19. Erratum in: Lancet. 2018;391(10119):430. PMID: 29056410.

Lim JJ, Lim YYE, Ng JY, Malipeddi P, Ng YT, Teo WY, Wong QYA, Matta SA, Sio YY, Wong YR, Teh KF, Rawanan Shah SM, Reginald K, Say YH, Liu MH, Chew FT. Burgers, fast foods, and increased associated risk for atopic dermatitis: a cross-sectional study of dietary habits among young Chinese adults in Singapore/Malaysia. Dermatology. 2024;240(1):77–84.

Ling Z, Li Z, Liu X, Cheng Y, Luo Y, Tong X, Yuan L, Wang Y, Sun J, Li L, Xiang C. Altered fecal microbiota composition associated with food allergy in infants. Appl Environ Microbiol. 2014;80(8):2546–54. https://doi.org/10.1128/AEM.00003-14. Epub 2014 Feb 14. PMID: 24532064; PMCID: PMC3993190.

Liu Y, Xu J, Chen D, et al. The association between air pollution and preterm birth and low birth weight in Guangdong China. BMC Public Health. 2019;19:3. https://doi.org/10.1186/s12889-018-6307-7.

Luo CH, Lai AC, Chang YJ. Butyrate inhibits Staphylococcus aureus-aggravated dermal IL-33 expression and skin inflammation through histone deacetylase inhibition. Front Immunol. 2023;16(14):1114699.

Mahmud MR, Akter S, Tamanna SK, Mazumder L, Esti IZ, Banerjee S, Akter S, Hasan MR, Acharjee M, Hossain MS, Pirttilä AM. Impact of gut microbiome on skin health: gut-skin axis observed through the lenses of therapeutics and skin diseases. Gut Microbes. 2022;14(1):2096995.

Messager S, Hann AC, Goddard PA, Dettmar PW, Maillard JY. Use of the 'ex vivo' test to study long-term bacterial survival on human skin and their sensitivity to antisepsis. J Appl Microbiol. 2004;97(6):1149–60.

Nadeau K, McDonald-Hyman C, Noth EM, Pratt B, Hammond SK, Balmes J, Tager I. Ambient air pollution impairs regulatory T-cell function in asthma. J Allergy Clin Immunol. 2010;126(4):845-852.e10. https://doi.org/10.1016/j.jaci.2010.08.008. PMID: 20920773.

Paller AS, Kong HH, Seed P, Naik S, Scharschmidt TC, Gallo RL, Luger T, Irvine AD. The microbiome in patients with atopic dermatitis. J Allergy Clin Immunol. 2019 Jan;143(1):26–35. https://doi.org/10.1016/j.jaci.2018.11.015. Epub 2018 Nov 23. Erratum in: J Allergy Clin Immunol. 2019;143(4):1660. PMID: 30476499; PMCID: PMC7163929.

Parrish A, Boudaud M, Kuehn A, Ollert M, Desai MS. Intestinal mucus barrier: a missing piece of the puzzle in food allergy. Trends Mol Med. 2022a;28(1):36–50.

Parrish A, Boudaud M, Grant ET, Willieme S, Neumann M, Wolter M, Craig SZ, De Sciscio A, Cosma A, Hunewald O, Ollert M, Desai MS. Akkermansia muciniphila exacerbates food allergy in fibre-deprived mice. Nat Microbiol. 2023;8(10):1863–79.

Parrish A, Grant E, Boudaud M, Hunewald O, Hirayama A, Ollert M, Fukuda S, Mahesh D. Dietary fibers boost gut microbiota-prodyced B vitamin pool an alter host immune landscape. Research Square, preprint 2022b. https://doi.org/10.21203/rs.3.rs-1563674/v1

Pawankar R, Canonica GW, Holgate ST, Lockey RF. Allergic diseases and asthma: a major global health concern. Curr Opin Allergy Clin Immunol. 2012;12(1):39–41.

Pessôa R, Clissa PB, Sanabani SS. The interaction between the host genome, epigenome, and the gut-skin axis microbiome in atopic dermatitis. Int J Mol Sci. 2023;24(18):14322.

Prunicki M, Cauwenberghs N, Lee J, et al. Air pollution exposure is linked with methylation of immunoregulatory genes, altered immune cell profiles, and increased blood pressure in children. Sci Rep. 2021;11:4067. https://doi.org/10.1038/s41598-021-83577-3.

Rachid R, Stephen-Victor E, Chatila TA. The microbial origins of food allergy. J Allergy Clin Immunol. 2021;147(3):808–13.

Sasaki M, Suaini NHA, Afghani J, Heye KN, O'Mahony L, Venter C, Lauener R, Frei R, Roduit C. Systematic review of the association between short chain fatty acids and allergic diseases. Allergy. 2024. https://doi.org/10.1111/all.16065.

Schwarz A, Bruhs A, Schwarz T. The short-chain fatty acid sodium butyrate functions as a regulator of the skin immune system. J Invest Dermatol. 2017;137(4):855–64.

Schwarz A, Philippsen R, Schwarz T. Induction of regulatory T cells and correction of cytokine disbalance by short-chain fatty acids: implications for psoriasis therapy. J Investig Derm. 2021;141(1):95–104. ISSN 0964-8305. https://doi.org/10.1016/S0964-8305(03)00090-8.rmatol.

Stefanovic N, Irvine AD, Flohr C. The role of the environment and exposome in atopic dermatitis. Curr Treat Options Allergy. 2021;8(3):222–241. https://doi.org/10.1007/s40521-021-00289-9. Epub 2021. PMID: 34055570; PMCID: PMC8139547.

Stein MM, Hrusch CL, Gozdz J, Igartua C, Pivniouk V, Murray SE, Ledford JG, Marques Dos Santos M, Anderson RL, Metwali N, Neilson JW, Maier RM, Gilbert JA, Holbreich M, Thorne PS, Martinez FD, von Mutius E, Vercelli D, Ober C, Sperling AI. Innate immunity and asthma risk in amish and hutterite farm children. N Engl J Med. 2016;375(5):411–21. https://doi.org/10.1056/NEJMoa1508749. PMID: 27518660; PMCID: PMC5137793.

Strachan DP. Hay fever, hygiene, and household size. BMJ. 1989;299(6710):1259–60. https://doi.org/10.1136/bmj.299.6710.1259.PMID:2513902;PMCID:PMC1838109.

Suellen Ferro de Oliveira C, Kekhasharú Tavaria F. The impact of bioactive textiles on human skin microbiota. Eur J Pharm Biopharm. 2023;188:66–77. https://doi.org/10.1016/j.ejpb.2023.05.004. Epub 2023. PMID: 37182552.

Szostak-Kotowa J. Biodeterioration of textiles. Int Biodeterior Biodegrad. 2004;53(3):165–170. ISSN 0964-8305. https://doi.org/10.1016/S0964-8305(03)00090-8

Teufel L, Pipal A, Schuster KC, Staudinger T, Redl B. Material-dependent growth of human skin bacteria on textiles investigated using challenge tests and DNA genotyping. J Appl Microbiol. 2010;108(2):450–61. https://doi.org/10.1111/j.1365-2672.2009.04434.x. Epub 2009 Jun 25 PMID: 19645767.

Thompson-Chagoyan OC, Fallani M, Maldonado J, Vieites JM, Khanna S, Edwards C, Doré J, Gil A. Faecal microbiota and short-chain fatty acid levels in faeces from infants with cow's milk protein allergy. Int Arch Allergy Immunol. 2011;156(3):325–32. https://doi.org/10.1159/000 323893. Epub 2011 Jun 29 PMID: 21720179.

US Environmental Protection Agency. Global Greenhouse Emissions 2014

US Environmental Protection Agency 2021

Van Herreweghen F, Amberg C, Marques R, Callewaert C. Biological and chemical processes that lead to textile malodour development. Microorganisms. 2020;8(11):1709. https://doi.org/10.3390/microorganisms8111709.

Venter C, Meyer RW, Greenhawt M, Pali-Schöll I, Nwaru B, Roduit C, Untersmayr E, Adel-Patient K, Agache I, Agostoni C, Akdis CA, Feeney M, Hoffmann-Sommergruber K, Lunjani N, Grimshaw K, Reese I, Smith PK, Sokolowska M, Vassilopoulou E, Vlieg-Boerstra B, Amara S, Walter J, O'Mahony L. Role of dietary fiber in promoting immune health-An EAACI position paper. Allergy. 2022;77(11):3185–98.

Virtanen H, Remitz A, Malmberg P, Rytilä P, Metso T, Haahtela T, Reitamo S. Topical tacrolimus in the treatment of atopic dermatitis–does it benefit the airways? A 4-year open follow-up. J Allergy Clin Immunol. 2007;120(6):1464–6.

Whelan K, Bancil AS, Lindsay JO, Chassaing B. Ultra-processed foods and food additives in gut health and disease. Nat Rev Gastroenterol Hepatol. 2024. https://doi.org/10.1038/s41575-024-00893-5.

World Health Organization. Air pollution. 2021

Yoshida M, Funasaka Y, Saeki H, Yamamoto M, Kanda N. Dietary fiber inulin improves murine imiquimod-induced psoriasis-like dermatitis. Int J Mol Sci. 2023;24(18):14197.

Zysk W, Mesjasz A, Trzeciak M, Horvath A, Plata-Nazar K. Gastrointestinal comorbidities associated with atopic dermatitis-a narrative review. Int J Mol Sci. 2024;25(2):1194.

Chapter 13
Oral Microbiome Products for the Treatment of Skin Diseases

Antti Lauerma

Abstract Skin and gut share parallel structures and functions, including barrier and immune responses. There is a well-established skin-gut-axis, where especially the gut has a significant effect on health. Microbiome, used synonymously here as microbiota, was found in 2009 and has been under intense investigation after that. Microbiome-related interventions to skin diseases such as atopic dermatitis and acne vulgaris, as well as skin aging, have been done. This chapter concentrates on available human data and its relevance in skin health.

Keywords Microbiome · Oral · Gut · Skin · Dermatology · Atopic dermatitis · Acne vulgaris · Psoriasis · Urticaria · Melasma · Skin aging

13.1 Introduction

Before the advent of next-generation sequencing techniques for the analysis of the microbiome, little was known about the structure and function of prokaryotes such as bacteria in the body. The technique of choice was bacterial culture, which is done in conditions resembling those in parenteral tissue, 100% humidity and 37 °C temperature. This is by no way an optimal approach especially in study of skin microflora, as skin is a dry habitat with varying temperature and multiple environmental factors. These new techniques revealed that > 99% of human skin bacteria were previously unknown (Grice et al 2009).

The most progress in human microbiome research has been done in the gut. This may be related to two reasons. Firstly, stool samples are easy to obtain and give therefore reliable data. Secondly, gut is an important set of organs with central importance in human health. The digestive tract is the most important interface between body tissues which usually quite devoid of bacteria, and gut content that has high proportion of bacteria in its own volume (Gabrayel et al. 2022).

A. Lauerma (✉)
Department of Dermatology, University of Helsinki, Helsinki, Finland
e-mail: antti.lauerma@helsinki.fi

© The Author(s), under exclusive license to Springer Nature Switzerland AG 2025
A. Lauerma et al. (eds.), *The Skin Microbiome Manual*,
https://doi.org/10.1007/978-3-031-82689-4_13

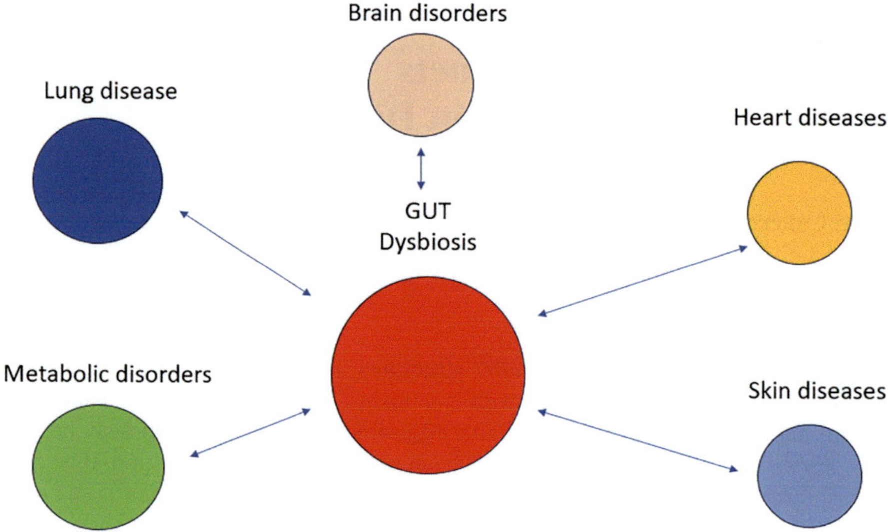

Fig. 13.1 A schematic representation of interaction between gut, gut microbiota and other organs, and their diseases

The gut has been shown to be driving several diseases, but the exact cause-effect relationship is not always clear. The only way to know this is through interventional studies, of which those available towards skin will be reviewed here. The gut has several axes between itself and other organs/processes, e.g. gut-brain axis, gut-lung axis, gut-skin axis, gut-heart axis, gut-metabolism axis (Fig. 13.1).

13.2 Manipulation of Gut Microbiota

Prebiotics are nutrients that are degraded by gut microbiota. They are considered safe, as they are not live or do not reproduce. Most important group is short-chain fatty acids (SCFA) that are related to high fiber content in food. SCFA's feature the most promising group of prebiotics. As opposed to prebiotics, *probiotics* are live bacteria. Despite potential of side-effects, they are widely available, and used widely. *Faecalibacterium prausnitzii* seems one of most promising probiotics. It also produces butyrate that effects the immune system (Gabrayel et al. 2022).

One promising approach has been *fecal microbial transplantation*. Despite a lot of promise, it seems to be most effective in treating antibiotic-associated diarrhea. Studies in other diseases are ongoing. Bacterial metabolites, especially CSFAs, are another promising avenue of research in manipulating gut microbiota. Other new techniques include *miRNA, hyaluronan and nanomedicine* (Gabrayel et al. 2022).

As there is a gut-skin axis in microbiota, the use of oral probiotics, prebiotics, postbiotics, and other manipulations above hold promise for the treatment of skin diseases. Related research has increased during recent years and several double-blind studies were published. Of note, there is a great variance and variability in the choice of distinct probiotics, ranging from one strain to multiple strains and the results of these intervention studies are just starting to arrive. Despite some scepticism, it seems that the field will move rapidly in next few years (De Almeida et al. 2023).

13.3 Atopic Dermatitis

Atopic dermatitis (AD) is a chronic inflammatory skin disease with unpredictable course. It is characterized by itch and dry sensitive skin, termed "atopic skin". AD is associated with several other atopic diseases, but despite its name, not all AD patients have atopy, termed as IgE-mediated allergy to common allergens such as animal epithelia and plant pollens. AD has significant effect on quality of life, and patients often suffer from anxiety and depression. Comorbidities, such as asthma and allergic conjunctivitis, add to the disease burden. In earlier decades treatment armarentum was limited to oral and topical corticosteroids, as well as oral methotrexate, azathioprine and cyclosporine, all with significant side effects. The advancement of topical calcineurin inhibitors and selective UVB therapy has greatly improved the situation. Surprisingly, there were no effective and safe biologics to AD before this decade, while for psoriasis they were available 15 years earlier (Paller et al. 2017). Dupilumab has good efficacy/safety balance, while now there are a total of four JAK kinase inhibitors that enter the market (Bieber et al. 2022; Kim 2022; Shih et al. 2023).

Given the great need, it is not surprising that oral microbial components have been tried in the treatment of AD repeatedly. Moreover, prevention of AD has been studied, with positive results in children (De Andrade et al. 2022). A recent systematic review on oral microbial products as add on to topical corticosteroids identified 21 studies, of which 20 met eligibility criteria. Most studies used lactobacillus products as oral supplements. Thirteen studies reported SCORAD scores, and overall microbial products were superior to topical corticosteroids in improving SCORAD. Twelve studies reported adverse events with no difference between groups. However, there was no effect on pruritus, quality of life or frequency of topical corticosteroid use (Xue et al. 2023).

The rapid advance in probiotics and also in microbial metabolites like SCFA suggests that there is a high likelihood for AD patients to find safe and effective new treatments in the near future. However, if there is no evidence of safety and efficacy, it would be harmful to patient to avoid more effective treatments, if for example the used oral microbial component product is not working. This is a fact that clinicians should note (Olabi and Williams 2021).

13.4 Acne Vulgaris

Acne vulgaris is a serious scarring inflammatory skin disease that is also associated with *Cutibacterium acnes*, a bacterium that has both anti- and proinflammatory mechanisms. For several decades there was no effective treatment for acne. The standard treatment was oral tetracyclines. Only after the introduction of oral isotretinoin there also was an effective medication for patients suffering from severe forms of acne vulgaris. Long lasting treatment with tetracyclins has been shown to be not only antimicrobial but also anti-inflammatory. Therefore, the pathogenic role of *Cutibacterium acnes* has not been certain. In addition the effect of *Cutibacterium* change on acne intensity differs between strains of cutibacteria (Nolan et al. 2023). Of note, the effect of diet has been suggested to be important in acne. High glycemic load activates androgenic receptor via insulin-like growth factor-1, and also insulin. This cascade has been shown to increase sebum production and keratinocyte proliferation *in vitro* (Sanchez-Pellicer et al. 2022).

Recently, there has been one published double-blind, placebo-controlled, randomized clinical trial on oral probiotic, that showed efficacy in acne scoring when probiotic mixture and botanical extract were used (Rinaldi et al. 2022). At this moment there are at least two more ongoing double-blind, placebo-controlled, randomized clinical trials going on with different probiotic combinations (Sanchez-Pellicer et al. 2022). The results of these studies will not only possibly provide new treatments, but also more insight towards the pathogenesis of acne vulgaris in general.

13.5 Psoriasis

Psoriasis vulgaris is a quite common chronic inflammatory skin disease. It is usually mild, but more severe cases are often associated with systemic comorbidities, such as diabetes, obesity and atherosclerosis. For the systemic treatment of moderate to severe psoriasis patients several effective and safe biologicals are currently available. The effective treatment of psoriasis lesions and symptoms is important since some comorbidities are related to lowered quality of life and lifestyle choices. Of note is that many aggravating factors in psoriasis are related to diet. Also is a gut microbiota composition in psoriasis patients' stool as compared to healthy people. (Xiao et al. 2023).

A systematic review on the effects of probiotic supplements was published (Zeng et al. 2021). The effect of probiotics was studied in three randomized clinical trials. In two of the trials PASI scores improved, whilst in one study proinflammatory factors such as interleukin (IL)-6, C-reactive protein (CRP) and tumor necrosis factor (TNF)-alpha cytokines decreased. Further studies are needed to validate whether microbial supplements may help psoriasis patients in larger trials (Zeng et al. 2021).

13.6   Urticaria

Urticaria is a debilitating histamine-mediated disease with high effect on quality of life. Next to high dose antihistamines, the standard treatment is nowadays the biological omalizumab, which is effective and well tolerated (Zuberbier et al. 2022). A systematic review on probiotics for urticaria was done, and a total of 9 studies were involved. There was no overall improvement with probiotic, even though one study showed improvement over antihistamine alone (Fu et al. 2023).

13.7   Melasma

Melasma is a benign skin hyperpigmentation that is especially usual in middle age and in darker skin color. It does not have good treatment alternatives, as hydroquinone, the earlier drug-of-choice, was discontinued in most countries because of likelihood of carcinogenesis. One research study from Thailand investigated synbiotic, a collection of 6 probiotics in melasma patients. Patients received synbiotic or placebo. The melasma score significantly improved (P = 0.0008). Hence oral probiotic supplements may have a role in reducing melasma (Piyavatin et al. 2021).

13.8   Skin Aging

Skin aging is a normal occurrence in life, but it involves several skin conditions such as thinning of skin. A review on oral microbial products found 6 studies, with some efficacy in wrinkles and skin hydration (Woolery-Royd et al. 2023).

13.9   Conclusions

The era of oral microbial supplements is beginning to unfold. Like earlier phases of development in other classes of treatments, the first trials are usually disappointments. However, with more systematic development of products, and recent insights into the metagenome, we will testify the potential of microbial component interventions in the upcoming decade.

References

Bieber T, Paller AS, Kabashima K, Feely M, Rueda MJ, Ross Terres JA, Wollenberg A. Atopic dermatitis: pathomechanisms and lessons learned from novel systemic therapeutic options. J Eur Acad Dermatol Venereol. 2022;36(9):1432–49.

De Almeida CV, Antiga E, Lulli M. Oral and topical probiotics and postbiotics in skincare and dermatological therapy: a concise review. Microorganisms. 2023;11(6):1420.

de Andrade PDSMA, Maria E Silva J, Carregaro V, Sacramento LA, Roberti LR, Aragon DC, Carmona F, Roxo-Junior P. Efficacy of probiotics in children and adolescents with atopic dermatitis: a randomized, double-blind placebo-controlled study. Front Nutr. 2022;8:833666

Fu HY, Yu HD, Bai YP, Yue LF, Wang HM, Li LL. Effect and safety of probiotics for treating urticaria: a systematic review and meta-analysis. J Cosmet Dermatol. 2023;22(10):2663–70.

Gebrayel P, Nicco C, Al Khodor S, Bilinski J, Caselli E, Comelli EM, Egert M, Giaroni C, Karpinski TM, Loniewski I, Mulak A, Reygner J, Samczuk P, Serino M, Sikora M, Terranegra A, Ufnal M, Villeger R, Pichon C, Konturek P, Edeas M. Microbiota medicine: towards clinical revolution. J Transl Med. 2022;20(1):111.

Grice EA, Kong HH, Conlan S, Deming CB, Davis J, Young AC, Bouffard GG, Blakesley RW, Murray PR, Green ED, Turner ML, Segre JA. Topographical and temporal diversity of the human skin microbiome. Science. 2009;324(5931):1190–2.

Kim HO. Targeting cytokines and signaling molecules related to immune pathways in atopic dermatitis: therapeutic implications and challenges. Arch Pharm Res. 2022;45(12):894–908.

Nolan ZT, Banerjee K, Cong Z, Gettle SL, Longenecker AL, Kawasawa YI, Zaenglein AL, Thiboutot DM, Agak GW, Zhan X, Nelson AM. Treatment response to isotretinoin correlates with specific shifts in Cutibacterium acnes strain composition within the follicular microbiome. Exp Dermatol. 2023;32(7):955–64.

Olabi B, Williams HC. Evidence-based management of eczema: five things that should be done more and five things that should be dropped. Curr Opin Allergy Clin Immunol. 2021;21(4):386–93.

Paller AS, Kabashima K, Bieber T. Therapeutic pipeline for atopic dermatitis: end of the drought? J Allergy Clin Immunol. 2017;140(3):633–43.

Piyavatin P, Chaichalotornkul S, Nararatwanchai T, Bumrungpert A, Saiwichai T. Synbiotics supplement is effective for Melasma improvement. J Cosmet Dermatol. 2021;20(9):2841–50.

Rinaldi F, Marotta L, Mascolo A, Amoruso A, Pane M, Giuliani G, Pinto D. Facial acne: a randomized, double-blind, placebo-controlled study on the clinical efficacy of a symbiotic dietary supplement. Dermatol Ther (Heidelb). 2022;12(2):577–89.

Sánchez-Pellicer P, Navarro-Moratalla L, Núñez-Delegido E, Ruzafa-Costas B, Agüera-Santos J, Navarro-López V. Acne, microbiome, and probiotics: the gut-skin axis. Microorganisms. 2022;10(7):1303.

Shih PY, Li CJ, Yong SB. Emerging trends in clinical research on Janus kinase inhibitors for atopic dermatitis treatment. Int Immunopharmacol. 2023;124(Pt B): 111029.

Woolery-Lloyd H, Andriessen A, Day D, Gonzalez N, Green L, Grice E, Henry M. Review of the microbiome in skin aging and the effect of a topical prebiotic containing thermal spring water. J Cosmet Dermatol. 2023;22(1):96–102.

Xiao X, Hu X, Yao J, Cao W, Zou Z, Wang L, Qin H, Zhong D, Li Y, Xue P, Jin R, Li Y, Shi Y, Li J. The role of short-chain fatty acids in inflammatory skin diseases. Front Microbiol. 2023;13:1083432.

Xue P, Qin H, Qin D, Liu H, Li J, Jin R, Xiao X. The efficacy and safety of oral microecological agents as add-on therapy for atopic dermatitis: a systematic review and meta-analysis of randomized clinical trials. Clin Transl Allergy. 2023;13(12): e12318.

Zeng L, Yu G, Wu Y, Hao W, Chen H. The effectiveness and safety of probiotic supplements for psoriasis: a systematic review and meta-analysis of randomized controlled trials and preclinical trials. J Immunol Res. 2021;2021:7552546.

Zuberbier T, Abdul Latiff AH, Abuzakouk M, Aquilina S, Asero R, Baker D, Ballmer-Weber B, Bangert C, Ben-Shoshan M, Bernstein JA, Bindslev-Jensen C, Brockow K, Brzoza Z, Chong

Neto HJ, Church MK, Criado PR, Danilycheva IV, Dressler C, Ensina LF, Fonacier L, Gaskins M, Gáspár K, Gelincik A, Giménez-Arnau A, Godse K, Gonçalo M, Grattan C, Grosber M, Hamelmann E, Hébert J, Hide M, Kaplan A, Kapp A, Kessel A, Kocatürk E, Kulthanan K, Larenas-Linnemann D, Lauerma A, Leslie TA, Magerl M, Makris M, Meshkova RY, Metz M, Micallef D, Mortz CG, Nast A, Oude-Elberink H, Pawankar R, Pigatto PD, Ratti Sisa H, Rojo Gutiérrez MI, Saini SS, Schmid-Grendelmeier P, Sekerel BE, Siebenhaar F, Siiskonen H, Soria A, Staubach-Renz P, Stingeni L, Sussman G, Szegedi A, Thomsen SF, Vadasz Z, Vestergaard C, Wedi B, Zhao Z, Maurer M. The international EAACI/GA^{2}LEN/EuroGuiDerm/APAAACI guideline for the definition, classification, diagnosis, and management of urticaria. Allergy. 2022;77(3):734–66.

Chapter 14
Topical Microbiome Products for Treatment of Skin Diseases

Ville Salo, Antti Lauerma, and Alexander Salava

Abstract Frequent observations about disease-characteristic alterations in the cutaneous microbiome of skin diseases have led to an increasing clinical interest to find microbiome-targeting treatment strategies, especially topical products. In recent years, topical microbiome products have been explored as novel therapeutic options, however, the used microbial composition (e.g., lactobacilli), underlying therapeutic strategy (e.g., postbiotics) and topical formulations (e.g., emollient creams) have varied substantially and limited their comparability. Significant heterogeneity also accounts for reported efficacy, tolerability, and adverse effects. Atopic dermatitis has been studied most deeply, but latest research indicates that topical microbiome products may be useful in large number of other relevant chronic skin disorders, e.g., acne vulgaris and skin barrier dysfunction. The underlying theoretical concepts and preliminary clinical data suggest that they may contain a high potential as novel treatment and prevention options in chronic skin diseases.

Keywords Microbiome · Therapy · Topical microbiome · Prebiotic · Probiotic · Postbiotics · Atopic dermatitis · Acne vulgaris · Skin diseases

14.1 Introduction

Novel sequencing methods have had a substantial impact on our understanding of the cutaneous microbiome and its role and specific pathophysiological changes in skin diseases (Smythe and Wilkinson 2023; Fyhrquist et al. 2016). There have been frequent observations about disease-characteristic alterations of the cutaneous microbiome in different skin-related disorders. These observations have led to an increasing clinical interest to find useful and practicable microbiome-targeting treatment strategies, especially topical microbiome products (Chen et al. 2023).

Unfortunately, there has only been a limited amount of well conducted research regarding this topic and our current understanding still lacks larger clinical studies

V. Salo · A. Lauerma (✉) · A. Salava
Department of Dermatology, University of Helsinki, Helsinki, Finland
e-mail: antti.lauerma@helsinki.fi

with control groups and randomization. Microbiome-targeting therapies have been studied based on the underlying theoretical concepts (e.g., directly targeting the skin microbiome) and possible application modes (e.g., topical formulations), but topical microbiome products remain the most used and studied to date (Boxberger et al. 2021). The physiological microbiome of healthy human skin is already characterized quite well and in a growing number of skin diseases our knowledge and understanding of the microbiome. Its role in pathophysiological changes is steadily increasing (Byrd et al. 2018, Dréno et al. 2020). Regarding the use of topical microbiome-targeting therapies the most experience we have is in atopic dermatitis, one of the most frequent chronic skin diseases in the general population with a very relevant disease-related as well as socioeconomic burden (Harris-Tryon and Grice 2023, Salava and Lauerma 2014). In addition, in other skin diseases, e.g., acne, topical treatment strategies have been explored to modify the cutaneous microbiome (Dréno et al. 2020).

Topical therapy including microbiome products possesses many advances when compared to systemically applied drugs. First, the risk for systemic adverse effects is very limited and thus the safety profile is often better. Regarding topical microbiome products there has been only a small number of reports of adverse effects but the potential of cutaneous infections (e.g., by the product itself or indirectly by shifts in the cutaneous microbiome) should be acknowledged (Gelmetti et al. 2023). Second, topical products can be applied directly to the skin and the treatment can be concentrated only to the affected skin sites, thus reducing the treated skin surface and amount of topical therapy. For example, in acne the treatment sites are usually limited to the facial areas (Wongtada et al. 2023). And third, since the cutaneous microbiome is localized mostly on and in between the skin's superficial layers (epidermis), topical microbiome products ensure sufficient contact and microbial concentrations of the microbiome-targeted treatment strategy (Herbert et al. 2023).

In this chapter we would like to present the current status of research regarding topical microbiome products in the treatment of skin diseases. The chapter "The skin microbiome: potential for novel diagnostic and therapeutic strategies" of this book deals with microbiome-targeted treatment strategies more in general.

14.2 Atopic Dermatitis

Atopic dermatitis (AD) is a chronic inflammatory skin disease affecting patients of all age groups. Typical symptoms include dry itchy skin and lichenification. There are no curative treatments available at the moment, but the symptoms can be managed with proper treatment. AD can be associated with several other atopy-linked diseases such as asthma, allergic rhinoconjunctivitis and different IgE-mediated allergies (animal epithelia and pollen). As a chronic disease that may involve recurrent relapses and treatment fatigue, anxiety and depression are common in AD and worsen the quality of life of patients.

The pathogenesis of AD is not yet completely understood. Three major factors causing AD has been identified: Firstly, epidermal barrier dysfunction and gene mutations connected to it (Rodríguez et al. 2009), secondly, hereditary predisposition and immunological changes (Patrick et al. 2021), and thirdly changes in the skin microbiome (Salava and Lauerma 2014 and Kong et al. 2012).

Treatment of atopic dermatitis consists of basic emollients, topical corticosteroids, topical calcineurin inhibitors, short courses of oral antibiotics in superinfection, antiviral herpes medications when needed, antifungal treatment in selected patients, narrowband UVB light therapy, PUVA (psoralen, UVA) treatment when needed, avoidance of triggering factors such as exacerbating allergens, irritation, psychological stress, smoking, evaluation of dietary triggering factors, and patient education (Wollenberg et al. 2022b). As systemic treatments, antihistamines are not recommended. Systemic treatments are recommended for patients above SCORAD score of 50, including azathioprine, ciclosporine in selected patients, corticosteroids as short term rescue therapy, methotreaxate, dupilumab, tralokinumab, baricitinib, upadacitinib and alitretinoin in selected patients with recalcitrant hand eczema, First-line treatment of AD is topical corticosteroids or calcineurin inhibitors with concomitant emollient creams. (Wollenberg et al. 2022a).

Skin microbiome manipulation with topical probiotics offers a novel route to managing atopic dermatitis symptoms. The most common vehicle for introducing probiotic bacteria to the skin has been emollient cream. Live and dead bacteria have been used as well as bacterial lysate. Probiotics are believed to maintain a normal microbial flora and prevent colonization with pathogenic microbes (colonization resistance). Various probiotic bacteria have been used with different *Lactobacillus* strains being most common (Xie et al. 2023; Butler et al. 2020.) Other used bacteria include *Streptococci, Vitreoscilla, Staphylococci epidermidis, Roseomonas,* and *Bifidobateria* (Gueniche et al. 2008; Szöllösi et al. 2017; Herbert et al. 2023).

14.2.1 Clinical Studies

Most clinical studies demonstrated statistically significant improvements in SCORAD or EASI and pruritus (Table 14.1). Moreover, improved TEWL and skin capacitance (Park et al. 2014), significant decrease in *Staphylococcus aureus* abundance (Nakatsuji et al. 2017 and Blanchet-Rethore et al. 2017), significant decrease in topical corticosteroid use (Myles et al. 2018) and significant improvement in keratinocyte re-epithelization rate (Mohammadsaeed et al. 2015) have also been reported.

14.2.2 In Vitro-Studies

In vitro-studies have focused on more various topics (Table 14.2). It has been found that certain *Bifidobacterium longum* extracts increased the expression of differentiation markers, antimicrobial peptides, and wound healing-associated molecules in

Table 14.1 Relevant clinical studies investigating the use of topical microbiome products in the treatment of atopic dermatitis (selected by the authors)

Study	No. patients	Type of study	Results	Used probiotic	Additiona information
Di Marzio et al. 2003	11	Open-label, placebo controlled, split-body trial	Improvement in pruritus, ($p < 0.001$), erythema ($p < 0.001$) and scaling ($p = 0.003$) Increase in stratum coneum ceramide levels ($p = 0.002$)	*Streptococcus thermophilus*	Patient receiving placebo interrupted treatment within 4–5 d
Guéniche et al. 2006	13	Randomized, double-blind, vehicle controlled, split-body trial	Improved EASI index ($p = 0.012$) and pruritus ($p = 0.046$)	*Vitreoscilla filiformis*	
Guéniche et al. 2008	75	Randomized, double-blind, placebo-controlled trial	Improved SCORAD index ($p = 0.0044$) and pruritus ($p = 0.0174$)	*Vitreoscilla filiformis*	
Park et al. 2014	28	Randomized, double-blind, placebo-controlled, split-body trial	Improved pruritus ($p = 0.006$), TEWL ($p = 0.007$) and skin capacitance ($p = 0.001$)	*Lactobacillus sakei probio* 65	Concomitant use of topical corticosteroids in most cases
Nakatsuji et al. 2017	9	Randomized, double-blind, vehicle controlled, split-body trial	Significant decrease in *S. aureus* abundance ($p = 0.0402$)	*Staphylococcus epidermidis and S. hominis*	*S. aureus* abundence was measured only once, after 24 h of application
Blanchet-Rethore et al. 2017	21	Open-label trial	Improved SCORAD index ($p = 0.012$) Significant decrease in *S. aureus* abundance ($p < 0.05$)	*Lactobacillus johnsonii*	

(continued)

Table 14.1 (continued)

Study	No. patients	Type of study	Results	Used probiotic	Additiona information
Myles et al. 2018	10	Open-label trial	Improved SCORAD index (adult and children $p < 0.01$ and $p < 0.05$ respectively) Significant decrease in pruritus ($p < 0.01$) and topical steroid applications ($p < 0.05$)	*Roseomonas mucosa*	
Axt-Gadermann et al. 2021	22	Randomized, double-blind trial	Decrease in SCORAD index, pruritus and skin dryness	*Lactobacillus plantarum, L. gasseri, L. rhamnosus, L. paracasei, L. johnsonii, L. reuteri, Bifidobacterium longum, B. lactis and Streptococcus thermophilus*	No follow-up after 14 d period Statistical significance was not reported
Butler et al. 2020	36	Randomized, double-blind controlled trial	Improved SCORAD index ($p \leq 0.001$), no statistically significant improvement in skin dryness was observed	*Lactobacillus reuteri* DSM 17,938	
Mohammadsaeed et al. 2015	12	Open-label trial	Statistically significant improvement in keratinosyte re-epithelization rate with *L. rhamnosus* ($p = 0.003$) and *L. reuteri* ($p = 0.05$). L. plantarum had no effect and L. fermentum decreased keratinosyte re-epithelization rate ($p = 0.01$)	*Lactobacillus rhamnosus, L. reuteri, L. plantarum and L.fermentum lysate*	Epithelization rate was measured at 12 and 18 h Small number of patients per group (3)

cultured normal human epidermal keratinocytes, suggesting that they may enhance the barrier function and innate immunity of the skin (Szöllősi et al. 2017). Manipulation of certain pro-inflammatory pathways with *Lactococcus lactis* KR-050L has been shown to decrease TNF-α, IL-1β, IL-6, CCL17 and CCL22 gene expressions by down-regulation of p38 MAPK, STAT1 and NF-κB pathways in TNF-α/IFN-γ-stimulated keratinocytes (Jin et al. 2019).

Table 14.2 Relevant *in vitro*-studies investigating the use of topical microbiome products in the treatment of atopic dermatitis (selected by the authors)

Study	No. patients	Type of study	Results	Used probiotic	Additiona information
Szöllősi et al. 2017	*In vitro*		Increase in expression of keratinocyte differentiation markers and up-regulation of KRT1, KRT10 and TGM1. Increase in β defensin 1 and Cathepsins B, D and H	2 different *Bifidobacterium longum* strains and *B. longum reuter* extract	*In vitro*, p-values were not reported
Jin et al. 2019	30 mice		*In vitro*: decrease in TNF-α, IL-1β, IL-6, CCL17 and CCL22 gene expressions *In vivo*: significant reduction in ear dermal and epidermal thickening. Decrease in serum immunoglobulin, inflammatory cytokines and mast cell degranulation	*Lactococcus lactis* KR-050L	*In vitro* and *in vivo* murine model Cyclosporine A and tacrolimus were used as positive controls *in vivo* p < 0.05 was considered significant, p-values were not reported
Miyauchi et al. 2012	*In vitro*		Demostrated that some L. salivarius strains markedle reduce relocalization of tight-junction proteins in H_2O_2-induced barrier impaired epithelial cells	33 *different Lactobacillus salivarius* strains	*In vitro*: human intestinal epithelial Caco-2 cells Efficacy of different strains varied
Sultana et al. 2013	*In vitro*		All strains, excluding *L. fermentum*, markedly increased tight-junction barrier fuction within 24 h	*Bifidobacterium longum, Lactobacillus plantarum, L. reuteri, L. fermentum, L. rhamnosus* GG	*In vitro*: normal human epidermal keratonocytes

Tight-junctions in keratinocytes play an important role in skin barrier integrity. *Bifidobacterium longum* and *Lactococcus rhamnosus* GG lysates have been found to increase tight-junction protein expression. *B. longum*-induced effects are mediated by Toll-like receptor 2 (TLR2), while *L. rhamnosus* GG-induced effects are TLR2-independent (Sultana et al. 2013). The effect of different *Lactobacillus salivarius* strains on H_2O_2-treated human epithelial Caco-2 cells has shown that some studied strains markedly reduce relocalization of tight-junction proteins in H_2O_2-induced barrier impaired epithelial cells. The effective strains activated the extracellular signal-regulated kinase pathway in Caco-2 cells, whereas the ineffective strain activated the Akt and p38 pathways (Miyauchi et al. 2012).

14.3 Acne Vulgaris

Acne vulgaris is an inflammatory skin disease that is associated with *Cutibacterium acnes* (earlier name *Propionibacterium acnes*). For several decades there was no effective treatment for severe acne. The usual systemic treatment was oral tetracyclines. Only after the introduction of oral isotretinoin this situation changed and deleterious effects of severe acne such as scaring could be prevented. In addition, several topical products are used, with several showing antibacterial effects, e.g., lymecycline. However, as several antibiotics used have also anti-inflammatory properties, the role of *Cutibacterium acnes* in the pathogenesis of acne has not been very clear. It seems that different strains of cutibacteria exert differential effects. Recently, however, it has been shown that especially oral microbiota have an important role, especially when dysregulated due to a high glycemic index. There has now been a recurrence in interest in topical and systemic probiotic treatments in acne (De Alameida et al. 2023).

Cutibacterium acnes acts simultaneously as commensal increasing skin health and as immunomodulatory agent through the production of short-chain fatty acids (SCFA's) in sebum (Huang et al. 2022). As a commensal and pathogen it competes with other bacteria. Prebiotic or postbiotic components have been of interest therefore in controlling cutibacteria. It has been shown early that konjac glucomannan hydrosylates (GMH) inhibit cutibacteria growth *in vitro*, thus making it a candidate for probiotic acne vulgaris topical medication (Al-Ghazzewi and Tester 2010).

A recent study on *Lactiplantibacillus plantarum* has shown promise as topical treatment of acne vulgaris in the future. *Lactibacillus plantarum* was chosen to be studied after a thorough screening process of different strains. *Ex vivo*-studies with human skin models and *in vivo*-studies with skin of healthy human volunteers showed good viabilitity of the strain. Lactobacilli improved acne in skin disease models and reduced inflammation. It was shown that *Lactobacillus plantarum* counteracts *Cutibacterium acnes*, making it also a good candidate to topically treat acne vulgaris (Podrini et al. 2023).

14.4 Skin Aging and Barrier Repair

Skin aging causes several skin changes such as thinning. During aging, also skin barrier restoration slows down and there is a great need to have products that prevent or revert clinical signs of skin aging. Of separate interest is the effect of ultraviolet (UV) irradiation, that is a major causative factor in skin aging, and also keratinocyte skin cancers, such as basal cell carcinoma and spinous cell carcinoma (Woolery-Lloyd et al. 2023). Ceramides are major components of the skin's lipid barrier protecting from transepidermal waterloss and entry of pathogens such as viruses and bacteria, as well as biologically active components such as DNA, RNA and proteins, that may compromise normal cutaneous homeostasis. In an early study, bacterial sphingomyelinase from *Streptococcus thermophilus* was studied as topical product in human healthy volunteers. The study demonstrated that during a 2-week period, sphingomyelinase treatment led to a significant and relevant increase in stratum corneum ceramide levels improving the barrier skin function (Di Marzio et al. 2008).

An animal study to study the effect of ultraviolet irradiation B (UVB) in laboratory mice was performed with *Lactobacillus helveticus* NS8-fermented milk supernatant (NS8-FS). It was shown that NS8-FS improves symptoms of UVB-induced photo-damage, including epidermal thickness, transepidermal water loss and lipid peroxidation levels restoration. NS8-FS also diminished tanning effect of UVB, as well as stimulated Nrf2 protein and recovered antioxidant enzyme activities (Rong et al. 2017). In a separate study, products from *Lactobacíllus rhamnosus* restored UVB-induced effects in HaCaT cells such as upregulation of anti-oxidant components of cells (Shin et al. 2018).

Wrinkles are a phenomenon that is relatively easy and reliable to assess. *Nitrosonomas eutropha* was studied in a prospective human study and demonstrated that one week of topical treatment reduced the amount of wrinkles in human volunteers (Notay et al. 2020). Furthermore, *Lactobacillus acidophilus* reduced melanogenesis in a cell model (Lim et al. 2020). A proprietary dermo-cosmetic postbiotic product CLS022021 that features metabolites from probiotic bacterial cultures, but no live bacteria, improved both skin moisture, and reduced wrinkles, in a study involving 50 healthy volunteers (Catic et al. 2022).

14.5 Conclusions

In recent years, topical microbiome products have been explored as novel therapeutic options in the treatment of frequent chronic skin diseases. The topical formulations (e.g., emollient creams) used, the microbial composition (e.g., lactobacilli) (Caldwell et al. 2022), underlying therapeutic strategy (e.g., prebiotics, probiotics, postbiotics) (De Almeida et al. 2023) have, however, varied and limited the comparability of these studies. Significant heterogeneity also accounts for the reported efficacy, tolerability, and safety with partly conflicting results. Atopic dermatitis has been predominantly studied, but recent studies suggest that topical microbiome-targeting therapies may be useful in number of other, very relevant chronic skin disorders, e.g., acne, psoriasis, and chronic wounds (Baldwin et al. 2020). Most of the studies concerning topical microbiome-targeting therapies are based on small patient cohorts and report some benefit and good tolerability. However, there are yet very limited randomized and double-blinded studies available and there is clearly a need for more research regarding the role of topical microbiome products in the treatment of skin-related conditions. The underlying theoretical concepts and preliminary data of clinical studies suggest that they may contain a high potential as novel treatment and prevention options in chronic skin diseases.

References

Al-Ghazzewi FH, Tester RF. Effect of konjac glucomannan hydrolysates and probiotics on the growth of the skin bacterium Propionibacterium acnes in vitro. Int J Cosmet Sci. 2010;32(2):139–42.

Axt-Gadermann M, Chudomirova K, Noll M. Probiotische Teilbäder bei atopischer Dermatitis [Probiotic baths for atopic dermatitis]. Hautarzt. 2021;72(6):549–56.

Baldwin H, Aguh C, Andriessen A, Benjamin L, Ferberg AS, Hooper D, Jarizzo JL, Lio PA, Tlougan B, Woolery-Lloyd HC, Zeichner J. Atopic dermatitis and the role of the skin microbiome in choosing prevention, treatment, and maintenance options. J Drugs Dermatol. 2020;19(10):935–40.

Blanchet-Réthoré S, Bourdès V, Mercenier A, Haddar CH, Verhoeven PO, Andres P. Effect of a lotion containing the heat-treated probiotic strain Lactobacillus johnsonii NCC 533 on Staphylococcus aureus colonization in atopic dermatitis. Clin Cosmet Investig Dermatol. 2017;10:249–57.

Boxberger M, Cenizo V, Cassir N, La Scola B. Challenges in exploring and manipulating the human skin microbiome. Microbiome. 2021;9(1):125.

Butler É, Lundqvist C, Axelsson J. Lactobacillus reuteri DSM 17938 as a novel topical cosmetic ingredient: a proof of concept clinical study in adults with atopic dermatitis. Microorganisms. 2020;8(7):1026.

Byrd AL, Belkaid Y, Segre JA. The human skin microbiome. Nat Rev Microbiol. 2018;16(3):143–55.

Caldwell R, Zhou W, Oh J. Strains to go: interactions of the skin microbiome beyond its species. Curr Opin Microbiol. 2022;70: 102222.

Catic T, Pehlivanovic B, Pljakic N, Balicevac A. The Moisturizing efficacy of a proprietary dermo-cosmetic product(CLS02021) versus placebo in a 4-week application period. Med Arch. 2022;76(2):108–14.

Chen Y, Knight R, Gallo RL. Evolving approaches to profiling the microbiome in skin disease. Front Immunol. 2023;14:1151527.

De Almeida CV, Antiga E, Lulli M. Oral and topical probiotics and postbiotics in skincare and dermatological therapy: a concise review. Microorganisms. 2023;11(6):1420.

Di Marzio L, Centi C, Cinque B, et al. Effect of the lactic acid bacterium Streptococcus thermophilus on stratum corneum ceramide levels and signs and symptoms of atopic dermatitis patients. Exp Dermatol. 2003;12(5):615–20.

Di Marzio L, Cinque B, Cupelli F, De Simone C, Cifone MG, Giuliani M. Increase of skin-ceramide levels in aged subjects following a short-term topical application of bacterial sphingomyelinase from Streptococcus thermophilus. Int J Immunopathol Pharmacol. 2008;21(1):137–43.

Dréno B, Dagnelie MA, Khammari A, Corvec S. The skin microbiome: a new actor in inflammatory acne. Am J Clin Dermatol. 2020;21(Suppl 1):18–24.

Dréno B, Araviiskaia E, Berardesca E, Gontijo G, Sanchez Viera M, Xiang LF, Martin R, Bieber T. Microbiome in healthy skin, update for dermatologists. J Eur Acad Dermatol Venereol. 2016;30(12):2038–47.

Fyhrquist N, Salava A, Auvinen P, Lauerma A. Skin Biomes. Curr Allergy Asthma Rep. 2016;16(5):40.

Gelmetti C, Rigoni C, Cantù AM et al. Topical prebiotics/postbiotics and PRURISCORE validation in atopic dermatitis. International study of 396 patients. J Dermatolog Treat. 2023;34(1):2131703.

Guéniche A, Hennino A, Goujon C, Dahel K, Bastien P, Martin R, Jourdain R, Breton L. Improvement of atopic dermatitis skin symptoms by Vitreoscilla filiformis bacterial extract. Eur J Dermatol. 2006;16(4):380–4.

Guéniche A, Knaudt B, Schuck E, Volz T, Bastien P, Martin R, Röcken M, Breton L, Biedermann T. Effects of nonpathogenic gram-negative bacterium Vitreoscilla filiformis lysate on atopic dermatitis: a prospective, randomized, double-blind, placebo-controlled clinical study. Br J Dermatol. 2008;159(6):1357–63.

Gueniche A, Liboutet M, Cheilian S, Fagot D, Juchaux F, Breton L. Vitreoscilla filiformis extract for topical skin care: a review. Front Cell Infect Microbiol. 2021;11: 747663.

Harris-Tryon TA, Grice EA. Microbiota and maintenance of skin barrier function. Science. 2022;376(6596):940–5.

Herbert S, Haughton R, Nava J, Ji-Xu A, Le ST, Maverakis E. A review of topical probiotic therapy for atopic dermatitis. Clin Exp Dermatol. 2023;48(4):319–24.

Huang TY, Jiang YE, Scott DA. Culturable bacteria in the entire acne lesion and short-chain fatty acid metabolites of Cutibacterium acnes and Staphylococcus epidermidis isolates. Biochem Biophys Res Commun. 2022;622:45–9.

Jin M, Lee S, Choi YA, et al. Lactococcus lactis KR-050L extract suppresses house dust mite induced-atopic skin inflammation through inhibition of keratinocyte and mast cell activation. J Appl Microbiol. 2019;126(1):230–41.

Kong HH, Oh J, Deming C, et al. Temporal shifts in the skin microbiome associated with disease flares and treatment in children with atopic dermatitis. Genome Res. 2012;22(5):850–9.

Lim HY, Jeong D, Park SH, Shin KK, Hong YH, Kim E, Yu YG, Kim TR, Kim H, Lee J, Cho JY. Anti-wrinkle and Antimelanogenesis effects of Tyndallized Lactobacillus acidophilus KCCM12625P. Int J Mol Sci. 2020;21(5):1620.

Miyauchi E, O'Callaghan J, Buttó LF, et al. Mechanism of protection of transepithelial barrier function by Lactobacillus salivarius: strain dependence and attenuation by bacteriocin production. Am J Physiol Gastrointest Liver Physiol. 2012;303(9):G1029–41.

Mohammedsaeed W, Cruickshank S, McBain AJ, O'Neill CA. Lactobacillus rhamnosus GG lysate increases re-epithelialization of keratinocyte scratch assays by promoting migration. Sci Rep. 2015;5:16147.

Myles IA, Earland NJ, Anderson ED, et al. First-in-human topical microbiome transplantation with Roseomonas mucosa for atopic dermatitis. JCI Insight. 2018;3(9): e120608.

Nakatsuji T, Chen TH, Narala S, et al. Antimicrobials from human skin commensal bacteria protect against Staphylococcus aureus and are deficient in atopic dermatitis. Sci Transl Med. 2017;9(378):eaah4680.

Notay M, Saric-Bosanac S, Vaughn AR, Dhaliwal S, Trivedi M, Reiter PN, Rybak I, Li CC, Weiss LB, Ambrogio L, Burney W, Sivamani RK. The use of topical Nitrosomonas eutropha for cosmetic improvement of facial wrinkles. J Cosmet Dermatol. 2020;19(3):689–769.

Park SB, Im M, Lee Y, et al. Effect of emollients containing vegetable-derived lactobacillus in the treatment of atopic dermatitis symptoms: split-body clinical trial. Ann Dermatol. 2014;26(2):150–5.

Patrick GJ, Archer NK, Miller LS. Which way do we go? complex interactions in atopic dermatitis pathogenesis. J Invest Dermatol. 2021;141(2):274–84.

Podrini C, Schramm L, Marianantoni G, Apolinarska J, McGuckin C, Forraz N, Milet C, Desroches AL, Payen P, D'Aguanno M, Biazzo M. Topical administration of Lactiplantibacillus plantarum (SkinDuoTM) serum improves anti-acne properties. Microorganisms. 2023;11(2):417.

Rodríguez E, Baurecht H, Herberich E, et al. Meta-analysis of filaggrin polymorphisms in eczema and asthma: robust risk factors in atopic disease. J Allergy Clin Immunol. 2009;123(6):1361-70.e7.

Rong J, Shan C, Liu S, Zheng H, Liu C, Liu M, Jin F, Wang L. Skin resistance to UVB-induced oxidative stress and hyperpigmentation by the topical use of Lactobacillus helveticus NS8-fermented milk supernatant. J Appl Microbiol. 2017;123(2):511–23.

Salava A, Lauerma A. Role of the skin microbiome in atopic dermatitis. Clin Transl Allergy. 2014;4:33.

Shin D, Lee Y, Huang YH, Lim HW, Jang K, Kim DD, Lim CJ. Probiotic fermentation augments the skin anti-photoaging properties of Agastache rugosa through up-regulating antioxidant components in UV-B-irradiated HaCaT keratinocytes. BMC Complement Altern Med. 2018;18(1):196.

Smythe P, Wilkinson HN. The skin microbiome: current landscape and future opportunities. Int J Mol Sci. 2023;24(4):3950.

Sultana R, McBain AJ, O'Neill CA. Strain-dependent augmentation of tight-junction barrier function in human primary epidermal keratinocytes by Lactobacillus and Bifidobacterium lysates. Appl Environ Microbiol. 2013;79(16):4887–94.

Szöllősi A, Gueniche A, Jammayrac O, Szabó-Papp J, Blanchard C, Vasas N, Andrási M, Juhász I, Breton L, Bíró T. Bifidobacterium longum extract exerts pro-differentiating effects on human epidermal keratinocytes, in vitro. Bifidobacterium longum extract exerts pro-differentiating effects on human epidermal keratinocytes, in vitro. Exp Dermatol. 2017;26(1):92–4.

Wollenberg A, Kinberger M, Arents B, Aszodi N, Avila Valle G, Barbarot S, Bieber T, Brough HA, Calzavara Pinton P, Christen-Zäch S, Deleuran M, Dittmann M, Dressler C, Fink-Wagner AH, Fosse N, Gáspár K, Gerbens L, Gieler U, Girolomoni G, Gregoriou S, Mortz CG, Nast A, Nygaard U, Redding M, Rehbinder EM, Ring J, Rossi M, Serra-Baldrich E, Simon D, Szalai ZZ, Szepietowski JC, Torrelo A, Werfel T, Flohr C. European guideline (EuroGuiDerm) on atopic eczema: part I—systemic therapy. J Eur Acad Dermatol Venereol. 2022a;36(9):1409–31.

Wollenberg A, Kinberger M, Arents B, Aszodi N, Avila Valle G, Barbarot S, Bieber T, Brough HA, Calzavara Pinton P, Christen-Zäch S, Deleuran M, Dittmann M, Dressler C, Fink-Wagner AH, Fosse N, Gáspár K, Gerbens L, Gieler U, Girolomoni G, Gregoriou S, Mortz CG, Nast A, Nygaard U, Redding M, Rehbinder EM, Ring J, Rossi M, Serra-Baldrich E, Simon D, Szalai ZZ, Szepietowski JC, Torrelo A, Werfel T, Flohr C. European guideline (EuroGuiDerm) on atopic eczema—part II: non-systemic treatments and treatment recommendations for special AE patient populations. J Eur Acad Dermatol Venereol. 2022b;36(11):1904–2192.

Wongtada C, Prombutara P, Asawanonda P, Noppakun N, Kumtornrut C, Chatsuwan T. Distinct skin microbiome modulation following different topical acne treatments in mild acne vulgaris patients: a randomized, investigator-blinded exploratory study. Exp Dermatol. 2023;32(6):906–14.

Woolery-Lloyd H, Andriessen A, Day D, Gonzalez N, Green L, Grice E, Henry M. Review of the microbiome in skin aging and the effect of a topical prebiotic containing thermal spring water. J Cosmet Dermatol. 2023;22(1):96–102.

Xie A, Chen A, Chen Y, et al. Lactobacillus for the treatment and prevention of atopic dermatitis: clinical and experimental evidence. Front Cell Infect Microbiol. 2023;13:1137275.

Chapter 15
Skin Microbiome Manipulations

Chris Callewaert

Abstract The skin microbiome has become a focal point in the study of various skin diseases, and its potential for medical and cosmetic applications has gained significant attention. Skin microbiome manipulations have arisen as a new and exciting approach to combat skin conditions and to revolutionize skin care. Promising approaches include skin microbiome transplantation, skin bacteriotherapy, and the use of prebiotics, probiotics and postbiotics. Skin microbiome transplantation involves transferring a healthy individual's microbiome to another person's skin to improve their skin condition. Similarly, skin bacteriotherapy utilizes selected cultivated microorganisms applied to the skin to yield positive effects for the host. Prebiotics are also widely adopted, as they have the ability to stimulate the growth of health-enhancing microbes on the skin. In recent years, these approaches have shown promise in combating common skin disorders and restoring skin health associated with microbiome imbalances. Research in this area has led to successful applications of complete microbiome transplants and single-strain treatments with favorable therapeutic outcomes. Nevertheless, challenges persist, and ongoing research aims to optimize these strategies for more effective and precise skin microbiome interventions. As knowledge grows, the manipulation of the skin microbiome will likely lead to transformative therapies and improved skin health.

Keywords Bacteriotherapy · Fecal microbiome transplant FMT · Atopic dermatitis · Probiotics · Postbiotics · Prebiotics · Skin health · Body odor

C. Callewaert (✉)
Ghent University, Frieda Saeysstraat 1, 9052 Gent, Belgium
e-mail: chris.callewaert@ugent.be

DrArmpit BV, Kortrijksepoortstraat 279, 9000 Gent, Belgium

© The Author(s), under exclusive license to Springer Nature Switzerland AG 2025
A. Lauerma et al. (eds.), *The Skin Microbiome Manual*,
https://doi.org/10.1007/978-3-031-82689-4_15

15.1 Introducing the Symbiotic Journey of Human Skin Microbiome

The human body is not an isolated entity but rather a thriving ecosystem cohabiting with trillions of microorganisms. This newfound understanding of the symbiotic relationship between us and our microbial companions has revolutionized our perception of human health. It has become evident that harmony within this microbial system is crucial, and any disruption can lead to dysbiosis, setting the stage for potential diseases.

Probiotics, an age-old practice dating back to ancient times when fermented milk was used as a remedy, have evolved into modern nutritional supplements and even advanced drug products (McCall et al. 2020). With some probiotics currently undergoing phase III clinical trials, the future for these beneficial microorganisms looks promising.

Technological breakthroughs, particularly next-generation sequencing and bioinformatics, have propelled our ability to study the microbiome to new heights (Knight et al. 2018). These cutting-edge tools have provided us with unprecedented insights into the intricate composition of our microbial world.

A recent exciting development involves genetically engineered probiotics, precisely designed to perform specific health-enhancing tasks. These engineered bacterial strains have shown immense potential in tackling various health conditions, from type II diabetes to phenylketonuria (Zhou et al. 2020; Takiishi et al. 2012; Robert et al. 2014).

The intricate link between gastrointestinal health and skin health has been the focus of extensive research (Pessemier et al. 2021). Imbalances in the gut microbiome can contribute to common skin conditions prevalent in Western societies, underscoring the significance of the gut-skin connection (Greuter et al. 2017; O'Neill et al. 2016).

Beyond the gut, researchers are exploring the microbiomes of other body parts, including the skin, vagina, mouth, lungs, and eyes. Among these, the skin stands out as the largest organ, serving as a formidable shield against environmental factors and pathogens (Segre 2006). Its unique microenvironment presents an array of challenges that its inhabitants, comprising both human and bacterial cells, must navigate (Naik et al. 2012; Nakatsuji et al. 2017).

Remarkably, different skin areas host diverse microbial populations, making the skin an accessible organ for studying and manipulating the microbiome. As a result, the skin emerges as an ideal environment for pioneering microbiome research and potential interventions, offering a plethora of opportunities to unlock the mysteries of this fascinating ecosystem. The skin microbiome has emerged as a fascinating subject, capturing attention for its potential therapeutic and cosmetic applications. Imbalances in the skin microbiome are closely linked to various skin conditions, spurring the exploration of innovative strategies to manipulate this complex microbial ecosystem. In this book chapter, we delve into the cutting-edge world of skin microbiome manipulation, where exciting new paths for therapy have been opened.

15.2   The Intricate World of Human Skin Microbiome

The skin microbiome refers to the microorganisms that live on the surface of the skin and play an important role in maintaining skin health. The human skin is a diverse ecosystem, comprising moist, dry, and sebaceous sites, each with its own unique microorganism community (Grice and Segre 2011). Despite these variations, there are common bacterial and fungal species shared across these sites, such as *Cutibacterium, Corynebacterium, Staphylococcus* and *Malassezia* (Byrd et al. 2018). The sebaceous areas are dominated by cutibacteria and staphylococci, while moist regions are predominantly inhabited by *Corynebacterium* and *Staphylococcus* species (Grice et al. 2009). Dry skin, although containing fewer bacteria, exhibits the highest diversity, with *Corynebacterium, Cutibacterium, Staphylococcus* and various Proteobacteria present (Byrd et al. 2018).

Surprisingly, the skin microbiome is relatively stable over time. Research revealed that the newly developed skin microbiome after skin removal resembles the deeper layers' microbiome more closely than the initial surface microbiome, suggesting that the core skin microbiome originates from within the skin (Zeeuwen et al. 2012). Nevertheless, the dynamics of the skin microbiome differ depending on the skin site. Sebaceous and moist skin sites exhibit greater stability, while dry skin sites experience more fluctuations due to factors such as limited nutrients and external influences.

The healthy skin microbiome demonstrates remarkable biogeographical and individual variations in microbial abundance, diversity, and functionality (Oh et al. 2014). These differences play a significant role in microbial, fungal, or viral stability on the human skin and have provided valuable insights into site-specific skin conditions.

Recent advancements in sequencing technologies have shed light on the importance of strain-level differences among microorganisms. It has become evident that strains of the same species can have varying effects on the host, with some being beneficial and others pathogenic. Disease pathogenicity is often not driven by a single strain but rather by changes in the abundance of specific strains or organisms (Byrd et al. 2017).

Understanding the intricacies of the human skin microbiome, including its diverse sites, stability over time, and the significance of strain-level differences, opens new avenues for exploring skin health and developing targeted interventions to address skin conditions.

15.3   Tackling the Microbial Imbalance in Skin Conditions

Skin dysbiosis occurs in specific areas of the skin, leading to conditions like atopic dermatitis, rosacea, acne vulgaris, and psoriasis (Picardo and Ottaviani 2014; Dréno et al. 2018; Fyhrquist et al. 2019). Although psoriasis and atopic dermatitis are distinct diseases influenced by the immune system, their dysbiosis at a global level appears quite similar, characterized by increased *S. aureus* and decreased *C. acnes* and other commensals of the skin (Chang et al. 2018).

In atopic dermatitis, an autoimmune disease driven by overexpressed IL-24 and IL-13 cytokines, the *Staphylococcus* population's strain level differences seem closely tied to flare-ups. Higher abundances of *Staphylococcus aureus* during flares suggest a link with disease severity (Kong et al. 2012). Remarkably, treatments that suppress the immune response in atopic dermatitis show reduced *S. aureus* abundances, leading to clinical improvement (Callewaert et al. 2020a).

In psoriasis, an autoimmune disease with an overexpression of IL-23 and IL-17 cytokines, no direct link between skin microbiome imbalance and disease pathology has been established (Benhadou et al. 2018). However, recent findings have hinted at the potential involvement of fungi, urging further investigation (Hurabielle et al. 2020).

Acne vulgaris, affecting sebaceous skin areas, has been linked to specific strains of *Cutibacterium acnes*. Genetic markers differentiating between health and disease-associated strains have been proposed (Dréno et al. 2018).

Dandruff on the scalp is usually associated with fungi like *Malassezia furfur* and *Malassezia globosa*, causing inflammation due to excess oleic acid production (Dawson 2007). A bacterial impact, with an imbalance in *Cutibacterium* and *Staphylococcus* species, has also been suggested (Xu et al. 2016).

Body odor, though not commonly considered a pathology, is associated with the microbiome. Certain bacteria (*Corynebacterium, Anaerococcus, Peptoniphilus, Staphylococcus hominis*) can lead to malodorous volatiles in apocrine sweat, especially in individuals with specific gene alleles (Troccaz et al. 2015).

Rosacea has also been linked to skin microbiome dysbiosis, with increased *Demodex* mites observed in the condition. Some research has explored the microbiota of *Demodex* mites, but conclusive results are pending (Murillo et al. 2014).

Skin cancers like Squamous cell carcinomas and Actinic Keratosis show dysbiosis with increased *S. aureus* and reduced skin commensals like *C. acnes*. Interestingly, *C. acnes* was found to potentially protect against UV-induced DNA damage, while certain *S. epidermidis* strains could inhibit tumor cell proliferation (Allhorn et al. 2016).

Though impressive evidence exists, it remains challenging to determine whether microbiome dysbiosis is the cause or consequence of the diseases mentioned above. To definitively address this question, we must directly change a diseased microbiome to a healthy state and observe improvements in the disease. The skin offers an ideal experimental area, where existing microbiomes can be reduced with topical disinfectants before applying new bacteria and monitoring their behavior. Encouraging results from multiple studies attempting to change the skin microbiome have emerged.

15.4 Methods of Transferring Skin Microbiota

Various approaches can be employed to modify the skin microbiome. Each of these methods possesses its own set of benefits and drawbacks. Presently, various scientific investigations are underway utilizing these methods to address prevalent skin disorders.

15.4.1 Skin Microbiome Transplantation

A first technique is the technique of skin microbiome transplantation. Although not entirely novel, this method draws inspiration from the well-known fecal microbiota transplantation (FMT), widely used to treat gastric *Clostridium difficile* infections (Borody et al. 2004).

In skin microbiome transplantation, the approach involves transferring a healthy individual's skin microbiome to the cleansed and/or disinfected skin area of another person, with the aim of improving their skin condition (Callewaert et al. 2021). A notable advantage of this method lies in its ability to preserve the microbiome's natural environment. Bacteria are cultured on the skin and pre-cultivated in a sugar-rich solution, maintaining their original ecological setting.

One of the most common methods of transplantation is through the use of skin swabs, which are taken from a healthy donor and applied to the affected skin of the recipient. This allows the transfer of healthy microorganisms to the recipient, which can help restore the balance of the skin microbiome. Studies have shown that skin microbiota transplantation can lead to significant improvements in skin health, including reduced inflammation and improved skin hydration. Additionally, this method has been found to be safe and effective in treating a variety of skin conditions.

However, like any technique, skin microbiome transplantation comes with limitations and challenges. One prominent drawback is the limited quantity of harvested bacteria available for the recipient's skin. To overcome this hurdle, a culturing step is typically required to obtain a sufficient number of bacterial species for transplantation. This additional step adds complexity and time to the process.

Other challenges are the difficulty in selecting appropriate donors and the potential for the transfer of harmful microorganisms. As a result, the scalability and applicability of skin microbiome transplantation to industrial settings remain uncertain. As the method heavily relies on individualized donor-recipient pairs, implementing it on a larger scale poses practical challenges. Standardization becomes an issue, and the process may become less feasible when applied to a broader population. Another critical concern is the lack of clarity surrounding the specific microorganisms transmitted to the recipient's skin during transplantation. It remains unclear whether potential pathogenic taxa could also be transferred, raising safety considerations. Further research is needed to fully understand the mechanisms behind the success of this treatment and to develop standardized protocols for its use.

Despite these challenges, skin microbiome transplantation represents an intriguing avenue in the quest for innovative skin interventions. As research continues to unravel the complexities of the skin microbiome, refining and optimizing this technique may unlock its full potential in promoting healthy skin and treating various skin conditions. Moreover, collaborations between scientists, dermatologists, and industry experts may lead to breakthroughs in making skin microbiome transplantation more accessible and effective for a broader range of individuals.

15.4.2 Skin Bacteriotherapy

A second method to modify the skin microbiome is by means of skin bacteriotherapy. In this approach, one or multiple pure cultures of microorganisms with beneficial health properties are applied to the washed and disinfected skin area of an individual. The primary goal is to enhance skin health and address various skin conditions effectively.

This approach involves the application of various types of microbiota, each serving a unique purpose. First, we have live probiotics, which are defined as living microorganisms administered in sufficient quantities to confer advantageous effects for the host (Zendeboodi et al. 2020). Second, there are postbiotics, also known as thermo-killed or tyndallized bacteria, where bacterial cell structures, enzymes, and excreted factors are introduced, although bacterial replication ceases (Collado et al. 2019). Third, we have cell lysates or physically killed bacteria, which also fall under the category of postbiotics, wherein the bacteria are destroyed, but their beneficial cell contents and walls are present in the solution. Additionally, purified enzymes, either as single entities or groups of bacterial enzymes, can be extracted and added to the skin. Lastly, fermentation products or supernatants can be utilized, where the bacteria themselves are not applied, but their supernatants containing beneficial substances are employed.

The advantages of skin bacteriotherapy are noteworthy. Scalability and industry-applicability are among the major strengths, as substantial quantities of bacteria can be administered, resulting in heightened efficacy (Ito and Amagai 2022). Furthermore, the strains utilized in the process are well-defined, ensuring a targeted and specific approach to address skin conditions. Incorporating these beneficial pro- or postbiotics into various skin products, such as emollients, creams, or suitable skin mediums, facilitates their practical use and accessibility for individuals.

Nevertheless, some challenges are encountered in the pursuit of effective skin bacteriotherapy. Bacteria cultivated in sugar-rich media may face difficulties adapting to the sebum-rich skin environment, necessitating further investigation to optimize their performance. Additionally, the engraftment of applied bacteria into the skin is not straightforward, as they must compete with the resident microbiome of the deeper skin layers. Striking the right balance of applied bacteria is crucial, as an excess might trigger adverse skin immune reactions and lead to irritation and side-effects. Safety is a paramount concern, and ongoing research aims to provide clear INCI names and safety sheets for these substances, ensuring their safe and responsible use in skincare products (Callewaert et al. 2021).

In conclusion, skin bacteriotherapy holds immense promise as an innovative approach to enhance skin health and combat various skin conditions. As research progresses, addressing the challenges and optimizing the application of beneficial microorganisms will undoubtedly pave the way for a brighter and healthier future for skincare.

15.4.3 Skin Prebiotics

A notable approach gaining traction is prebiotic stimulation. This innovative technique involves introducing prebiotics to the skin, with the intent of fostering the growth of specific health-enhancing microbes. A prebiotic refers to an ingredient with bio-selective activity that bestows beneficial effects on the host, aiming to improve the host's health (Gibson and Roberfroid 1995). Prebiotic stimulation offers several advantages. One key benefit is that it does not involve the introduction of live bacteria, thereby reducing the likelihood of eliciting a skin immune reaction. Instead, it operates indirectly, leveraging the influence of prebiotics on the existing microbial ecosystem. Prebiotics are typically well-defined compounds with thoroughly studied side-effects, ensuring their safety for use. Moreover, they come with standardized International Nomenclature of Cosmetic Ingredients (INCI) names and safety data sheets, providing additional reassurance to both consumers and researchers.

However, it is crucial to acknowledge the limitations and challenges associated with prebiotic stimulation. As an indirect approach, its effects may not manifest as immediately as some other interventions, requiring patience and consistent application (Maguire and Maguire 2017). Additionally, the complex interplay of skin microbiome, physiology, and individual immune responses introduces an element of unpredictability in the outcomes of prebiotic interventions. These variations among individuals necessitate careful consideration when designing and evaluating prebiotic-based interventions. Moreover, the interaction between prebiotics and the skin microbiome can be intricate, potentially leading to unintended stimulation of non-targeted, low-abundant bacteria. This phenomenon underscores the need for thorough investigation and understanding of specific prebiotics and their impacts on the skin ecosystem (Callewaert et al. 2021).

Despite these challenges, prebiotic stimulation remains a promising avenue in the quest to promote skin health through microbiome manipulation. As research in this field advances, refining prebiotic formulations and tailoring them to individual skin types will likely enhance their efficacy and safety, paving the way for innovative therapeutic applications. Continued exploration of prebiotics and their impact on skin health holds great potential in shaping the future of dermatological interventions.

15.5 Human Skin Microbiome Manipulation Efforts

15.5.1 Transplanting Microbes from One Body Site to Another Within the Same Subject

In their study, Costello et al. investigated whether alterations in microbial communities resulted from environmental influences or historical exposures. To address this inquiry, bacterial communities from the tongue were transplanted to the forehead or volar forearm, and vice versa. Subsequent samples were collected at intervals of 2, 4, and 8 h. The results revealed that transplantation from tongue to forearm resulted in the engraftment of tongue bacteria, whereas transplantation from tongue to forehead had minimal impact on the original native microbiome composition. Similarly, transplantations between the forearm and forehead, in either direction, exhibited communities akin to the native state (Costello et al. 2009).

15.5.2 Transplanting Skin Microbes from One Skin Site to Another Within the Same Subject

Numerous publications have underscored the significance of syntrophy in upholding metabolic interplay between species (Hoek and Merks 2017; Morris et al. 2013). While most studies have focused on the transfer of individual bacterial phylogenetic groups without considering potential cross-feeding, a few investigations have explored the transplantation of the entire naive skin microbiome from one skin site to another.

For instance, Leyden et al. (1981) conducted a study where they transferred underarm odor-causing bacteria to the forearm of subjects to ascertain the reproduction of malodor. Samples with two types of diphtheroids incubated on the forearm produced a strong odor, demonstrating the transferability of odor-causing bacteria from the armpit to the forearm (Leyden et al. 1981).

Similarly, Perin et al. (2019) performed a microbiome swab transfer from the arm to the upper back of the same individual. The microbiome composition of the antecubital fossa (inner elbow) exhibited higher diversity in contrast to the back. While the back predominantly housed abundant *Cutibacterium*, the inner elbow showcased comparable levels of *Staphylococcus*, *Streptococcus*, and *Corynebacterium*. Despite the challenges in sampling and transferring the complete community, particularly the Gram-negative species, after 24 h, a median of 4 arm-only species persisted in the transplanted area. These species mainly belonged to the taxa *Gardnerella*, *Brachybacterium*, *Janthinobacterium*, *Actinomyces*, *Anaerococcus*, *Microbacteriaceae* and Dermabacteriaceae (Perin et al. 2019).

15.5.3 S. epidermidis *Application on Facial Skin*

A double-blinded randomized clinical study was conducted wherein *S. epidermidis* strains were initially isolated from individual participants. These isolated strains were subsequently cultured and applied twice per week for a total of 4 weeks on the same subjects' facial skin. In comparison to the control group, the application of *S. epidermidis* demonstrated an increase in relative lipid and water content while reducing water evaporation from the skin. Moreover, the skin acidity, as measured by pH, decreased in patients with applied *S. epidermidis*, reaching a pH of 5 instead of 5.5. This decline in acidity might be attributed to the elevated presence of lactic acid and propionic acid in the patients. The study effectively showcased the favorable impact of *S. epidermidis* application on human facial skin, highlighting its potential as a cosmetic ingredient (Nodake et al. 2015).

15.5.4 *Armpit Microbial Transplants and Bacteriotherapy to Treat Body Odor*

In a clinical study, a group of siblings participated, where one sibling suffered from heavy body odor, while the other didn't (Callewaert et al. 2016). Recognizing the crucial role of bacteria in body odor, the researchers successfully attempted to establish the skin microbiome of the non-smelly sibling to that of the one with strong body odor. A trained odor panel detected a reduction in body odor accompanied by a new equilibrium of microbiota, characterized by an increased presence of staphylococci and a decreased presence of corynebacteria. To enhance the establishment of the applied strains, the recipient's skin was disinfected before the introduction of the new bacteria. Furthermore, the application of pure cultures of *S. epidermidis* yielded improved odor scores compared to the baseline (unpublished data). These promising results are currently further developed in a startup from Ghent University and their first product will be a probiotic deodorant to treat heavy underarm odor.

15.5.5 *Gram-Positive Bacteriotherapy to Treat Atopic Dermatitis*

S. aureus has been associated with dysbiosis in patients with Atopic Dermatitis (AD), and it has been hypothesized that a deficiency in antimicrobial peptides (AMPs) produced by skin cells might contribute to the loss of protection against *S. aureus* growth (Sieprawska-Lupa et al. 2004). Nakatsuji et al. demonstrated that certain members of the healthy microbiome can offer selective protection against *S. aureus* by secreting Sh-lantibiotics (Nakatsuji et al. 2017). Their study compared the microbiome of lesional skin with that of patients colonized or non-colonized by *S. aureus*, revealing reduced taxonomic diversity in those colonized by *S. aureus*. Additionally, they observed a tenfold increase in relative colony-forming units (rCFU) compared to live colony counting in normal skin, suggesting the presence of an inactive antimicrobial defense system in lesional AD patients. Coagulase-negative *Staphylococcus* (CoNS) species, such as *S. epidermidis* and *S. hominis*, were found to have the potential to produce AMPs. Accordingly, CoNS strains were isolated from subjects with Atopic Dermatitis, capable of inhibiting *S. aureus* growth. These strains were subsequently amplified and applied to the subjects' skin through autologous transplantation. The reported outcome was a reduction in *S. aureus* colonization, although clinical symptom measurement was not undertaken (Nakatsuji et al. 2016).

These findings led to the establishment of the company Matrisys Bioscience, which is currently pursuing further development. The ultimate goal is to obtain a single strain that can be applied to numerous patients, aiming to address the challenges associated with *S. aureus* colonization in AD effectively.

15.5.6 Gram-Negative Bacteriotherapy to Treat Atopic Dermatitis

Myles et al. investigated the protective function of skin microbiota from healthy individuals as treatment against AD (Myles et al. 2016). The researchers collected culturable Gram-negative bacteria from the skin of healthy individuals and AD patients. They studied the effects of these bacteria on immune, epithelial, and bacterial functions in both cell cultures and animal models of AD. The findings revealed that Gram-negative bacteria from healthy individuals improved barrier function, activated innate immunity, and helped control *S. aureus* in the AD mouse model. This suggests that using live bacteria as a treatment approach could hold promise for managing AD. The researchers observed that when they killed the *Roseomonas mucosa* isolate, its efficacy decreased, indicating that live bacteria might be necessary for the treatment's success. Based on these preclinical results, a series of clinical trials were conducted with adult and pediatric patients (Myles et al. 2018). Treatment with *Roseomonas* resulted in significant improvements in disease severity, reduced need for topical steroids, and decreased *S. aureus* levels, with no adverse events or complications. These promising results supported further investigation of *Roseomonas* therapy on AD patients. The Gram-negative skin commensals play a role in normalizing skin homeostasis in AD, and sheds light on a potential new approach to managing this challenging skin condition. These findings led to the establishment of the company Forte Biosciences and went on to become a stock-listed company on Nasdaq in 2020. Several clinical trials were conducted, but the end results were not as promising as initially hoped. The company said that "the primary endpoint was achieved by 58% of subjects on the *Roseomonas* treatment, compared with 60% of subjects on placebo". As the results were not significantly different from the placebo group, the company decided to no longer pursue the *Roseomonas* treatment in AD, but rather invest in other early-stage biotech efforts. They were one of the first companies to develop skin bacteriotherapy for skin conditions and have faced the many difficulties that are associated with it.

15.5.7 Skin Microbiome Modulation to Treat Acne Vulgaris

Paetzold et al. conducted a study where they isolated whole microbiome samples from two individuals and also utilized mixtures of specific *C. acnes* species for transplantation to account for potential synergistic effects between species (Paetzold et al. 2019). These samples were transplanted onto different individuals' sebaceous-rich skin sites. The analysis revealed five distinct dermatotypes of *C. acnes*. Remarkably, engraftment occurred merely after three days and persisted even after the application was discontinued for several days. Specific mixtures of *C. acnes* were found to engraft better than whole microbiome samples, especially at a concentration of 10^8 CFU/mL. Additionally, mixtures containing multiple *C. acnes* species demonstrated superior engraftment compared to single *C. acnes* species. Donor skin microbiota with a higher proportion of *C. acnes* species relative to *Staphylococcus* species appeared more suitable for transplantation.

In an extension of this experiment, Karoglan et al. applied mixtures of *C. acnes* strains to individuals with acne vulgaris (Karoglan et al. 2019). Prior to this treatment, the autochthonous skin microbiome was reduced using a benzoyl peroxide treatment. After this initial disinfection, a bacterial mix containing two or four live *C. acnes* strains was applied twice daily for 5 weeks. In this open-label study, a statistically significant reduction in lesion count was observed. However, the clinical relevance of this finding still requires confirmation through a double-blinded randomized placebo-controlled trial. Notably, the applied bacteria were detected after the treatment in approximately 50% of the study participants. Surprisingly, no advantage in terms of engraftment effect was observed for the four-strain solution over the two-strain solution. These promising findings are further developed by the company S-Biomedic, which was recently acquired by the multinational Beiersdorf.

15.5.8 Application of Non-commensal Bacteria on Skin

AOBiome has successfully completed a series of clinical trials involving their lead strain, *Nitrosomonas eutropha*. Interestingly, this bacterial species is not typically found on normal Western skin. The argument put forth is that we have lost this species, which is naturally abundant in soil and sewage plants, due to heightened hygiene practices. While the positive outcomes of a clinical trial were announced in a press release, these results have not yet been made publicly available. Furthermore, AOBiome has initiated additional trials exploring the effects of *Nitrosomonas eutropha* in pruritus associated with atopic dermatitis and rosacea, and the findings from these trials are expected to be released in future. AOBiome is recognized as one of the pioneering companies to pave the way in skin microbiome manipulations, both for cosmetic and pharmaceutical treatments. Their spinoff company Mother Dirt has been crucial in educating the main public and was sold to the multinational S.C. Johnson, where the live bacterial product later phased out.

15.5.9 Genetically Modified Bacteria as Topical Therapeutics

An intriguing approach involves the genetic engineering of skin commensals, such as *S. epidermidis* or *C. acnes*, to produce and secrete active biotherapeutics. Potential biotherapeutics include Fillaggrin, LEKTI, IL-10, anti-inflammatory somatotropin, as well as other growth factors and hormones. Azitra, a company pioneering this method, has already conducted a clinical trial using their bacterial chassis organism, and the results are eagerly awaited. Similarly, the company ILYA is currently conducting a phase I clinical trial using *Lactobacillus reuteri* as a chassis to secrete CXCL12, a short-lived human cytokine, with the aim of enhancing wound healing. The main advantage of this approach lies in the efficient delivery of an active substance with a short half-life directly to the site of action, potentially improving the effectiveness of the biotherapeutic intervention. As these clinical trials progress, they hold great promise for advancing the field of genetic engineering in skin commensals and its therapeutic applications.

15.6 Application of *Lactobacillus* and Other Gut Probiotics on Skin

In recent years, numerous companies have begun incorporating established probiotics or their derivatives into products designed for topical application. In 2009, a pioneering group explored the use of *Lactobacillus plantarum* in wound treatment (Peral et al. 2009). Whether this probiotic acts through similar or distinct pathways as the more recent findings (Domizio et al. 2020) remains to be fully understood and requires further investigation.

Concurrently, many cosmetic companies have embraced the use of probiotic derivatives, such as extracts or postbiotics, in their products. Lactobacilli, as a group of bacteria, are particularly intriguing due to their well-established safety and long history of use as probiotics for gut health. However, up until now, only a few companies have taken on the technical challenge of incorporating live bacteria directly into their products. This cautious approach is likely due to the complexities involved in ensuring the stability and efficacy of live probiotics in topical formulations. Nevertheless, ongoing research in this area holds the potential to unlock exciting opportunities for the application of live bacteria in skincare products.

15.7 Challenges, Promises and Outlook for Manipulating the Skin Microbiome

Changing the skin microbiome by applying live bacteria has become a hot topic of interest. Researchers are finding more and more links between specific types of microbes and various skin diseases. However, many studies struggle to fully unravel the cause-and-effect mystery. To get solid answers, we need to transform a diseased skin microbiome into a healthy one, but that's easier said than done. The skin's microbiome, with its easy accessibility and safety, makes it an ideal place to tackle these questions. Bacteria can be easily applied to targeted areas, and if any issues arise, we can remove the applied bacteria with a disinfection treatment.

Yet, making the applied bacteria stick to the skin is a major challenge. Even with initial disinfection, getting rid of the subcutaneous microbiota is tough. As a result, the newly applied microbiota on the skin's surface will compete with the deeper skin layers. This competition, known as engraftment, is a big hurdle not just for skin researchers but also for those studying the gut microbiome. Early data suggests that different bacterial strains might work together in harmony (Paetzold et al. 2019) or refuse to cooperate with each other (Christensen et al. 2016). Unfortunately, there are only a few publicly available studies reporting on the transfer of strains between individuals. In most cases, very few subjects accept the new strains, and we haven't yet figured out the clear reasons behind it. We need more intensive research to identify subjects more likely to successfully accept the applied bacteria. One interesting idea is to combine the classic culture-independent analysis with a culture-based approach. By testing isolated cultures against each other, we might uncover their ecological interactions.

Once we understand how these bacteria interact with each other, we can delve into the relationship between the microbiome and the skin's host. In earlier studies, we found certain bacterial strains that seem to establish themselves on the skin more easily. However, we're not sure if this means they're just more metabolically fit than other strains or if the skin's host simply tolerates them better. To get a clearer picture, we need more systematic studies. Are certain hosts limited to tolerating only a specific subset of strains, or can any native bacterial strain successfully colonize the skin in a given environment?

Another challenge arises when dealing with pure cultures of bacteria. The culturing process usually involves growing the bacteria in sugar-rich media, and they're then lyophilized and covered in a sugar coating. These bacteria become adapted to the sugar-rich environment where they were cultured. However, when we apply them to someone's skin, which is low in sugars and nutrients but rich in lipids, the bacteria struggle to adapt to the new environment. To address this, we need to choose the right culture media so the applied bacteria can easily thrive in the skin environment.

Over the past century, our lifestyle has drastically changed, especially with the industrial revolution. Unfortunately, this has also led to a rise in auto-immune skin conditions. Many of these skin conditions are treated with antimicrobial or anti-inflammatory approaches. While these treatments may bring temporary relief, they can lead to imbalances and an increase in multi-resistant strains. Anti-inflammatory treatments might soothe local issues, but often, the real solution lies in the deeper realms of systems biology. To truly understand and address skin conditions, we need a more holistic approach.

The diversity of the Western skin microbiome has considerably declined in comparison to Indigenous skin (Callewaert et al. 2020b). This shift is a consequence of Western hygiene practices, involving frequent use of skin cosmetics and detergents that strip away skin lipids and alter the skin's microbial composition. In contrast, Indigenous, non-urbanized populations, and farmers possess a more diverse skin microbiome, which may explain their lower susceptibility to skin allergies, acne, and other skin disorders (Lehtimäki et al. 2017). It appears that lifestyle and environment play a significant role in maintaining a healthy skin microbiome. Consequently, studying the microbiome of Western individuals without skin conditions may provide insights into whether their microbiome is better suited to a Western lifestyle, offering answers to unresolved questions.

While research has predominantly focused on bacteria, it is crucial to acknowledge that the skin harbors not only bacteria but also fungi, phages, and micro-eukaryotes, which likely contribute to maintaining skin homeostasis. Exploring the manipulation of these various inhabitants could hold valuable potential in addressing skin conditions.

Amidst the challenges and hurdles, the future of skin microbiome modulation in treating skin conditions appears bright, with initial study outcomes already displaying significant promise. The pioneering work of the past decade has uncovered a series of hurdles to be taken to successfully alter and manipulate the skin microbiome to combat skin conditions. Ongoing clinical trials are expected to yield a wealth of scientific data in the coming years. Recognizing the paramount importance of the skin microbiome for skin health, the presence of "good" species plays a pivotal role in safeguarding and sustaining a healthy skin state.

References

Allhorn M, Arve S, Brüggemann H, Lood R. A novel enzyme with antioxidant capacity produced by the ubiquitous skin colonizer Propionibacterium acnes. Sci Rep [Internet]. 2016;6(1):36412. Available from: https://doi.org/10.1038/srep36412

Benhadou F, Mintoff D, Schnebert B, Thio HB. Psoriasis and microbiota: a systematic review. Dis (Basel, Switzerland). 2018;6(2).

Borody TJ, Warren EF, Leis SM, Surace R, Ashman O, Siarakas S. Bacteriotherapy using fecal flora—toying with human motions. J Clin Gastroenterol. 2004;38(6):475–83.

Byrd AL, Belkaid Y, Segre JA. The human skin microbiome. Nat Rev Microbiol. 2018;16(3):143–55.

Byrd AL, Deming C, Cassidy SKB, Harrison OJ, Ng W-I, Conlan S, et al. Staphylococcus aureus and Staphylococcus epidermidis strain diversity underlying pediatric atopic dermatitis. Sci Transl Med. 2017;9(397).

Callewaert C, Nakatsuji T, Knight R, Kosciolek T, Vrbanac A, Kotol P, et al. IL-4Rα blockade by dupilumab decreases staphylococcus aureus colonization and increases microbial diversity in atopic dermatitis. J Invest Dermatol. 2020a;140(1):191-202.e7.

Callewaert C, Ravard Helffer K, Lebaron P. Skin microbiome and its interplay with the environment. Am J Clin Dermatol. 2020;21(Suppl 1):4–11

Callewaert C, Lambert J, Van de Wiele T. Towards a bacterial treatment for armpit malodour. Exp Dermatol [Internet]. 2016 Nov 28 [cited 2017 Jan 6]. Available from: http://www.ncbi.nlm.nih.gov/pubmed/27892611

Callewaert C, Knödlseder N, Karoglan A, Güell M, Paetzold B. Skin microbiome transplantation and manipulation: Current state of the art. Comput Struct Biotechnol J [Internet]. 2021;19:624–31. Available from: https://www.sciencedirect.com/science/article/pii/S2001037021000052

Chang H-W, Yan D, Singh R, Liu J, Lu X, Ucmak D, et al. Alteration of the cutaneous microbiome in psoriasis and potential role in Th17 polarization. Microbiome. 2018;6(1):154.

Christensen GJM, Scholz CFP, Enghild J, Rohde H, Kilian M, Thürmer A, et al. Antagonism between staphylococcus epidermidis and propionibacterium acnes and its genomic basis. BMC Genomics. 2016;17:152.

Collado MC, Vinderola G, Salminen S. Postbiotics: facts and open questions. A position paper on the need for a consensus definition. Benef Microbes. 2019;10(7):711–9.

Costello EK, Lauber CL, Hamady M, Fierer N, Gordon JI, Knight R. Bacterial community variation in human body habitats across space and time. Science (80). 2009;326(5960):1694–7.

Dawson TLJ. Malassezia globosa and restricta: breakthrough understanding of the etiology and treatment of dandruff and seborrheic dermatitis through whole-genome analysis. J Investig Dermatology Symp Proc. 2007;12(2):15–9.

Di Domizio J, Belkhodja C, Chenuet P, Fries A, Murray T, Mondéjar PM, et al. The commensal skin microbiota triggers type I IFN-dependent innate repair responses in injured skin. Nat Immunol. 2020;21(9):1034–45.

De Pessemier B, Grine L, Debaere M, Maes A, Paetzold B, Callewaert C. Gut–skin axis: current knowledge of the interrelationship between microbial dysbiosis and skin conditions. Microorganisms. 2021;9.

Dréno B, Pécastaings S, Corvec S, Veraldi S, Khammari A, Roques C. Cutibacterium acnes (Propionibacterium acnes) and acne vulgaris: a brief look at the latest updates. J Eur Acad Dermatol Venereol. 2018;32 Suppl 2:5–14

Fyhrquist N, Muirhead G, Prast-Nielsen S, Jeanmougin M, Olah P, Skoog T, et al. Microbe-host interplay in atopic dermatitis and psoriasis. Nat Commun. 2019;10(1):4703.

Gibson GR, Roberfroid MB. Dietary modulation of the human colonic microbiota: introducing the concept of prebiotics. J Nutr. 1995;125(6):1401–12.

Greuter T, Navarini A, Vavricka SR. Skin Manifestations of inflammatory bowel disease. Clin Rev Allergy Immunol. 2017;53(3):413–27.

Grice EA, Segre JA. The skin microbiome. Nat Rev Microbiol [Internet]. 2011;9(4):244–53. Available from: http://www.nature.com/nrmicro/journal/v9/n4/pdf/nrmicro2537.pdf

Grice EA, Kong HH, Conlan S, Deming CB, Davis J, Young AC, et al. Topographical and temporal diversity of the human skin microbiome. Science (80). 2009;324(5931):1190–2.

Hurabielle C, Link VM, Bouladoux N, Han S-J, Merrill ED, Lightfoot YL, et al. Immunity to commensal skin fungi promotes psoriasiform skin inflammation. Proc Natl Acad Sci [Internet]. 2020;117(28):16465 LP–74. Available from: http://www.pnas.org/content/117/28/16465.abstract

Ito Y, Amagai M. Controlling skin microbiome as a new bacteriotherapy for inflammatory skin diseases. Inflamm Regen [Internet]. 2022;42(1):26. Available from: https://doi.org/10.1186/s41232-022-00212-y

Karoglan A, Paetzold B, Pereira de Lima J, Brüggemann H, Tüting T, Schanze D, et al. Safety and efficacy of topically applied selected cutibacterium acnes strains over five weeks in patients with acne vulgaris: an open-label, pilot study. Acta Derm Venereol. 2019;99(13):1253–7.

Knight R, Vrbanac A, Taylor BC, Aksenov A, Callewaert C, Debelius J, et al. Best practices for analysing microbiomes. Nat Rev Microbiol. 2018.

Kong HH, Oh J, Deming C, Conlan S, Grice EA, Beatson MA, et al. Temporal shifts in the skin microbiome associated with disease flares and treatment in children with atopic dermatitis. Genome Res. 2012;22(5):850–9.

Lehtimäki J, Karkman A, Laatikainen T, Paalanen L, von Hertzen L, Haahtela T, et al. Patterns in the skin microbiota differ in children and teenagers between rural and urban environments. Sci Rep. 2017;7:45651.

Leyden JJ, McGinley KJ, Holzle E, Labows JN, Kligman AM. The microbiology of the human axilla and its relationship to axillary odor. J Invest Dermatol. 1981;77(5):413–6.

Maguire M, Maguire G. The role of microbiota, and probiotics and prebiotics in skin health. Arch Dermatol Res [Internet]. 2017;309(6):411–21. Available from: https://doi.org/10.1007/s00403-017-1750-3

McCall L-I, Callewaert C, Zhu Q, Song SJ, Bouslimani A, Minich JJ, et al. Home chemical and microbial transitions across urbanization. Nat Microbiol [Internet]. 2020;5(1):108–15. Available from: https://doi.org/10.1038/s41564-019-0593-4

Morris BEL, Henneberger R, Huber H, Moissl-Eichinger C. Microbial syntrophy: interaction for the common good. FEMS Microbiol Rev. 2013;37(3):384–406.

Murillo N, Aubert J, Raoult D. Microbiota of Demodex mites from rosacea patients and controls. Microb Pathog. 2014;71–72:37–40.

Myles IA, Williams KW, Reckhow JD, Jammeh ML, Pincus NB, Sastalla I, et al. Transplantation of human skin microbiota in models of atopic dermatitis. JCI insight. 2016;1(10).

Myles IA, Earland NJ, Anderson ED, Moore IN, Kieh MD, Williams KW, et al. First-in-human topical microbiome transplantation with Roseomonas mucosa for atopic dermatitis. JCI insight. 2018;3(9).

Naik S, Bouladoux N, Wilhelm C, Molloy MJ, Salcedo R, Kastenmuller W, et al. Compartmentalized control of skin immunity by resident commensals. Science (80) [Internet]. 2012;337(6098):1115 LP–9. Available from: http://science.sciencemag.org/content/337/6098/1115.abstract

Nakatsuji T, Chen TH, Two AM, Chun KA, Narala S, Geha RS, et al. Staphylococcus aureus exploits epidermal barrier defects in atopic dermatitis to trigger cytokine expression. J Invest Dermatol. 2016;136(11):2192–200.

Nakatsuji T, Chen TH, Narala S, Chun KA, Two AM, Yun T, et al. Antimicrobials from human skin commensal bacteria protect against Staphylococcus aureus and are deficient in atopic dermatitis. Sci Transl Med [Internet]. 2017;9(378). Available from: http://stm.sciencemag.org/content/9/378/eaah4680.abstract

Nodake Y, Matsumoto S, Miura R, Honda H, Ishibashi G, Matsumoto S, et al. Pilot study on novel skin care method by augmentation with Staphylococcus epidermidis, an autologous skin microbe–A blinded randomized clinical trial. J Dermatol Sci. 2015;79(2):119–26.

O'Neill CA, Monteleone G, McLaughlin JT, Paus R. The gut-skin axis in health and disease: a paradigm with therapeutic implications. BioEssays. 2016;38(11):1167–76.

Oh J, Byrd AL, Deming C, Conlan S, Kong HH, Segre JA. Biogeography and individuality shape function in the human skin metagenome. Nature. 2014;514(7520):59–64.

Paetzold B, Willis JR, Pereira de Lima J, Knödlseder N, Brüggemann H, Quist SR, et al. Skin microbiome modulation induced by probiotic solutions. Microbiome [Internet]. 2019;7(1):95. Available from: https://doi.org/10.1186/s40168-019-0709-3

Peral MC, Martinez MAH, Valdez JC. Bacteriotherapy with Lactobacillus plantarum in burns. Int Wound J. 2009;6(1):73–81.

Perin B, Addetia A, Qin X. Transfer of skin microbiota between two dissimilar autologous microenvironments: a pilot study. PLoS ONE. 2019;14(12): e0226857.

Picardo M, Ottaviani M. Skin microbiome and skin disease: the example of rosacea. J Clin Gastroenterol. 2014;48 Suppl 1:S85-6

Robert S, Gysemans C, Takiishi T, Korf H, Spagnuolo I, Sebastiani G, et al. Oral delivery of glutamic acid decarboxylase (GAD)-65 and IL10 by Lactococcus lactis reverses diabetes in recent-onset NOD mice. Diabetes. 2014;63(8):2876–87.

Segre JA. Epidermal barrier formation and recovery in skin disorders. J Clin Invest. 2006;116(5):1150–8.

Sieprawska-Lupa M, Mydel P, Krawczyk K, Wójcik K, Puklo M, Lupa B, et al. Degradation of human antimicrobial peptide LL-37 by Staphylococcus aureus-derived proteinases. Antimicrob Agents Chemother. 2004;48(12):4673–9.

Takiishi T, Korf H, Van Belle TL, Robert S, Grieco FA, Caluwaerts S, et al. Reversal of autoimmune diabetes by restoration of antigen-specific tolerance using genetically modified Lactococcus lactis in mice. J Clin Invest. 2012;122(5):1717–25.

Troccaz M, Gaïa N, Beccucci S, Schrenzel J, Cayeux I, Starkenmann C, et al. Mapping axillary microbiota responsible for body odours using a culture-independent approach. Microbiome [Internet]. 2015;3(1):1–15. Available from: https://doi.org/10.1186/s40168-014-0064-3

van Hoek MJA, Merks RMH. Emergence of microbial diversity due to cross-feeding interactions in a spatial model of gut microbial metabolism. BMC Syst Biol. 2017;11(1):56.

Xu Z, Wang Z, Yuan C, Liu X, Yang F, Wang T, et al. Dandruff is associated with the conjoined interactions between host and microorganisms. Sci Rep [Internet]. 2016;6(1):24877. Available from: https://doi.org/10.1038/srep24877

Zeeuwen PLJM, Boekhorst J, van den Bogaard EH, de Koning HD, van de Kerkhof PMC, Saulnier DM, et al. Microbiome dynamics of human epidermis following skin barrier disruption. Genome Biol Novemb Issue. 2012;13(11):R101.

Zendeboodi F, Khorshidian N, Mortazavian AM, da Cruz AG. Probiotic: conceptualization from a new approach. Curr Opin Food Sci [Internet]. 2020;32:103–23. Available from: https://www.sciencedirect.com/science/article/pii/S221479932030028X

Zhou Z, Chen X, Sheng H, Shen X, Sun X, Yan Y, et al. Engineering probiotics as living diagnostics and therapeutics for improving human health. Microb Cell Fact. 2020;19(1):56.

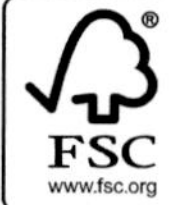